Health Information for International Travel

2005-2006

Health Information for International Travel

2005-2006

Edited by
Paul M. Arguin
Phyllis E. Kozarsky
Ava W. Navin

U.S. DEPARTMENT OF HEALTH AND HUMAN SERVICES
Public Health Service
Centers for Disease Control and Prevention
National Center for Infectious Diseases
Division of Global Migration and Quarantine
Atlanta, Georgia

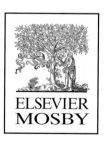

ELSEVIER
MOSBY

ELSEVIER
MOSBY

The Curtis Center
170 S Independence Mall W 300E
Philadelphia, Pennsylvania 19106

Published by Elsevier Inc.

HEALTH INFORMATION FOR
INTERNATIONAL TRAVEL 2005-2006

Elsevier is proud to pay a portion of their sales for this book to the CDC Foundation. Chartered by Congress, the CDC Foundation began operations in 1995 as an independent, non-profit organization fostering support for CDC through public-private partnerships. Further information about the Foundation can be found at www.cdcfoundation.com. The CDC Foundation did not prepare any portion of this book and is not responsible for its contents.

Suggested Citation
Centers for Disease Control and Prevention. Health Information for International Travel 2005–2006. Atlanta: US Department of Health and Human Services, Public Health Service, 2005.

Disclaimer
Both generic and trade names are used in this text. In all cases, the decision to use one or the other was made based on recognition factors and was done for the convenience of the intended audience. Therefore, the use of trade names in this publication is for identification only and does not imply endorsement by the U.S. Department of Health and Human Services, Public Health Service, or Centers for Disease Control and Prevention.

For additional copies, please contact Elsevier:
Order online at www.elsevierhealth.com
Ordering within the U.S.: 1-800-545-2522
UK, Germany, Italy and Spain: 1-800-460-3110
All other countries: 1-314-453-7095

Acquisitions Editor: Tom Hartman
Editorial Assistant: Dennis DiClaudio
Publishing Services Manager: Frank Polizzano
Marketing Manager: Megan Carr

ISBN-13: 978-0-323-03716-7
ISBN-10: 0-323-03716-X

Printed in China

Last digit is the print number: 9 8 7 6 5 4 3 2

Working together to grow libraries in developing countries

www.elsevier.com | www.bookaid.org | www.sabre.org

ELSEVIER   BOOK AID
International   Sabre Foundation

>>Preface

One of the important responsibilities of the Centers for Disease Control and Prevention (CDC) is to provide up-to-date and comprehensive information on immunization requirements and recommendations for international travelers. This publication is one of the methods employed to help fulfill that responsibility.

The Travelers' Health Section of the Division of Global Migration and Quarantine, National Center for Infectious Diseases, gratefully acknowledges the contributions of all internal and external writers and reviewers. Without their valuable assistance, this publication would not have been possible.

Readers are invited to send comments and suggestions regarding this publication to—

Centers for Disease Control and Prevention
National Center for Infectious Diseases
Division of Global Migration and Quarantine (E-03)
Attention: Travelers' Health Section
Atlanta, Georgia 30333

Centers for Disease Control and Prevention
Julie L. Gerberding, MD, MPH, *Director*

National Center for Infectious Diseases
James M. Hughes, MD, *Director*

Division of Global Migration and Quarantine
Martin S. Cetron, MD, *Director*
Paul M. Arguin, MD, *Acting Chief, Geographic Medicine Branch*
Christie Reed, MD, *Chief, Travelers' Health*
Phyllis E. Kozarsky, MD, *Expert Travel Health Consultant*
Ava W. Navin, MA, *Health Communicator*

>>CDC Contributors

Addiss, David G.
Alexander, Jim
Alexander, Lorraine N.
Anderson, Larry J.
Ansari, Armin
Arguin, Paul M.
Ashford, David A.
Averhoff, Francisco
Barber, Ann M.
Batts-Osborne, Dahna
Beach, Michael J.
Belay, Ermias D.
Bell, Beth P.
Bell, Michael
Bern, Caryn
Blackburn, Brian
Brooks, John T.
Cetron, Martin S.
Clark, Gary G.
Clark, Thomas
Cortese, Margaret M.
Cox, Chad
Dasch, Gregory A.
Eidex, Rachel Barwick
Eremeeva, Marina
Fiore, Anthony E.
Fisk, Tamara A.
Gage, Kenneth L.
Guris, Dalya
Harper, Scott

Hayes, Edward B.
Henderson, Alden
Herwaldt, Barbara
Hochberg, Natasha
Iademarco, Michael F.
Jumaan, Aisha
Juranek, Dennis D.
Kim, David
Koppaka, Ram
Kozarsky, Phyllis
Lau, Eileen
Luby, Stephen
Maguire, James
Mali, Sonja
Malilay, Josephine
Maloney, Susan
Marfin, Anthony A.
Marin, Mona
Massoudi, Mehran S.
Mead, Paul
Miller, Charles W.
Mintz, Eric D.
Moore, Anne
Moore, Matthew
Moran, John S.
Morgan, Juliette
Nasci, Roger S.
Nicolls, Deborah
Papania, Mark
Parashar, Umesh D.

Parise, Monica
Posey, Drew
Quick, Robert
Ranney, Megan
Reed, Christie
Reef, Susan E.
Richards, Frank O. Jr
Rigau, José
Rollin, Pierre
Roper, Martha
Rosenstein, Nancy
Rotz, Lisa
Rupprecht, Charles E.
Russell, Michelle
Schonberger, Lawrence B.
Sejvar, James
Shealy, Katherine
Simone, Patricia
Soriano-Gabarró, Montse
Steele, Stefanie
Sutton, Madeline
Tiwari, Tejpratap
Uhde, Kristin
Watkins, Margaret
Weinberg, Michelle
Weinberg, Nicholas
Whitney, Cynthia
Widdowson, Marc-Alain
Workowski, Kimberly

>>External Contributors

Bunning, Michael, *United States Air Force, Fort Collins, CO*
Connor, Bradley A., *Weill Medical College of Cornell University, New York, NY*
Freedman, David O., *University of Alabama, Birmingham, AL*
Gubler, Duane, *University of Hawaii, Honolulu, HI*
Keystone, Jay, *University of Toronto, Toronto, Canada*
Monath, Thomas, *Acambis, Cambridge, United Kingdom*
Nord, Daniel A., *Divers Alert Network, Durham, NC*
Shlim, David, *Jackson Hole Travel and Tropical Medicine, Jackson Hole, WY*
Teuwen, Dirk E., *Aventis Pasteur SA, Lyon, France*
Wilson, Mary E., *Harvard University, Boston, MA*

All contributors have signed a statement indicating that they have no conflicts of interest with the subject matter or materials discussed in the document(s) that they have written or reviewed for this book and that the information that they have written or reviewed for this book is objective and free from bias.

>>Contents

Disclaimer iv
Preface v
Contributors vi
List of Tables xii
List of Maps xiii

Chapter 1–Introduction
Introduction 2
General Recommendations for Vaccination
and Immunoprophylaxis 8

**Chapter 2–Pre- and Post-travel General Health
        Recommendations**
Planning for Healthy Travel 20
Protection Against Mosquitoes and Other Arthropods 24
Risks from Food and Drink 29
Travelers' Health Kit 35
Seeking Health Care Abroad 37
The Post-Travel Period 43

**Chapter 3–Geographic Distribution of Potential Health
        Hazards to Travelers**
Introduction: Goals and Limitations 48

Chapter 4–Prevention of Specific Infectious Diseases
Acquired Immunodeficiency Syndrome (AIDS) 96
African Trypanosomiasis (African Sleeping Sickness) 100
Amebiasis 102
American Trypanosomiasis (Chagas' Disease) 104
Bovine Spongiform Encephalopathy and Variant
Creutzfeld-Jakob Disease 106
Cholera 109
Coccidioidomycosis 111
Cryptosporidiosis 114
Cyclosporiasis 116
Dengue 117
Diphtheria, Tetanus, & Pertussis 123

Chapter 4–Prevention of Specific Infectious Diseases–cont'd

Encephalitis, Japanese 131
Encephalitis, Tickborne 140
Filariasis, Lymphatic 144
Giardiasis 146
Haemophilus influenzae Type b Meningitis and Invasive Disease 148
Hepatitis, Viral, Type A 151
Hepatitis, Viral, Type B 159
Hepatitis, Viral, Type C 167
Hepatitis, Viral, Type E 169
Histoplasmosis 171
Influenza 174
Legionellosis 180
Leishmaniasis 183
Leptospirosis 185
Lyme Disease 187
Malaria 189
Measles (Rubeola) 212
Meningococcal Disease 219
Mumps 226
Norovirus Infection 228
Onchocerciasis (River Blindness) 231
Plague 233
Streptococcus pneumoniae (Pneumococcal) Disease 236
Poliomyelitis 242
Rabies 247
Rickettsial Infections 253
Rubella 263
Schistosomiasis 266
Severe Acute Respiratory Syndrome 270
Sexually Transmitted Diseases (STDs) 273
Smallpox 276
Travelers' Diarrhea 278
Tuberculosis 288
Typhoid Fever 291
Varicella (Chickenpox) 295
Viral Hemorrhagic Fevers 302
Yellow Fever 308

**Chapter 5—Yellow Fever Vaccine Requirements
and Information on Malaria Risk, by Country** 326

Chapter 6—Non-Infectious Risks During Travel
Jet Lag 374
Motion Sickness. 376
Sunburn 378
Temperature Extremes. 382
Altitude Illness 385
Swimming and Recreational Water Safety 389
Scuba Diving 390
Food Poisoning from Marine Toxins 394
Natural Disasters and Environmental Hazards 399
Injuries 402
Animal-Associated Hazards. 408

Chapter 7—Conveyance and Transportation Issues
Air Travel 414
Cruise Ship Travel 420
Death Overseas 424
Animal Importation and Reentry. 426

**Chapter 8—International Travel with Infants
and Young Children**
Traveling Safely with Infants and Children 434
Vaccine Recommendations for Infants and Children . . . 447
Breastfeeding and Travel 459
International Adoptions. 464

Chapter 9—Advising Travelers with Specific Needs
The Immunocompromised Traveler 474
Preconceptional Planning, Pregnancy and Travel 484
International Travelers with Disabilities. 499
VFRs: Recent Immigrants Returning "Home" To Visit
Friends and Relatives. 501

Index 505

>>List of Tables

Table 1-1.   Revaccination (booster) schedules 11

Table 1-2.   Recommended intervals between administration of antibody-containing products and measles-containing vaccine or varicella vaccine 12

Table 2-1.   Travel notice definitions 22

Table 2-2.   Treatment of water with tincture of iodine 33

Table 3-1.   Disease distribution 50

Table 4-1.   Risk of Japanese encephalitis, by country, region, and season 133

Table 4-2.   Japanese encephalitis vaccine 139

Table 4-3.   Recommended *Haemophilus influenzae* type b (Hib) routine vaccination schedule 150

Table 4-4.   Licensed schedule for HAVRIX 155

Table 4-5.   Licensed schedule for VAQTA 155

Table 4-6.   Licensed schedule for TWINRIX 155

Table 4-7.   Immune globulin for protection against viral Hepatitis A 157

Table 4-8.   Recommended doses of currently licensed Hepatitis B vaccines 164

Table 4-9.   Drugs used in the prophylaxis of malaria 200

Table 4-10.   Pediatric prophylactic doses of atovaquone/proguanil 205

Table 4-11.   Presumptive self-treatment of malaria 211

Table 4-12.   Meningococcal vaccine 224

Table 4-13.   Recommended regimens for use of pneumococcal conjugate vaccine in children <5 years of age 239

Table 4-14.   Countries and political units reporting no indigenous cases of rabies during 2003 248

Table 4-15.   Criteria for preexposure immunization for rabies . . 250

Table 4-16.   Preexposure immunization for rabies 252

Table 4-17.   Postexposure immunization for rabies 252

Table 4-18.   Epidemiologic features and symptoms of rickettsial diseases 255

Table 4-19.   Composition of WHO Oral Rehydration Solution (ORS) for diarrheal illness 286

Table 4-20.   Dosage and schedule for typhoid fever vaccination 294

Table 4-21.   Common adverse reactions to typhoid
               fever vaccines   294
Table 4-22.   Countries in the yellow fever-endemic zone   309
Table 4-23.   Countries that require proof of vaccination
               against yellow fever   321
Table 6-1.   Dosages of anti-motion sickness medications   377
Table 7-1.   Requirements for entry of pet dogs into the
               United States   428
Table 8-1.   Assessment of dehydration levels in infants.   437
Table 8-2.   Recommended childhood and adolescent
               immunization schedule – United States, 2005.   448
Table 8-3.   Recommended childhood and adolescent
               immunization schedule – United States, 2005.
               For children and adolescents who start late or
               who are >1 month behind   449
Table 8-4.   Human milk storage for healthy infants   461
Table 8-5.   Vaccination of breastfeeding mothers   462
Table 9-1.   Vaccination of immunocompromised adults   478
Table 9-2.   Potential contraindications to international travel
               during pregnancy   486
Table 9-3.   Half-lives of selected antimalarial drugs   492
Table 9-4.   Vaccination during pregnancy   494

>>List of Maps

Map 3-1.   Regions—Africa and the Middle East   57
Map 3-2.   Regions—North America, Mexico and Central
            America, and the Caribbean.   67
Map 3-3.   Regions—South America   69
Map 3-4.   Regions—Asia.   75
Map 3-5.   Regions—Western Europe   85
Map 3-6.   Regions—Eastern Europe and Northern Asia   87
Map 3-7.   Regions—Australia and the South Pacific Islands . . .   91
Map 4-1.   Distribution of dengue, Western Hemisphere   119
Map 4-2.   Distribution of dengue, Eastern Hemisphere.   120
Map 4-3.   Geographic distribution of Japanese encephalitis . . .   137
Map 4-4.   Geographic distribution of Hepatitis A
            prevalence, 2005   153

Map 4-5.   Geographic distribution of Hepatitis B
             prevalence, 2005   161
Map 4-6.   Malaria-endemic countries in the
             Western Hemisphere   192
Map 4-7.   Malaria-endemic countries in the
             Eastern Hemisphere   193
Map 4-8.   Geographic distribution of mefloquine-resistant
             malaria   202
Map 4-9.   Areas with frequent epidemics of meningococcal
             meningitis   221
Map 4-10.   Geographic distribution of schistosomiasis 267
Map 4-11.   Areas of risk for travelers' diarrhea 281
Map 4-12.   Yellow fever–endemic zones in Africa, 2005   310
Map 4-13.   Yellow fever–endemic zones in the Americas, 2005 . . . 311

CHAPTER 1

Introduction

>>Introduction

The Division of Global Migration and Quarantine (formerly the Division of Quarantine), National Center for Infectious Diseases, Centers for Disease Control and Prevention (CDC), is pleased to present the 2005 – 2006 edition of *Health Information for International Travel.* The Yellow Book has been written, edited, published, compiled, and disseminated for over a quarter of a century. First published as a small pamphlet with sets of recommendations for the prevention of illnesses such as smallpox, the Yellow Book has become a trusted reference for travelers worldwide. In recent years, it has been written biennially, and it remains the standard set of recommendations for health maintenance and prevention of illness among US travelers. It is written primarily for health-care providers, including physicians, nurses, and pharmacists, although the public will find the book an excellent resource as well. The travel industry, multinational corporations, missionary and volunteer organizations, and families who vacation abroad can all find a wealth of information within this text. Although this information is also provided on CDC's Travelers' Health website (www.cdc.gov/travel), many readers find that this handy text is user-friendly enough to have on their shelves in their offices or at home.

The increase in global travel and the recognition of the specialty of Travel Medicine have resulted in a growing body of knowledge in the field, and an accompanying increase in research and evidence-based guidelines. The reader will immediately note that this is the first edition in which important references have been listed at the end of each section. This new feature will enable readers to quickly find additional and supporting data for the recommendations made.

This edition has been completely revised and updated. The contents have been reorganized, as have many of the chapters. Vaccine requirements have been clarified, and the maps have been improved. The "yellow pages" (Chapter 5) remain a quick reference for areas of the world where yellow fever vaccine is required or recommended and where malaria chemoprophylaxis is recommended. Sections that have been enhanced substantially include those covering immunosuppressed travelers, disabled travelers, cruise ship travel, and children who travel. New sections have been added on air travel, norovirus infection, SARS, and legionellosis. Although the authors of most sections are subject-matter experts at CDC, travel health experts from outside the agency have also made substantial contributions.

A new partnership between CDC and Elsevier publishing house to produce the Yellow Book was launched with this edition. Elsevier, publishers of numerous authoritative texts on infectious diseases and travel medicine, will collaborate with CDC to bring the Yellow Book to the public, institutions involved in health and travel, and to an even greater number of health-care providers, especially those who occasionally counsel travelers but have not had any formal training in travel medicine.

OTHER SOURCES OF TRAVEL HEALTH INFORMATION FROM CDC

- "Yellow Book" online: The online version of the "Yellow Book" may be found on the CDC Internet website at www.cdc.gov/travel/yb/index.htm. It is searchable by destination country, disease, vaccination, type of traveler (e.g., pregnant or special needs), or other topics. The "Yellow Book" may also be accessed through the travelers' health home page.
- Travelers' Health home page: The CDC Travelers' Health home page (www.cdc.gov/travel) is an important way of accessing the most current travel health information. It contains information about outbreaks and links to information about specific diseases, emergency preparedness and response, cruise ship sanitation, air travel health recommendations, emerging infections, vaccine requirements and recommendations, and medications for prevention and treatment of common travel-related problems. In addition, there are valuable links to other websites, such as the World Health Organization, the Pan American Health Organization, and the U.S. State Department, as well as state and local health departments.
- Travelers' Health Fax Information: The Travelers' Health Hotline for faxed information remains active, particularly for those who do not have access to the Internet. Information is periodically updated but may not be as current as that in this text or online. Access is toll-free at 1-888-232-3299.
- Travelers' Health Electronic Mail: E-mail queries, comments, and suggestions for Travelers' Health, including comments about this

book, may be made through a link from the Travelers' Health home page. Urgent health questions from the public should be directed to a health-care provider, and those from health-care providers should be directed to the local or state health department, or to a medical center with a specialist in travel or tropical medicine (see Additional Sources of Travel Health Information).

■ Malaria Information: CDC's Malaria Branch has published a brochure, which may be accessed and downloaded from the Travelers' Health website. In addition, specific malaria prevention and case management questions can be addressed to the CDC's Malaria Branch Telephone Hotline at 770-488-7788 during business hours. After hours and on weekends, a Malaria Branch clinician may be reached by calling 770-488-7100.

■ Yellow Fever Vaccine Registry: In an effort to assist health-care providers and the public in locating a site for yellow fever vaccination and a proof-of-vaccine certificate, a registry of licensed yellow fever vaccine sites in the 50 states and U.S. territories has been added to the Travelers' Health website and is linked to the home page.

■ National Immunization Program (NIP): CDC's vaccine program provides information on their website (www.cdc.gov/nip/default) about vaccines, their recommended schedules in adults and children, and adverse events.

ADDITIONAL SOURCES OF TRAVEL HEALTH INFORMATION

■ The International Society of Travel Medicine (ISTM): The ISTM website (www.istm.org) contains a list of travel health clinics both in the United States and worldwide. The ISTM primarily focuses on pre-travel health education and migration medicine.

■ The American Society of Tropical Medicine and Hygiene (ASTM&H): The ASTM&H website (www.astmh.org) includes a directory of clinicians, primarily within the United States, who specialize in clinical tropical medicine and travelers' health. These health-care providers are available for evaluation of returning travelers who are ill.

■ The World Health Organization (WHO): The WHO website (www.who.int) provides global health information and links to various other international sites. It also includes WHO's online travel health information, entitled International Travel and Health. In some instances, travel health recommendations from the WHO may vary from CDC guidelines. Variability in access to different vaccines and drugs, as well as some differences in expert opinion regarding the prevention of illness, may contribute to the occasional differences.

- The Pan American Health Organization (PAHO): PAHO is a regional office of WHO. For travelers visiting other countries in the Western Hemisphere, the PAHO website (www.paho.org) includes information about outbreaks, disease trends, some country-specific health statistics, and disease control efforts in the Americas.
- The United States Department of State: This website (www.state.gov/travel) is very valuable for both travelers and those living abroad. It contains information about safety and security throughout the world, US consulate information, a list of companies that specialize in travel insurance and medical evacuation, and issues public announcements and travel warnings when there is a threat to the security of travelers. The U.S. Department of State also has a new secure online travel registration site (https://travel registration.state.gov/ibrs/) for American citizens to record information about their trip abroad so that the Department of State can provide assistance in the case of an emergency.
- U.S. Central Intelligence Agency (CIA): The CIA website (www.odci.gov/cia/publications/pubs; select World Factbook) contains useful information for travelers.

In addition to those listed above, a number of commercial travel health information resources may be accessed through health-care providers who subscribe to them. Many are quite useful and have excellent information.

THE WHO INTERNATIONAL HEALTH REGULATIONS (IHR)

The purpose of the WHO IHR is to ensure maximum security against the international spread of diseases, with minimum interference with world traffic. Its origins date back to the mid-19th century when cholera epidemics spread throughout Europe. Epidemics were catalysts for intensive multilateral cooperation in public health. In 1948, the WHO constitution came into being, and the first International Sanitary Regulations were adopted in 1951. These were renamed the International

Health Regulations in 1969; they were modified in 1973 and 1981 and will again be updated to reflect our changing world in 2006. As a member state of the WHO, the United States adheres to the IHR and participates in their development.

The IHR were originally intended to help monitor and control six serious infectious diseases: cholera, plague, yellow fever, smallpox, relapsing fever and typhus. Today, only cholera, plague and yellow fever are notifiable diseases. For the purposes of the IHR, the incubation periods of the quarantinable diseases are 5 days for cholera, 6 days for plague, and 6 days for yellow fever.

Most immunizations are not required under the IHR but may be recommended to protect the health of the traveler. However, an International Certificate of Vaccination against yellow fever is required by some countries as a condition for entry (Chapter 5). Because some countries require vaccination against yellow fever only if travelers arrive from a country where the disease is present, current information must be taken into consideration in determining whether vaccinations are required. Although this text includes the most up-to-date information regarding these requirements at publication, the Travelers' Health website may be accessed for additional information.

PRE-TRAVEL HEALTH MEASURES

Although the information in this book can guide the health-care provider and public toward more healthy and safe travel, a risk assessment of every traveler should be performed. To determine the best health advice, it is not adequate to merely know the destination country. Numerous other factors help determine the risk of illness: the entire itinerary; the destination city, town, or village; the style of travel; the length of stay; and the season of travel. The underlying health of the traveler is equally important: medical problems, previous vaccinations, adverse events, current prescription and over-the-counter medications, previous travel, immune problems, and pregnancy issues are just some of these. Thus, travel health advice needs to be tailored both to the individual and to the itinerary. Many primary-care practitioners are comfortable in giving some pre-travel health advice and are encouraged to learn the basics; for the more complicated travel itineraries or for the traveler with multiple medical problems, it is advisable to refer to a travel health specialist.

In general, the risk of becoming ill during international travel depends on the region of the world visited, as well as the many factors listed above. Travelers to developing countries are at greater risk than those who travel to developed countries (e.g., Canada, Australia, New Zealand, Japan, and Western Europe) where the risk to the health of the traveler is no greater than that incurred in the United States. Travelers visiting urban tourist areas and staying in first-class accommodations may have a lower risk for exposure to infectious diseases. Consequently, additional vaccines and protective measures may be recommended for the more adventuresome travelers. Additionally, children, the elderly, pregnant women, and immunocompromised travelers may be particularly vulnerable to certain problems while traveling and may require more specialized counseling.

Health-care providers have available to them a number of vaccinations for protection of travelers. In addition, providers should take the opportunity, while giving advice to travelers, to update them on routine vaccinations as needed, such as diphtheria/tetanus and measles. Other vaccines that may be recommended include pertussis, poliomyelitis, hepatitis A, hepatitis B, varicella, Japanese B encephalitis, meningococcal meningitis, rabies, and typhoid. For diseases for which no vaccines are available, specific preventive behaviors or medications that may be helpful are detailed in this book. Chapters are also included that address the specific needs of potentially high-risk travelers.

International travelers should contact health-care providers who provide pre-travel health advice at least 4-6 weeks before departure for current health information and to obtain vaccinations and prophylactic medications. Being a responsible traveler means taking care of oneself as well as being sensitive to the cultural variability and fragility of the environment in a world that has been made smaller by our ability to travel from one end of the globe to the other in a matter of hours. The goal of CDC's travel health information is to better enable individuals to enjoy their international travels safely.

—STEFANIE STEELE AND PHYLLIS KOZARSKY

>>General Recommendations for Vaccination and Immunoprophylaxis

Recommendations for immunization are developed by the Advisory Committee on Immunization Practices (ACIP), and these guidelines assist CDC in its role in the ongoing education of health-care providers and the public. To achieve optimal levels of protection against vaccine-preventable diseases, the recommendations are based on scientific evidence of benefits and risks, and, where there are little or no data, on expert opinion. The recommendations include information on general immunization issues and the use of specific vaccines. When these recommendations are issued or revised, they are published in the Morbidity and Mortality Weekly Report (www.cdc.gov/mmwr).

Vaccinations against diphtheria, tetanus, pertussis, measles, mumps, rubella, varicella, poliomyelitis, hepatitis B, *Haemophilus influenzae* type b, and pneumococcal invasive disease are routinely administered in the United States, usually in childhood. If travelers do not have a history of adequate protection against these diseases, immunizations appropriate to their age and previous immunization status should be obtained, whether or not international travel is planned. The fact that a person is seeing a travel health provider or a primary provider for immunizations for travel should be a signal to take the opportunity and vaccinate where there are gaps in routine coverage.

The childhood vaccination schedule changes annually, and recommendations for adolescents and adults change often. Vaccine providers should obtain the most current schedules from the National Immunization Program website, http://www.cdc.gov/nip/. The text and Tables 1–1, 1–2, 4–1 through 4–8, 4–12 through 4–17, 4–20 through 4–23, 8–2 through 8–4, 9–1, and 9–4 of this publication present recommendations for the use, number of doses, dose intervals, adverse reactions, precautions, and contraindications of vaccines and toxoids that may be indicated for travelers. For specific vaccines and toxoids, additional details on background, adverse reactions, precautions, and contraindications are found in the respective ACIP statements.

SPACING OF IMMUNOBIOLOGICS

Simultaneous Administration

All commonly used vaccines can safely and effectively be given simultaneously (that is, on the same day) without impairing antibody responses or increasing rates of adverse reactions. This knowledge is particularly helpful for international travelers for whom exposure to several infectious diseases might be imminent.

In general, inactivated vaccines may be administered simultaneously at separate sites. However, when vaccines commonly associated with local or systemic reactions are given simultaneously, reactions can be accentuated.

Simultaneous administration of acellular pertussis (DTaP); inactivated poliovirus (IPV); *Haemophilus influenzae* type b (Hib); measles, mumps, and rubella (MMR); varicella; pneumococcal conjugate; and hepatitis B vaccines is encouraged for persons who are the recommended age to receive these vaccines and for whom no contraindications exist.

Yellow fever vaccine may be administered simultaneously with all other currently available vaccines.

Limited data suggest that the immunogenicity and safety of Japanese encephalitis (JE) vaccine are not compromised by simultaneous administration with DTaP or whole-cell pertussis (DTP) vaccine. No data exist on the effect of concurrent administration of other vaccines, drugs (e.g., chloroquine or mefloquine), or biologicals on the safety and immunogenicity of JE vaccine.

Inactivated vaccines generally do not interfere with the immune response to other inactivated or live-virus vaccines. An inactivated vaccine may be given either simultaneously or at any time before or after a different inactivated vaccine or a live-virus vaccine.

The immune response to an injected live-virus vaccine (e.g., MMR, varicella, or yellow fever) might be impaired if administered within 28 days of another live virus vaccine. Whenever possible, injected live-virus vaccines administered on different days should be given at least 28 days apart. If two injected live-virus vaccines are not administered on the same day but <28 days apart, the second vaccine should be readministered at least 4 weeks later.

Live-virus vaccines can interfere with a person's response to tuberculin testing. Tuberculin testing, if otherwise indicated, can be done either on the day that live-virus vaccines are administered or 4-6 weeks later.

Missed Doses and Boosters

Persons will often forget to return for a follow-up dose of vaccine or booster at the specified time. It is unnecessary in these cases to restart the interrupted series or to add any extra doses. This is true for all vaccines except for the oral typhoid vaccine. Most products require periodic booster doses to maintain protection (See Table 1–1).

Immune Globulin Preparations

When MMR and varicella vaccines are given with immune globulin (IG, also called immune serum globulin and immunoglobulin) preparations, antibody response can be diminished. IG preparations do not interfere with the immune response to yellow fever vaccine. The duration of inhibition of MMR and varicella vaccines is related to the dose of IG. Administration of MMR or its components and of varicella vaccines should be delayed 3-11 months after IG administration (Table 1–2).

IG administration may become necessary for another indication after MMR or its individual components or varicella vaccines have been given. In such a situation, the IG may interfere with the immune response to the MMR or varicella vaccines. Vaccine virus replication and stimulation of immunity usually occur 2–3 weeks after vaccination. If the interval between administration of one of these vaccines and the subsequent administration of an IG preparation is 14 days or more, the vaccine need not be readministered. If the interval is <14 days, the vaccine should be readministered after the interval shown in Table 1–2, unless serologic testing indicates that antibodies have been produced. If administration of IG becomes necessary, MMR or its components or varicella vaccines can be administered simultaneously with IG, with the recognition that vaccine-induced immunity can be compromised. The vaccine should be administered in a body site different from that chosen for the IG injection. Vaccination should be repeated after the interval noted in Table 1–2, unless serologic testing indicates antibodies have been produced.

TABLE 1-1. REVACCINATION (BOOSTER) SCHEDULES

VACCINE	RECOMMENDATION
Cholera	No longer available in U.S.
Japanese encephalitis	Full duration of protection unknown. Neutralizing antibodies may persist at least 2 years after primary immunization.
Hepatitis A (HAV)	Booster not recommended for adults and children who complete primary series (2 doses)
Hepatitis B (HBV)	Booster doses of vaccine are not recommended for adults and children who completed primary series according to routine schedule.[1] Booster is recommended at least 6 months after the start of the accelerated schedule.
Influenza	1 annual dose
Measles, Mumps, Rubella (MMR)	1 dose if measles, mumps, or rubella vaccination history is unreliable and person did not have these illnesses; 2 doses for persons with occupational or other indications
Meningococcal Quadrivalent A, C, Y, W-135	Full duration of protection is unknown; immunity may persist at least 3 years in adults
Pneumoccocal (polysaccharide)	One-time revaccination 5 years after original dose for persons >65 years of age or who have immunosuppressive conditions
Polio (IPV)	For adults who have completed primary series, a single lifetime booster
Rabies Preexposure vaccine	No serologic testing or boosters recommended for travelers. For persons in higher risk groups, such as rabies laboratory workers, serologic testing and booster doses are recommended. See Table 4-15.
Tetanus/diphtheria (Td)	Booster every 10 years
Typhoid Oral	Booster every 5 years
Typhoid IM	Booster every 2 years
Varicella	Booster not recommended after completion of primary series.
Yellow fever	Booster every 10 years. Note that there are age-related risks for severe adverse reactions.

[1]Booster dosing may be appropriate for certain populations, such as hemodialysis patients.

TABLE 1-2. RECOMMENDED INTERVALS BETWEEN ADMINISTRATION OF ANTIBODY-CONTAINING PRODUCTS AND MEASLES-CONTAINING VACCINE OR VARICELLA VACCINE[1]

INDICATION	DOSE	RECOMMENDED INTERVAL BEFORE MEASLES OR VARICELLA VACCINATION
Tetanus (TIG)	250 units (10 mg IgG/kg) IM[2]	3 months
Hepatitis A (IG), duration of international travel		
<3-month stay	0.02 mL/kg (3.3 mg IgG/kg) IM	At least 5 months for varicella At least 3 months for measles
>3-month stay	0.06 mL/kg (10 mg IgG/kg) IM	At least 5 months for varicella At least 3 months for measles
Hepatitis B prophylaxis (HBIG)	0.06 mL/kg (10 mg IgG/kg) IM	At least 3 months
Rabies prophylaxis (HRIG)	20 IU/kg (22 mg IgG/kg) IM	At least 3 months
Varicella prophylaxis (VZIG)	125 units/10 kg (20-40 mg IgG/kg) IM (maximum 625 units)	At least 5 months
Measles prophylaxis (IG)		
Immunocompetent contact	0.25 mL/kg (40 mg IgG/kg) IM	3-5 months
Immunocompromised contact	0.50 mL/kg (80 mg IgG/kg) IM	6 months
Blood transfusion		
Red blood cells (RBCs), washed	10 mL/kg negligible IgG/kg) IV	None
RBCs, adenine-saline added	10 mL/kg (10 mg IgG/kg) IV	At least 5 months for varicella At least 3 months for measles
Packed RBCs (Hct 65%)[3]	10 mL/kg (60 mg IgG/kg) IV	At least 5 months for varicella At least 5 months for measles
Plasma/platelet products	10 mL/kg (160 mg IgG/kg) IV	At least 5 months for varicella At least 7 months for measles

This table is adapted from the AAP Committee on Infectious Diseases. Recommended timing of routine measles immunization for children who have recently received immune globulin preparations. Pediatrics. 1994.

[1]This table is not intended for determining the correct indications and dosage for the use of IG preparations. Unvaccinated people may not be fully protected against measles during the entire recommended interval, and additional doses of IG or measles vaccine may be indicated after measles exposure. Concentrations of measles antibody in an IG preparation can vary by manufacturer's lot. For example, fourfold or greater variation in the amount of measles antibody titers has been demonstrated in different IG preparations. Rates of antibody clearance after receipt of an immune globulin preparation can also vary. Recommended intervals are extrapolated from an estimated half-life of 30 days for passively acquired antibody and an observed interference with the immune response to measles vaccine for 5 months after a dose of 80 mg IgG/kg.

TABLE 1–2. RECOMMENDED INTERVALS BETWEEN ADMINISTRATION OF ANTIBODY-CONTAINING PRODUCTS AND MEASLES-CONTAINING VACCINE OR VARICELLA VACCINE-CONT'D

INDICATION	DOSE	RECOMMENDED INTERVAL BEFORE MEASLES OR VARICELLA VACCINATION
Cytomegalovirus prophylaxis (CMV IGIV)	Variable	At least 3 months
Respiratory syncytial virus (RSV) monoclonal antibody (Synagis)[4]	15 mg/kg IM	No data (or unknown)
RSV prophylaxis (RSV IGIV)	750 mg/kg	9 months
Intravenous immune globulin (IVIG)		
Replacement therapy	300-400 mg/kg IV	8 months
Immune thrombocytopenic purpura (ITP)	400 mg/kg IV	8 months
ITP	1 gm/kg IV	10 months
ITP or Kawasaki disease	1.6 gm/kg IV - 2 gm	11 months

[2]IG, immune globulin; IM, intramuscular; IV, intravenous
[3]Assumes a serum IgG concentration of 16 mg/mL.
[4]Contains only antibody to respiratory syncytial virus.

When IG is given with the first dose of hepatitis A vaccine (HAV), the proportion of recipients who develop protective levels of antibody is not affected, but antibody concentrations are lower. Because the final concentrations of anti-HAV are many times higher than those considered protective, this reduced immunogenicity is not expected to be clinically important. IG preparations interact minimally with other inactivated vaccines and toxoids. Therefore, other inactivated vaccines may be given simultaneously or at any time interval after or before an antibody-containing blood product is used. However, such vaccines should be administered at different sites from the IG (not from each other).

Vaccination of Persons with Acute Illnesses
Every opportunity should be taken to provide appropriate vaccinations. The decision to delay vaccination because of a current or recent acute illness depends on the severity of the symptoms and their cause.

Although a moderate or severe acute illness is sufficient reason to postpone vaccination, minor illnesses (such as diarrhea, mild upper respiratory infection with or without low-grade fever, or other low-grade febrile illness) are not contraindications to vaccination. Antimicrobial therapy is not a contraindication to vaccination, except with oral typhoid vaccine (Ty21a). People with moderate or severe acute illness with or without fever should be vaccinated as soon as the condition has improved. This precaution is to avoid superimposing adverse effects from the vaccine on underlying illness or mistakenly attributing a manifestation of underlying illness to the vaccine.

Routine physical examinations or temperature measurements are not prerequisites for vaccinating anyone who appears to be in good health. Asking if a person is ill, postponing a vaccination for someone with moderate or severe acute illness, and vaccinating someone without contraindications are appropriate procedures in immunization programs.

Vaccination Scheduling for Last-Minute Travelers
In general, as noted above under "Simultaneous Administration," most vaccine products can be given during one visit for those anticipating imminent travel. Unless the vaccines given are boosters of those typically given during childhood, every vaccine has a time period necessary for the host to develop sufficient antibodies, and this period of time may vary depending on the vaccine. This information is found in the Food and Drug Administration (FDA) drug information insert that accompanies each product.

Some vaccines require more than one dose for best protection. The use of multiple reduced doses or doses given at less than minimum intervals can lessen the antibody response. Because some travelers visit their health-care providers without ample time for administration of the several vaccine doses recommended for optimal protection against certain diseases, studies have been performed and others are ongoing to determine whether accelerated scheduling is adequate. This concern is primarily the case for hepatitis B vaccine or the combined hepatitis A and B vaccine (See Chapter 4). With imminent travel, a clinician may opt to accelerate these vaccine schedules, with the understanding that such administration has not been FDA approved and thus not endorsed by CDC. However, many travel medicine experts are using shortened schedules, feeling that they may provide better protection than the administration of just one dose of vaccine before travel. It is unclear what level of protection any given traveler will have if a full series of vaccination is not completed when more than one dose is recommended.

Hypersensitivity to Vaccine Components

Vaccine components can cause allergic reactions in some recipients. These reactions can be local or systemic and can include anaphylaxis or anaphylactic-like responses. The vaccine components responsible can include the vaccine antigen, animal proteins, antibiotics, preservatives (e.g., thimerosal), or stabilizers (e.g., gelatin). The most common animal protein allergen is egg protein in vaccines prepared by using embryonated chicken eggs (influenza and yellow fever vaccines). Generally, people who can eat eggs or egg products safely may receive these vaccines, while people with histories of anaphylactic allergy (e.g., hives, swelling of the mouth and throat, difficulty breathing, hypotension, or shock) to eggs or egg proteins ordinarily should not. Screening people by asking whether they can eat eggs without adverse effects is a reasonable way to identify those who might be at risk from receiving yellow fever and influenza vaccines. Recent studies have indicated that other components in vaccines in addition to egg proteins (e.g., gelatin) may cause allergic reactions, including anaphylaxis in rare instances. Protocols have been developed for testing and vaccinating people with anaphylactic reactions to egg ingestion.

Some vaccines contain preservatives or trace amounts of antibiotics to which people might be allergic. Those administering the vaccine(s) should carefully review the information provided in the package insert before deciding if the rare person with such an allergy should receive the vaccine(s). Thimerosal in trace quantities may be found in the meningococcal polysaccharide vaccine (groups A, C, Y, and W-125 combined) and the Japanese encephalitis vaccines, as well as in a few others. For a listing of preservatives used and the vaccines in which they are found, see www.fda.gov/cber/vaccine/thimerosal.htm. No currently recommended vaccine contains penicillin or penicillin derivatives. Some vaccines (e.g., MMR and its individual component vaccines, IPV, varicella, rabies) contain trace amounts of neomycin or other antibiotics; the amount is less than would normally be used for the skin test to determine hypersensitivity. However, people who have experienced anaphylactic reactions to the antibiotic generally should not receive these vaccines. Most often, neomycin allergy is a contact dermatitis—a manifestation of a delayed-type (cell-mediated) immune response—rather than anaphylaxis. A history of delayed-type reactions to neomycin is not a contraindication to receiving these vaccines.

Reporting Adverse Events Following Immunization

Modern vaccines are extremely safe and effective. Benefits and risks are associated with the use of all immunobiologics—no vaccine is completely effective or completely free of side effects. Adverse events following immunization have been reported with all vaccines, ranging from frequent, minor, local reactions to extremely rare, severe, systemic illness such as that associated with yellow fever vaccine. Information on side effects and adverse events following specific vaccines and toxoids are discussed in detail in each ACIP statement. Health-care providers are required by law to report selected adverse events occurring after vaccination with tetanus vaccine in any combination, pertussis in any combination, measles and rubella alone or in any combination, OPV, IPV, hepatitis B, varicella, *Haemophilus influenzae* type b (conjugate), pneumococcal conjugate, and yellow fever vaccines. Reportable events are generally those requiring the recipient to seek medical attention and are stated on the Vaccine Adverse Events Reporting System (VAERS) web site (www.vaers.org/reportable.htm). VAERS is a cooperative program for vaccine safety of the CDC and the FDA. Information about vaccine safety and reporting may be found on their homepage at www.vaers.org.

Bibliography

Ada, G. "Vaccines and vaccination." *N Engl J Med.* 2001;345(14):1042–53.

American Academy of Pediatrics. Pickering LK, ed. *Red Book: 2003 Report of the Committee on Infectious Diseases.* 26th ed. Elk Grove Village, IL: American Academy of Pediatrics, 2003.

American Academy of Pediatrics Committee on Infectious Diseases. "Recommended timing of routine measles immunization for children who have recently received immune globulin preparations." *Pediatrics.* 1994;93:682–5.

American Academy of Pediatrics. Committee on Infectious Diseases and Committee on Fetus and Newborn: Respiratory Syncytial Virus Immune Globulin Intravenous: Indications for Use. *Pediatrics.* 1997;99:645–50.

CDC. Epidemiology and Prevention of Vaccine-Preventable Diseases. [monograph on the internet] Atlanta: Centers for Disease Control and Prevention; 2004 [cited 2004 Nov 2]. Available from: http://www.cdc.gov/nip/publications/pink/default.htm

Feldman S. Interchangeability of vaccines. *Pediatr Infect Dis J.* 2001;20(11 Suppl):S23–9.

Plotkin SA. Immunologic correlates of protection induced by vaccination. *Pediatr Infect Dis J.* 2001;20(1):63–75.

Plotkin SA, Orenstein WA, editors. Vaccines. 4th ed. Philadelphia: W.B. Saunders; 2004.

Varricchio F, Iskander J, Destefano F, et al. Understanding vaccine safety information from the Vaccine Adverse Event Reporting System. *Pediatr Infect Dis J.* 2004;23(4):287–94.

–PHYLLIS KOZARSKY, PAUL ARGUIN, AND STEFANIE STEELE

CHAPTER 2

Pre- and Post-Travel General Health Recommendations

>>Planning for Healthy Travel

International travelers can take a number of simple steps to avoid potential health problems before and during travel. International travelers should contact their physicians, local health departments, or private or public agencies that advise international travelers at least 4 to 6 weeks before departure to schedule an appointment to receive current health information on the countries they plan to visit, obtain vaccinations and prophylactic medications as indicated, and address any special needs.

It is wisest for persons to postpone travel if they are not feeling well, particularly if they have febrile illnesses. By delaying travel, persons who are ill avoid potential emergencies and are courteous toward other travelers who may not wish to be exposed to someone with a transmissible illness. Trip cancellation insurance is available from a variety of sources.

Handwashing is one of the most important practices in preventing illness from infections while traveling. Travelers should wash their hands often with soap and water or an alcohol-based hand rub to remove potentially infectious materials from the skin and help prevent disease transmission.

New risks to international travelers may arise that are not detailed in this book. These new risks may result from unanticipated outbreaks of infectious diseases in an international travel destination or emerging infectious diseases.

Emerging infectious diseases are diseases of infectious origin the incidence of which in humans has increased within the past two decades or threatens to increase in the near future. Many factors or combinations of factors can contribute to disease emergence and outbreaks. New infectious diseases can emerge from genetic changes in existing organisms; known diseases can spread to new geographic areas and populations; and previously unknown diseases can appear in humans living or working in changing ecologic conditions that increase their exposure to insect vectors, animal reservoirs, or environmental sources of novel pathogens. A good example is the emergence of the severe acute respiratory syndrome (SARS). SARS is a viral respiratory illness caused by a coronavirus

(SARS-CoV). SARS was recognized as a global threat in March 2003, after first appearing in Southern China in November 2002. Over the next few months, the illness spread to more than two dozen countries in North America, South America, Europe, and Asia. Although the 2003 global outbreak was contained, person-to-person transmission of SARS-CoV may recur. Although there is no evidence that direct contact with civets or other wild animals from live-food markets has led to cases of SARS, viruses very similar to SARS-CoV have been found in these animals. In addition, some persons working with these animals have evidence of infection with SARS-CoV or a very similar virus.

Reemergence can occur because of the development of antimicrobial resistance in existing infections (e.g., gonorrhea, malaria, and pneumococcal disease) or breakdowns in public health measures for previously controlled infections (e.g., cholera, tuberculosis, and pertussis).

Travelers should be aware of the occurrence of any disease outbreaks in their international destinations. Current travel notices on diseases of international concern are posted on the Travelers' Health home page on the CDC website at www.cdc.gov/travel.

CDC issues different types of notices for international travelers. As of May 20, 2004, these definitions were refined to make the announcements more easily understood by travelers, health-care providers, and the general public (Table 2–1). Each type of notice describes the level of risk for the traveler and recommended preventive measures. Guidance is posted on the CDC Travelers' Health website as outbreaks occur, in four levels:

> *In The News,* the lowest level of notice, will provide information about sporadic cases of disease or an occurrence of a disease of public health significance affecting a traveler or travel destination. The risk for an individual traveler does not differ from the usual risk in that area.
> *Outbreak Notice* provides information about a disease outbreak in a limited geographic area or setting. The risk to travelers is defined and limited, and the notice will remind travelers about standard or enhanced travel recommendations, such as vaccination.
> *Travel Health Precaution* provides specific information to travelers about a disease outbreak of greater scope and over a larger geographic area so they can take measures to reduce the risk of infection.

TABLE 2-1. TRAVEL NOTICE DEFINITIONS

TYPE OF NOTICE/ LEVEL OF CONCERN	SCOPE[1]	RISK FOR TRAVELERS[2]	PREVENTIVE MEASURES	EXAMPLE OF NOTICE	EXAMPLE OF RECOMMENDED MEASURES
In the News	Reports of sporadic cases	No increased risk over baseline for travelers observing standard recommendations	Keeping travelers informed and reinforcing standard prevention recommendations	Report of cases of dengue in Mexico, 2001	Reinforced standard recommendations for protection against insect bites
Outbreak Notice	Outbreak in limited geographic area or setting	Increased but definable and limited to specific settings	Reminders about standard and enhanced recommendations for the region	Outbreak of yellow fever in a state in Brazil in 2003	Reinforced enhanced recommendations, such as vaccination
Travel Health Precaution	Outbreak of greater scope affecting a larger geographic area	Increased in some settings, along with risk for spread to other areas	Specific precautions to reduce risk during the stay, and what to do before and after travel[3]	Outbreak of avian influenza among poultry and humans in several countries in Southeast Asia in early 2004	Recommended specific precautions including avoiding areas with live poultry, such as live animal markets and poultry farms; ensuring poultry and eggs are thoroughly cooked; monitoring health

[1]The term "scope" incorporates the size, magnitude, and rapidity of spread of an outbreak.
[2]Risk for travelers is dependent on patterns of transmission, as well as severity of illness.
[3]Preventive measures other than the standard advice for the region may be recommended depending on the circumstances (e.g., travelers may be requested to monitor their health for a certain period after their return, or arriving passengers may be screened at ports of entry).

TABLE 2-1. TRAVEL NOTICE DEFINITIONS-cont'd

TYPE OF NOTICE/ LEVEL OF CONCERN	SCOPE[1]	RISK FOR TRAVELERS[2]	PREVENTIVE MEASURES	EXAMPLE OF NOTICE	EXAMPLE OF RECOMMENDED MEASURES
Travel Health Warning	Evidence that outbreak is expanding outside the area or populations initially affected	Increased because of evidence of transmission outside defined settings and/or inadequate containment measures	In addition to the specific precautions cited above, **postpone nonessential travel**[3]	SARS outbreak in Asia in 2003	Recommended travelers to postpone nonessential travel because of level of risk

[3]Preventive measures other than the standard advice for the region may be recommended depending on the circumstances (e.g., travelers may be requested to monitor their health for a certain period after their return, or arriving passengers may be screened at ports of entry).

The precaution also provides guidance to travelers about what to do if they become ill while in the area. CDC does not recommend against travel to a specific area but may recommend limiting exposure to a defined setting, such as poultry farms or health-care settings.

Travel Health Warning recommends against nonessential travel to an area because a disease of public health concern is expanding outside the areas or populations that were initially affected. The purpose of a travel warning is to reduce the volume of traffic to affected areas, thus limiting the risk of spreading the disease to unaffected areas.

A complete description of the definitions and criteria for issuing and removing travel notices can also be found at www.cdc.gov/travel.

–PATRICIA M. SIMONE

>>Protection against Mosquitoes and Other Arthropods

Although vaccines or chemoprophylactic drugs are available against important vector-borne diseases such as yellow fever and malaria, travelers still should be advised to use repellents and other general protective measures against biting arthropods.

The effectiveness of malaria chemoprophylaxis is variable, depending on patterns of resistance and compliance with medication, and no similar preventive measures exist for other mosquito-borne diseases such as dengue. For many vector-borne diseases, no specific preventives are available.

GENERAL PREVENTIVE MEASURES

The principal approach to prevention of vector-borne diseases is avoidance. Tick- and mite-borne infections characteristically are diseases of "place;" whenever possible, known foci of disease transmission should be avoided. Although many vector-borne infections can be prevented by avoiding rural locations, certain mosquito- and midge-borne arboviral and parasitic infections are transmitted seasonally, and simple changes in itinerary can greatly reduce risk for acquiring them.

Travelers should be advised that exposure to arthropod bites can be minimized by modifying patterns of activity or behavior. Some vector mosquitoes are most active in twilight periods, at dawn and dusk or in the evening. Avoidance of outdoor activity during these periods can reduce risk of exposure. Wearing long-sleeved shirts, long pants, and hats minimizes areas of exposed skin. Shirts should be tucked in. Repellents applied to clothing, shoes, tents, mosquito nets, and other gear will enhance protection.

When exposure to ticks or biting insects is a possibility, travelers should be advised to tuck their pants into their socks and to wear boots, not sandals. Permethrin-based repellents applied as directed (see the following section, "Repellents") will enhance protection. Travelers should be advised to inspect themselves and their clothing for ticks, both during outdoor activity and at the end of the day. Ticks are detected more easily on light-colored or white clothing. Prompt removal of attached ticks can prevent some infections.

When accommodations are not adequately screened or air conditioned, bed nets are essential to provide protection and comfort. Bed nets should be tucked under mattresses and can be sprayed with a repellent such as permethrin. The permethrin will be effective for several months if the bed net is not washed. Aerosol insecticides can help to clear rooms of mosquitoes.

REPELLENTS

Travelers should be advised that permethrin-containing repellents (e.g., Permanone) are recommended for use on clothing, shoes, bed nets, and camping gear, and are registered by the U.S. Environmental Protection Agency for this use. Permethrin is highly effective both as an insecticide and as a repellent. Permethrin-treated clothing repels and kills ticks, mosquitoes, and other arthropods and retains this effect after repeated laundering. There appears to be little potential for toxicity from permethrin-treated clothing. The insecticide should be reapplied after every five washings.

The U.S. Environmental Protection Agency has registered several active ingredients for use in personal repellents applied to skin. EPA registration of repellent active ingredients indicates the materials have been reviewed and approved for efficacy and human safety if applied according to the instructions on the label. These active ingredients are DEET (N,N-diethylmetatoluamide), Picaridin (KBR 3023), MGK-326, MGK-264, IR 3535, oil of citronella, and p-Menthane 3,8-diole (Oil of Lemon Eucalyptus).

All the EPA-registered active ingredients have some repellent activity, but most authorities recommend repellents containing DEET (N,N-diethylmetatoluamide) as the most reliable and long-lasting. DEET repels mosquitoes, ticks, and other arthropods when applied to the skin. In general, the more DEET a repellent contains, the longer time it can protect against mosquito bites. However, there appears to be no added benefit of concentrations >50%. A microencapsulated, sustained-release formulation can have a longer period of activity than liquid formulations at the same concentrations. Length of protection also varies with ambient temperature, amount of perspiration, any water exposure, abrasive removal, and other factors. DEET-based repellents applied according to label instructions may be used with sunscreen with no reduction in repellent activity.

No definitive studies have been published about what concentration of DEET is safe for children. No serious illness has been reported from use of DEET according the manufacturer's recommendations. DEET formulations as high as 50% are recommended for both adults and children >2 months of age. Lower concentrations are not as long lasting, offering short-term protection only and necessitating more frequent reapplication. Repellent products that do not contain DEET are not likely to offer the same degree of protection from mosquito bites as products containing DEET. Other types of repellents have not necessarily been as thoroughly studied as DEET and may not be safer for use on children. Parents should choose the type and concentration of repellent to be used by taking into account the amount of time that a child will be outdoors, exposure to mosquitoes, and the risk of mosquito-transmitted disease in the area. The recommendations for DEET use in pregnant women do not differ from those for nonpregnant adults.

DEET is toxic when ingested and may cause skin irritation in sensitive persons. High concentrations applied to the skin can cause blistering. However, because DEET is so widely used, a great deal of testing has been done, and over the long history of DEET use, very few confirmed incidents of toxic reactions to DEET have occurred when the product is used properly.

Travelers should be advised that the possibility of adverse reactions to DEET will be minimized if they take the following precautions:

- Use enough repellent to cover exposed skin. Do not apply repellent to skin that is under clothing. Heavy application is not necessary to achieve protection.
- Do not apply repellent to cuts, wounds, or irritated skin.
- After returning indoors, wash treated skin with soap and water.
- Do not spray aerosol or pump products in enclosed areas; do not inhale the aerosol.
- Do not apply aerosol or pump products directly to the face. Spray your hands and then rub them carefully over the face, avoiding eyes and mouth.
- When using repellent on a child, apply it to your own hands and then rub them on the child. Avoid the child's eyes and mouth and apply sparingly around the ears.
- Do not apply repellent to children's hands. (Children tend to put their hands in their mouths.)
- Do not allow children <10 years old to apply insect repellent to themselves; have an adult do it for them. Keep repellents out of reach of children.
- Protect infants ≤2 months of age by using a carrier draped with mosquito netting with an elastic edge for a tight fit.
- Bed nets, repellents containing DEET, and permethrin should be purchased before traveling and can be found in hardware, camping, sporting goods, and military surplus stores. Overseas, permethrin or a similar insecticide, deltamethrin, may be purchased to treat bed nets and clothes.

Useful Links

U.S. Environmental Protection Agency. How to Use Insect Repellents Safely http://www.epa.gov/pesticides/factsheets/insectrp.htm

Centers for Disease Control and Prevention: Insect Repellent Use and Safety http://www.cdc.gov/ncidod/dvbid/westnile/qa/ insect_repellent.htm

Bibliography

Barnard DR, Bernier UR, Posey KH, et al. Repellency of IR3535, KBR3023, para-menthane-3,8-diol, and DEET to black salt marsh mosquitoes (Diptera: Culicidae) in the Everglades National Park. *J Med Entomol.* 2002;39:895–9.

Barnard DR, Xue RD. Laboratory evaluation of mosquito repellents against *Aedes albopictus, Culex nigripalpus,* and *Ochlerotatus triseriatus* (Diptera: Culicidae). *J Med Entomol.* 2004;41:726–30.

Chou JT, Rossignol PA, Ayres JW. Evaluation of commercial insect repellents on human skin against *Aedes aegypti* (Diptera: Culicidae). *J Med Entomol.* 1997;34:624–30.

Fradin MS. Mosquitoes and mosquito repellents: a clinician's guide. *Ann Intern Med.* 1998;128:931–40.

Fradin MS, Day JF. Comparative efficacy of insect repellents against mosquito bites. *N Engl J Med.* 2002;347:13–8.

Koren G, Matsui D, Bailey B. DEET-based insect repellents: safety implications for children and pregnant and lactating women. *CMAJ.* 2003;169:209–12.

McGready R, Hamilton KA, Simpson JA, et al. Safety of the insect repellent N,N-diethyl-M-toluamide (DEET) in pregnancy. *Am J Trop Med Hyg.* 2001;65:285–9.

Murphy ME, Montemarano AD, Debboun M, et al. The effect of sunscreen on the efficacy of insect repellent: a clinical trial. *J Am Acad Dermatol.* 2000;43(2 Pt 1):219–22.

Rutledge LC, Gupta RK, Mehr ZA, et al. Evaluation of controlled-release mosquito repellent formulations. *J Am Mosq Control Assoc.* 1996;12:39–44.

Sudakin DL, Trevathan WR. DEET: a review and update of safety and risk in the general population. *J Toxicol Clin Toxicol.* 2003;41:831–9.

—ROGER NASCI

>>Risks from Food and Water

Contaminated food and drink are common sources for the introduction of infection into the body. Among the more common infections that travelers can acquire from contaminated food and drink are *Escherichia coli* infections, shigellosis or bacillary dysentery, giardiasis, cryptosporidiosis, noroviruses, and hepatitis A. Other less common infectious disease risks for travelers include typhoid fever and other salmonelloses, cholera, rotavirus infections, and a variety of protozoan and helminthic parasites (other than those that cause giardiasis and cryptosporidiosis). Many infectious diseases transmitted in food and water can also be acquired directly through the fecal-oral route.

FOOD

To avoid illness, travelers should be advised to select food with care. All raw food is subject to contamination. Particularly in areas where hygiene and sanitation are inadequate, the traveler should be advised to avoid salads, uncooked vegetables, and unpasteurized milk and milk products such as cheese, and to eat only food that has been cooked and is still hot or fruit that has been washed in clean water and then peeled by the traveler personally. Undercooked and raw meat, fish, and shellfish can carry various intestinal pathogens. Cooked food that has been allowed to stand for several hours at ambient temperature can provide a fertile medium for bacterial growth and should be thoroughly reheated before serving. Consumption of food and beverages obtained from street vendors has been associated with an increased risk of illness.

The easiest way to guarantee a safe food source for an infant <6 months of age is to have the infant breastfeed. If the infant has already been weaned from the breast, formula prepared from commercial powder and boiled water is the safest and most practical food.

Cholera cases have occurred in people who ate crab brought back from Latin America by travelers. Travelers should be advised not to bring perishable seafood with them when they return to the United States from high-risk areas. Moreover, travelers may assume incorrectly that food and water aboard commercial aircraft are safe. Food and water may be obtained in the country of departure, where items may be contaminated.

WATER

Swimming

A variety of infections (e.g., skin, ear, eye, respiratory, neurologic, and diarrheal infections) have been linked to wading or swimming in the ocean, freshwater lakes and rivers, and swimming pools, particularly if the swimmer's head is submerged. Water may be contaminated by other people and from sewage, animal wastes, and wastewater run-off. Diarrhea and other serious waterborne infections can be spread when disease-causing organisms from human or animal feces are introduced into the water. Travelers who swim should be advised to avoid beaches that may be contaminated with human sewage or dog feces.

Accidentally swallowing small amounts of fecally contaminated water can cause illness. Travelers should be warned to try to avoid swallowing water while engaging in aquatic activities. Generally, for infectious disease prevention, pools that contain chlorinated water can be considered safe places to swim if the disinfectant levels and pH are properly maintained. However, some organisms (e.g., *Cryptosporidium*, *Giardia*, hepatitis A, and Norovirus) have moderate to very high resistance to chlorine levels commonly found in chlorinated swimming pools, so travelers also should avoid swallowing chlorinated swimming pool water. All travelers who have diarrhea should refrain from swimming to avoid contaminating recreational water.

Travelers should be advised to avoid swimming or wading with open cuts or abrasions that might serve as entry points for pathogens. In certain areas, fatal primary amebic meningoencephalitis has occurred after swimming in warm freshwater lakes or rivers, thermally polluted areas around industrial complexes, and hot springs, so travelers should avoid submerging the head and should wear nose plugs when entering untreated water to prevent water getting up the nose. Travelers should also be advised to avoid wading or swimming in freshwater streams, canals, and lakes in schistosomiasis-endemic areas of the Caribbean, South America, Africa, and Asia (see Map 4–10, Geographic distribution of schistosomiasis), or in bodies of water that may be contaminated with urine from animals infected with *Leptospira*.

Drinking

Water that has been adequately chlorinated according to the minimum recommended water treatment standards used in the United States will afford substantial protection against viral and bacterial waterborne diseases. However, chlorine treatment alone, as used in the routine disinfection of water, may not kill some enteric viruses and the parasitic organisms that cause giardiasis, amebiasis, and cryptosporidiosis. In areas where chlorinated tap water is not available or where hygiene and sanitation are poor, travelers should be advised that only the following may be safe to drink:

- Beverages, such as tea and coffee, made with boiled water.
- Canned or bottled beverages, including water, carbonated mineral water, and soft drinks.
- Beer and wine.

Where water might be contaminated, travelers should be advised that ice should also be considered contaminated and should not be used in beverages. If ice has been in contact with containers used for drinking, travelers should be advised to clean the containers thoroughly, preferably with soap and hot water, after the ice has been discarded.

It is safer to drink a beverage directly from the can or bottle than from a questionable container. However, water on the outside of beverage cans or bottles may also be contaminated. Therefore, travelers should be advised to dry wet cans or bottles before they are opened and to wipe clean surfaces with which the mouth will have direct contact. Where water may be contaminated, travelers should be advised to avoid brushing their teeth with tap water.

Treatment of Drinking Water

Travelers should be advised of the following methods for treating water to make it safe for drinking and other purposes.

Boiling

Boiling is by far the most reliable method to make water of uncertain purity safe for drinking. Water should be brought to a vigorous rolling boil for 1 minute and allowed to cool to room temperature; ice should not be added. This procedure will kill bacterial and parasitic causes of diarrhea at all altitudes and viruses at low altitudes. To kill viruses at altitudes >2,000 m (6,562 ft), water should be boiled for 3 minutes or chemical disinfection should be used after the water has boiled for 1 minute. Adding a pinch of salt to each quart or pouring the water several times from one clean container to another will improve the taste.

Chemical Disinfection

Chemical disinfection with iodine is an alternative method of water treatment when it is not feasible to boil water. However, this method cannot be relied on to kill *Cryptosporidium*. Two well-tested methods for disinfection with iodine are the use of tincture of iodine (Table 2–2) and tetraglycine hydroperiodide tablets (e.g., Globaline, Potable-Aqua, or Coghlan's). These tablets are available from pharmacies and sporting goods stores. The manufacturer's instructions should be followed. If water is cloudy, the number of tablets used should be doubled; if water is extremely cold (<5° C; <41° F), an attempt should be made to warm the water, and the recommended contact time should be increased to achieve reliable disinfection. Cloudy water should be strained through a clean cloth into a container to remove any sediment or floating matter, and then the water should be boiled or treated with iodine. Iodine treatment of water is intended for short-term use only. When the only water available is iodine treated, it should be used for only a few weeks.

Chlorine, in various forms, can also be used for chemical disinfection. However, its germicidal activity varies greatly with the pH, temperature, and organic content of the water to be purified; therefore, it can produce less consistent levels of disinfection in many types of water.

Water Filters

Portable filters currently on the market will provide various degrees of protection against microbes. Reverse-osmosis filters provide protection against viruses, bacteria, and protozoa, but they are expensive and larger than most filters used by backpackers, and the small pores on this type of filter are rapidly plugged by muddy or cloudy water. In addition, the membranes in some filters can be damaged by chlorine in water. Microstrainer filters with pore sizes in the 0.1- to 0.3-μm range can remove bacteria and protozoa from drinking water, but they do not remove viruses. To kill viruses, travelers using microstrainer filters should be advised to disinfect the water with iodine or chlorine after filtration, as described

TABLE 2-2. TREATMENT OF WATER WITH TINCTURE OF IODINE

TINCTURE OF IODINE	DROPS[1] TO BE ADDED PER QUART OR LITER	
	CLEAR WATER	COLD OR CLOUDY WATER[2]
2%	5	10

[1]One drop = 0.05 mL. Water must stand for a minimum of 30 minutes before it is safe to use.
[2]Very turbid or cold water can require prolonged contact time; if possible, such water should be allowed to stand several hours before use. To ensure that *Cryptosporidium* is killed, water must stand for 15 hours before drinking.

previously. Some filtration kits come with an additional filter effective against viruses. Filters with iodine-impregnated resins are most effective against bacteria, and the iodine will kill some viruses; however, the contact time with the iodine in the filter is too short to kill the protozoa *Cryptosporidium* and, in cold water, *Giardia*.

Filters that are designed to remove *Cryptosporidium* and *Giardia* carry one of the four messages below—verbatim—on the package label.

- Reverse osmosis
- Absolute pore size of ≤1 micron
- Tested and certified by NSF International (formerly the National Sanitation Foundation) Standard 53 or NSF Standard 58 for cyst removal
- Tested and certified by NSF Standard 53 or NSF Standard 58 for cyst reduction

Filters may not be designed to remove *Cryptosporidium* and *Giardia* if they are labeled only with these words:

- *Nominal* pore size of ≤1 micron
- One-micron filter
- Effective against *Giardia*
- Effective against parasites
- Carbon filter
- Water purifier
- Environmental Protection Agency (EPA)-approved (Caution: EPA does not approve or test filters.)
- EPA-registered (Caution: EPA does not register filters for *Cryptosporidium* removal)

- Activated carbon
- Removes chlorine
- Ultraviolet light
- Pentiodide resins
- Water softener

Filters collect organisms from water. Anyone changing cartridges should wash hands afterwards. Filters may not remove *Cryptosporidium* as well as boiling does, because even good brands of filters may sometimes have manufacturing flaws that allow small numbers of organisms to pass through the filter. In addition, poor filter maintenance or failure to replace filter cartridges as recommended by the manufacturer can cause a filter to fail.

A travelers' guide to buying water filters for preventing cryptosporidiosis and giardiasis can be found at URL: www.cdc.gov/ncidod/dpd/parasites/cryptosporidiosis/factsht_crypto_prevent_water.htm. These two organisms are either highly *(Cryptosporidium)* or moderately *(Giardia)* resistant to chlorine; so conventional halogen disinfection may be ineffective. Boiling water or filtration can be used as an alternative to chemical disinfection.

Proper selection, operation, care, and maintenance of water filters are essential to producing safe water. The manufacturers' instructions should be followed. NSF International, an independent testing company, tests and certifies water filters for their ability to remove protozoa, but not for their ability to remove bacteria or viruses. Few published scientific reports have evaluated the efficacy of specific brands or models of filters against bacteria and viruses in water. Until such information becomes available, CDC cannot identify which specific brands or models of filters are most likely to remove bacteria and viruses. To find out if a particular filter is certified to remove *Cryptosporidia,* contact NSF International by calling 1-877-867-3435; by fax to 313-769-0109; or by writing to 789 North Dixboro Road, P.O. Box 130140, Ann Arbor, Michigan 48113-0140; or online at http://www.NSF.org/certified/DWTU/. Under "Reduction claims for drinking water treatment units—health effects," check the box in front of the words "Cyst Reduction."

As a last resort, if no source of safe drinking water is available or can be obtained, tap water that is uncomfortably hot to touch might be safer than cold tap water; however, proper disinfection, filtering, or boiling is still advised.

Bibliography

Backer H. Water disinfection for international and wilderness travelers. *Clin Infect Dis.* 2002;34:355–64.

Goodyer L, Behrens RH. Safety of iodine based water sterilization for travelers. *J Trav Med.* 2000;7:38.

Schlosser O, Robert C, Bourderioux C, et al. Bacterial removal from inexpensive portable water treatment systems for travelers. 2001; *J Travel Med.* 8:12–8.

Slifko TR, Smith HV, Rose JB. Emerging parasite zoonoses associated with water and food. *Int J Parasitol.* 2000;30:1379–93.

—ROBERT QUICK AND MICHAEL BEACH

>>Travelers' Health Kit

The purpose of a Travel Kit is twofold: to allow the traveler to take care of minor health problems as they occur and to treat exacerbations of pre-existing medical conditions. A variety of health kits is available commercially and may even be purchased over the internet (see below); however, similar kits can be assembled at home. The specific contents of the health kit are based on destination, duration of travel, type of travel, and the traveler's pre-existing medical conditions. Basic items that should be included are listed below. See also *Chapter 8: International Travel with Infants and Young Children* and *Chapter 9: Advising Travelers with Specific Needs* for additional suggestions that may be useful in planning the contents of the kit.

MEDICATIONS

- Personal prescription medications (copies of all prescriptions, including the generic names for medications, and a note from the prescribing physician on letterhead stationary for controlled substances and injectable medications should be carried)
- Antimalarial medications, if applicable
- Antidiarrheal medication (e.g., bismuth subsalicylate, loperamide)

- Antibiotic for self-treatment of moderate to severe diarrhea
- Antihistamine
- Decongestant, alone or in combination with antihistamine
- Antimotion sickness medication
- Acetaminophen, aspirin, ibuprofen, or other medication for pain or fever
- Mild laxative
- Cough suppressant/expectorant
- Throat lozenges
- Antacid
- Antifungal and antibacterial ointments or creams
- 1% hydrocortisone cream
- Epinephrine auto-injector (e.g., EpiPen), especially if history of severe allergic reaction. Also available in smaller-dose package for children.

OTHER IMPORTANT ITEMS

- Insect repellent containing DEET (up to 50%)
- Sunscreen (preferably SPF 15 or greater)
- Aloe gel for sunburns
- Digital thermometer
- Oral rehydration solution packets
- Basic first-aid items (adhesive bandages, gauze, ace wrap, antiseptic, tweezers, scissors, cotton-tipped applicators)
- Antibacterial hand wipes or alcohol-based hand sanitizer
- Moleskin for blisters
- Lubricating eye drops (e.g., Natural Tears)
- First Aid Quick Reference card

Other items that may be useful in certain circumstances

- Mild sedative (e.g., zolpidem) or other sleep aid
- Anti-anxiety medication
- High-altitude preventive medication
- Water purification tablets
- Commercial suture/syringe kits (to be used by local health-care provider. These items will also require a letter from the prescribing physician on letterhead stationary)
- Latex condoms
- Address and phone numbers of area hospitals or clinics

Commercial medical kits are available for a wide range of circumstances, from basic first aid to advanced emergency life support. Many outdoor sporting goods stores sell their own basic first aid kits. For more adventurous travelers, a number of companies produce advanced medical kits and will even customize kits based on specific travel needs. In addition, specialty kits are available for managing diabetes, dealing with dental emergencies, and handling aquatic environments. If travelers choose to purchase a health kit rather than assemble their own, they should be certain to review the contents of the kit carefully to ensure that it has everything needed; supplementation with additional items for comfort may be necessary.

Below is a list of websites supplying a wide range of medical kits. There are many suppliers, and this list is not meant to be all inclusive.

- Adventure Medical Kits: www.adventuremedicalkits.com
- Chinook Medical Gear: www.chinookmed.com
- Harris International Health Care: www.safetravel.com
- Travel Medicine, Inc.: www.travmed.com
- Wilderness Medicine Outfitters: www.wildernessmedicine.com

A final reminder: a health kit is useful only if it is available. It should be carried with the traveler at all times, e.g., in carry-on baggage and on excursions. All medications, especially prescription medications, should be stored in carry-on baggage, in their original containers with clear labels. With heightened airline security, sharp objects will have to remain in checked luggage.

–DEBORAH NICOLLS, TAMARA FISK, AND PHYLLIS KOZARSKY

>>Seeking Health Care Abroad

PREPARATION

In addition to ensuring that all necessary travel documents are complete before departure, travelers should learn what medical services their health insurance will cover overseas, as well as any policy exclusions. While some major health insurance carriers in the United

States may provide coverage for emergencies that occur while traveling, most do not cover medical expenses due to exacerbations of pre-existing medical conditions while abroad. It is also important to know the insurance company's policy for "out-of-network" services, pre-authorization requirements, and need for a second opinion before obtaining treatment. Travelers should carry claim forms and a copy of their insurance policy card, if their insurance policy does provide coverage abroad. The Social Security Medicare program does not provide coverage for medical costs outside the United States. Furthermore, very few health insurance companies cover the cost of medical evacuation, which can vary widely, ranging from a few thousand dollars to over $100,000, depending on the circumstances. Travelers who will be outside the United States for an extended period of time, who have underlying illnesses, or who are participating in activities entailing risk for injury, are encouraged to consider a supplemental health insurance policy that provides guaranteed medical payments, assistance via a 24-hour physician-backed support center, and emergency medical transport, including repatriation. A list of travel insurance and medical evacuation companies is available at the U.S. Department of State website (travel.state.gov/travel/ index.html). A brief list of additional assistance companies is also included below; this list is not all-inclusive:

International SOS: www.internationalsos.com. International SOS offers comprehensive 24-hour physician-backed medical and security assistance, for which members pay a fee. Membership provides access to on-line services, including medical and safety travel advisories, pre-travel itinerary-based recommendations, and computerized medical records. Insurance policies include medical evacuation and repatriation coverage, access to international clinics that provide primary care, diagnostic, and emergency services, and voluntary patient support programs to assist with medication compliance while abroad.

MEDEX: www.medexassist.com. MEDEX travel assistance services include 24-hour access to coordinators who can help locate appropriate medical care providers, coordinate direct payment of covered medical expenses, and assist in other medical, legal or travel situations. Insurance policies include medical evacuation and repatriation services, emergency dental coverage, and assistance with replacement of medications. For an additional fee, subscribers also have access to itinerary-based destination reports, which cover practical topics from local transportation and cultural norms to medical and security alerts.

International Association for Medical Assistance to Travelers: www.iamat.org. IAMAT is a nonprofit organization established to provide medical information to travelers and to make competent medical care available to them worldwide. IAMAT maintains an international network of physicians, hospitals, and clinics who have agreed to treat IAMAT members in need of medical care while abroad. Membership is free, although a donation to support IAMAT efforts is appreciated. Members receive a directory of participating physicians and medical centers and have access to a variety of travel-related informational brochures.

Travelers with underlying medical conditions also should consider choosing a medical assistance company that allows them to store their medical history before departure, so it can be accessed worldwide if needed. Alternatively, they may carry a letter from their physician listing underlying medical conditions and current medications (including their generic names). Each travel insurance companies differ in their policies with regard to coverage for exacerbations of underlying medical conditions. Travelers are encouraged to research this carefully and understand the fine print. See also the Travel Health Kit section in this Chapter for more suggestions on travel preparation.

ILLNESS ABROAD

If an American citizen becomes seriously ill or is injured abroad, a U.S. consular officer can assist in locating appropriate medical services and notifying friends, family, or employer. Additional resources include the clinic where the traveler received pre-travel health advice and immunizations, embassies and consulates of other countries, hotel doctors, credit-card companies, and multinational corporations, which may offer health-care services for their employees. For informational purposes, *Travel Health Online* (www.tripprep.com/scripts) provides a list of travel medicine providers from around the world. Wherever they are posted, lists of providers are obtained from a variety of sources, and the quality of services and the expertise of the providers are not guaranteed. The International Society of Travel Medicine and the American Society of Tropical Medicine and Hygiene also have directories of travel clinics available at their websites (www.istm.org and www.astmh.org respectively). Although many of these clinics may only provide pre-travel services, some are located outside the United States and can see ill travelers.

The quality of health care from overseas medical centers can be variable, particularly in developing countries. Some foreign hospitals may have out-of-date facilities, while others have highly sophisticated diagnostic and therapeutic equipment similar to that found in the United States. Furthermore, physicians in other countries usually require payment in cash or credit card for services rendered rather than bill an insurance company. Travelers with health insurance coverage should carry their insurance card and claim forms and they should obtain copies of all bills and receipts. If one needs financial assistance, the U.S. consular office can assist with transferring funds from the United States. In extreme circumstances, they may even be able to approve small government loans until private funds are available. (See American Citizens Services and Crisis Management website: travel.state.gov/travel/overseas_whoweare.html.) Travelers must be aware, however, that they are responsible for paying all medical expenses they incur while abroad, including evacuation expenses.

In many developing countries, virtually any drug, including antibiotics and antimalarial medications, can be purchased without prescription. Travelers should be advised, however, not to buy these medications unless they are familiar with the products. The quality of these drugs may not meet U.S. standards and they may even be counterfeit or potentially hazardous due to contaminants. In addition, travelers requiring an injection overseas should consider bringing their own injection equipment (see Travel Health Kits section). At the very least, they should ask if the injection equipment is disposable and insist, if possible, that a new needle and syringe be used.

BLOOD TRANSFUSIONS

A blood transfusion can be a life-saving intervention when the blood supply has been appropriately screened and managed. For travelers, transfusion should be required only in rare and unexpected situations of massive hemorrhage, such as severe trauma, gynecologic and obstetric emergency, or gastrointestinal bleeding. Not all developing countries have accurate and systematic screening of all blood donations for infectious agents such as malaria, HIV, and hepatitis viruses, which can result in transfusion-related transmission of these infections. According to a WHO survey, 11%–21% of countries surveyed had inadequate screening of their blood supply for those infectious agents. Additionally, transfusion reactions can occur if the blood products are not adequately characterized for compatibility with the recipient before transfusion. Because of these inherent risks, transfusion should be prescribed only for conditions for which there is no other treatment. When blood transfusion cannot be avoided, travelers should make every effort to ensure that the blood has been screened for transmissible diseases, including HIV. In many cases, resuscitation can be achieved by use of colloid or crystalloid plasma expanders instead of blood. Once stabilized, travelers should consider urgent evacuation for additional management.

In the past, travelers planning international itineraries have requested to have their own blood or blood from their home country available to them in case of urgent need. There are no medical indications for travelers to take blood with them from their home countries. The international shipment of blood for transfusion is practical only when handled by agreement between two responsible organizations, such as national blood transfusion services. This mechanism is not useful for the emergency needs of individual travelers and should not be attempted by private travelers or organizations not operating recognized blood programs. The limited storage period of blood and the need for special equipment negate the feasibility of independent blood banking for individual travelers or small groups. Travelers should, however, carry a medical card or other document, showing their blood group and information about any current medical problems or treatment.

HEALTH-SEEKING TRAVEL

Traveling abroad for the purpose of improving one's physical, mental, and spiritual well-being is increasing in popularity. Such "health tourism" includes, but is not limited to, balneotherapy (treatment by baths), thalassotherapy (treatment based on the use of sea water), religious pilgrimages, and elective surgeries, including cosmetic surgery and organ transplantation.

Therapies that are considered "natural" are not without hazards. Mineral and "holy" waters may not be potable by U.S. standards and have been sources of infectious diseases. Moreover, pilgrims are subject to the same destination-associated risks as other travelers (e.g., heat and altitude-associated illnesses), but many may be traveling in ill-health. Outbreaks of meningitis due to *Neisseria meningitidis* have occurred in Hajj pilgrims, leading to the recommendation that all pilgrims participating in the Hajj be immunized before their departure (see Chapter 4, Meningococcal Disease section). With the shift in the timing of the Hajj to winter months, pilgrims may also be at increased risk for respiratory tract infections, such as influenza and adenovirus.

Furthermore, CDC has received a number of reports of nontuberculous mycobacterial infections after elective cosmetic surgery abroad. "Transplant Tourism" has been increasing as the number of available organs, especially kidneys, is decreasing relative to the increasing demand. A number of international transplantation rings have been discovered, in which people from developing countries are paid for donating organs. This practice is considered legal in only a few countries. Recently the World Health Assembly met to discuss the challenges of transplantation and to address international transplantation guidelines. It encouraged countries to protect those most vulnerable to such exploitation, but there is still no international consensus on incentives for organ donation. Regardless of the reason, people seeking health care abroad should understand that medical systems outside the United States may operate differently from those in the United States and are not subject to the same rules and regulations. Those who are considering seeking health care outside the United States should consult with their local physician before traveling.

Bibliography

CDC. Nontuberculous mycobacterial infections after cosmetic surgery — Santo Domingo, Dominican Republic, 2003–2004. *Morbid Mortal Wkly Rep MMWR.* 2004;53:509.

CDC. Serogroup W-135 meningococcal disease among travelers returning from Saudi Arabia — United States, 2000. *Morbid Mortal Wkly Rep MMWR.* 2000;49: 345–6.

El Bashir H, Haworth E, Zambon M, et al. Influenza among U.K. pilgrims to the Hajj, 2003 [letter]. *Emerg Infect Dis.* 2004;10:1882–3.

Jurado V, Ortiz-Martinez A, Gonzalez-del Valle M, et al. Holy water fonts are reservoirs of pathogenic bacteria. *Environ Microbiol.* 2002;4:617–20.

Kolars JC. Rules of the road: a consumer's guide for travelers seeking health care in foreign lands. *J Travel Med.* 2002;9:198–201.

Nullis-Kapp C. Organ trafficking and transplantation pose new challenges. *Bull World Health Organ.* 2004;82:639–718.

The Fifty-seventh World Health Assembly. Human organ and tissue transplantation [monograph on the Internet]. Geneva, Switzerland: World Health Organization; 2004. [cited 2004 Sept 17]. Available from: http://www.who.int/gb/ebwha/pdf_files/WHA57/A57_R18-en.pdf.

Zarocostas J. Blood donations must be safer in poor nations, says WHO. *Lancet.* 2004;363:2060.

—DEBORAH NICOLLS, PHYLLIS KOZARSKY, AND PAUL ARGUIN

>>The Post-Travel Period

The most frequent health problems in ill returned travelers are persistent gastrointestinal illness, 10%; skin lesions/rashes, 8%; respiratory infections, 5%–13% (depending on season of travel); and fever in up to 3%. Although gastrointestinal upset is the most frequent problem, febrile illness is the most serious since the infection may be life threatening to the patient (malaria) or a pose a serious public health hazard (viral hemorrhagic fever). The most frequent "tropical" causes of fever are malaria, dengue fever, invasive bacterial diarrhea, hepatitis A, typhoid fever, and rickettsial infections. However, nontropical entities such as respiratory or urinary tract infections account for a large proportion of febrile illnesses in returned travelers. The most frequent causes of persistent gastrointestinal illness are postinfectious irritable bowel syndrome and postinfectious lactose intolerance. The former often presents as intermittent diarrhea but may actually be a manifestation of constipation associated with episodic, rapid expulsions of loose stool. Although infections such as giardiasis or cyclosporiasis are often treated on the basis of clinical findings (without the benefit of laboratory confirmation), intestinal parasitic infections are uncommon causes of persistent diarrhea. Most post-travel skin ailments are insect bites, pyoderma, scabies, and cutaneous larva migrans.

Some diseases might not manifest themselves immediately on return. Most travelers infected abroad become ill within 12 weeks after returning to the United States. However, some diseases, such as malaria, may not cause symptoms for as long as 6–12 months after exposure. If travelers become ill after they return home, even many months after travel, they should be advised to tell their physician where they have traveled. Fever in a traveler returned from a malarious area should be considered a medical emergency; malaria should be evaluated urgently by appropriate laboratory tests, which should be repeated if the initial result is negative. Since most primary-care physicians have little expertise in tropical diseases, a newly returned, ill international traveler should be evaluated by an infectious disease or tropical medicine practitioner. For assistance in finding a provider who practices clinical tropical medicine, one may access the American Society of Tropical Medicine website for a listing by state at www.astmh.org/scripts/clinindex.asp.

It may be prudent for asymptomatic international travelers who have been abroad for many months or longer, particularly in developing countries, to be screened for certain diseases. The decision to screen for particular pathogens will depend on the travel and exposure history. For example, travelers who have engaged in unprotected sex or have received an injection, a body piercing, or a tattoo may be screened for HIV, hepatitis C and other STDs, and, if not immune, hepatitis B. Travelers who have been exposed to freshwater in areas endemic for schistosomiasis should be screened for this infection by serology and stool and/or urine tests. Eosinophilia in a returned traveler suggests the possibility of a helminth infection, of which the most important is strongyloidiasis. If left untreated, this infection may last for the lifetime of the host, and in an immunocompromised person it has the potential to disseminate. Serology is the most sensitive diagnostic test.

Bibliography

Spira AM. Assessment of travelers who return home ill. *Lancet.* 2003;361:1459–69.

Ryan ET, Wilson ME, Kain KC. Illness after international travel. *N Engl J Med.* 2002;347:505–16.

Wilson ME, Chen LH. Dermatologic infectious diseases in international travelers. *Curr Infect Dis Rep.* 2004;6:54–62.

Suh KN, Kozarsky PE, Keystone JS. Evaluation of fever in the returned traveler. *Med Clin North Am.* 1999;83:997–1017.

Connor BA, Landzberg BR. Persistent travelers' diarrhea. In: Keystone JS, Kozarsky PE, Freedman DO, Nothdurft H, Connor BA, eds. *Travel Medicine.* Philadelphia: Mosby; 2004. p. 503–15.

Leder K, Sundararajan V, Weld L, et al; GeoSentinel Surveillance Group. Respiratory tract infections in travelers: a review of the GeoSentinel surveillance network. *Clin Infect Dis.* 2003;36:399–406.

–JAY KEYSTONE

CHAPTER 3

Geographic Distribution of Potential Health Hazards for Travelers

>>Introduction: Goals and Limitations

This section provides information about which disease exposures are likely in different geographic regions of the world. It is intended to help the clinician provide useful region-specific education and other interventions to prospective travelers and assist in the evaluation of ill returned travelers. The data presented here have many limitations. The areas where an infection can be acquired may expand, contract, and shift over time. New diseases are recognized; old ones are sometimes eliminated, although sequelae in individuals may persist after active transmission has ceased. Humans move, sometimes carrying pathogens (and potential for transmission) with them. The data on which these descriptions are based may be incomplete, inaccurate, or out of date. Most infectious diseases are not notifiable; even when reported, the data typically reflect only a small fraction of actual cases. Reports may be withheld, delayed, or modified because of concerns about the economic impact of an infectious disease on travel and trade. Maps of disease distribution are usually based on infections in a local population, yet risk of clinical infection (e.g., hepatitis A or diarrhea) in a traveler to a region may be substantially higher than in a local resident (most of whom may be immune) or substantially lower (e.g., ascaris, hookworm, or filariasis) because of living conditions and duration of time spent in the area. Manifestations of the same infection in traveler and local resident may differ because of host factors.

Although we use country names to describe areas of risk, distributions of infection typically do not coincide with geopolitical boundaries. Adding to the complexity, countries may be split, boundaries may shift, and names may change, making tracking of data about distribution in a particular region over time more difficult.

Ideally, spatial (location of transmission) and temporal (seasons or years of risk) distribution and intensity of transmission would be displayed. Semiquantitative terms, such as common, uncommon, and rare, used to describe risk of infection have different meanings for different people and are used inconsistently. Portrayal of risk is often influenced by severity or lethality of infection and not just by the numbers of cases.

Host factors, duration of stay, accommodations, and specific activities influence types and level of risk. These summaries represent broad generalizations intended to provide some initial guidance to clinicians.

The information is displayed in different ways. Table 3–1 portrays 24 of the more common infections in travelers and allows a quick overview of disease risks for specific pathogens by region. Respiratory tract and diarrheal infections, among the most common infections in travelers, are caused by multiple different pathogens, many with a global distribution. For infections caused by specific pathogens, the level of risk (including history of epidemic activity or high-risk areas) is based on information in local populations. In the summary for each region, important infectious disease risks are described, organized by means of transmission. **Those marked by an asterisk (*) within the text have more than one mode of transmission.**

The reader should keep in mind that many microbes, such as influenza virus, cytomegalovirus, Epstein-Barr virus, HIV, *Toxoplasma*, *Streptococci*, *Streptococcus pneumoniae*, *Salmonella*, *Neisseria gonorrhoeae*, *Treponema pallidum* (syphilis), *Campylobacter*, the coliforms causing urinary tract infections, and many others are globally distributed and cause infections in travelers. Travelers may be at increased risk for some of these because of the conditions of travel (e.g., crowding, poor sanitation, and poor air quality) or activities during travel (e.g., sex with new partners). Most of these broadly distributed infections are not described specifically in the regional sections.

Most sections include a comment about more common infections that occur in travelers to the region and also note chronic and latent infections that may be seen in immigrants from the region.

The disease lists are by no means exhaustive. Infections that are preventable and treatable are more likely to be included. The materials in this section are intended to be used in conjunction with other sections of this book that provide maps and give more details about specific infections. Other useful materials can be found on the CDC and WHO websites and from other sources.

TABLE 3-1. DISEASE DISTRIBUTION

REGION	AMEBIASIS	ENDEMIC MYCOSES¹	DENGUE	FILARIASIS	HANTAVIRUSES	HEPATITIS A	HEPATITIS B	POLIO
North Africa	W	L	S	S		W	S	S
Central, E, W Africa	S	S, H	S, H	W	S	W	W, H	S, H
Southern Africa	S	S, H	S			S, H	W, H	L
North America	L	S, H	L		S, H	S, H	S	
Mexico, Central America	W	S, H	S, H		L	W	S	
Caribbean	S	S, H	S, H	S		S, H	S	
Tropical South America	W	S, H	S, H	S	S, H	W	W	
Temperate South America	S	S	L		S, H	S, H	S	
East Asia	S	L	S, H	S	W, H	W, H	W	
Southeast Asia	S	S	W, H	W	S	W, H	W	
South Asia	W	L	S, H	W	S	W	W	S
Middle East	W	L	S, H	S		W	W	
Western Europe	L	L			W, H	S, H	S	
Eastern Europe & Northern Asia	S	L			W, H	W, H	W	
Australia & South Pacific	L	L	S, H	S, H		S, H	S, H	

Key:
L   local transmission documented but rare
S   sporadic, focal, or seasonal transmission in region
W   widespread transmission
H   epidemic activity or high risk for infection in some areas
Blank   No reported cases (Does not necessarily mean that there is no risk)

¹Histoplasmosis, coccidioidomycosis, and paracoccidioidomycosis

TABLE 3-1. DISEASE DISTRIBUTION-CONT'D

REGION	DIPHTHERIA	HIV	JAPANESE ENCEPHALITIS	VIRAL HEMORRHAGIC FEVERS	LEPTOSPIROSIS	LEISHMANIASIS	MALARIA	PLAGUE
North Africa	S	S			S	W	S	S, H
Central, E, W Africa	S, H	W, H		S, H	W, H	W, H	W, H	W, H
Southern Africa	S	W, H			S	L	S, H	S, H
North America	L	S			S, H	L		S
Mexico, Central America	L	S			W, H	W	S	L
Caribbean	S	S			W, H	L	S	
Tropical South America	S, H	S		S, H	W, H	W, H	S, H	S, H
Temperate South America	L	S		S, H	S	S	S	L
East Asia	L	S	S, H		W	S	S	S, H
Southeast Asia	S, H	S, H	W, H		W, H	S	W	S, H
South Asia	S, H	S, H	W, H		W, H	W, H	W, H	S, H
Middle East	S	S		L	S	W, H	S	L
Western Europe	L	S			S	S		
Eastern Europe & Northern Asia	S, H	S, H	L		S	S	S	L
Australia & South Pacific	S, H	S	L		S		S, H	

TABLE 3-1. DISEASE DISTRIBUTION-CONT'D

REGION	DISEASE							
	RABIES	RICKETTSIAE	SCHISTOSOMIASIS	TICK-BORNE ENCEPHALITIS	TRYPANOSOMIASIS[2]	TUBERCULOSIS	TYPHOID & PARATYPHOID FEVER	YELLOW FEVER
North Africa	W	W	S, H			W, H	S, H	
Central, E, W Africa	W, H	W	W, H		S, H	W, H	S, H	S, H
Southern Africa	S	W, H	S, H		S	W, H	S	
North America	S	S				S	L	
Mexico, Central America	S	S			S	S	S, H	L
Caribbean	S	S	S			S, H	S	L
Tropical South America	W, H	S	S		S	S, H	S, H	S, H
Temperate South America	L	L			S	S	S	
East Asia	W	W	S			W	S	
Southeast Asia	W	W, H	W			W	W	
South Asia	W, H	W, H	L			W	W, H	
Middle East	W	S	S	S		W	S	
Western Europe	S	S		S, H		S	L	
Eastern Europe & Northern Asia	W	S		W, H		W, H	S, H	
Australia & South Pacific		S				S, H	S	

[2]Including African trypanosomiasis (sleeping sickness) and American trypanosomiasis (Chagas' disease)

AFRICA

North Africa

- Algeria
- Canary Islands
- Egypt
- Libya
- Madeira Islands
- Morocco
- Tunisia
- Western Sahara

Southern Africa

- Botswana
- Lesotho
- Namibia
- South Africa
- Swaziland
- Zimbabwe

Central Africa

- Angola
- Cameroon
- Central African Republic
- Chad
- Congo
- Democratic Republic of Congo (Zaire)
- Equatorial Guinea
- Gabon
- Sudan
- Zambia

East Africa

- Burundi
- Comoros
- Djibouti
- Eritrea
- Ethiopia

East Africa—cont'd

- Kenya
- Madagascar
- Malawi
- Mauritius
- Mayotte
- Mozambique
- Réunion
- Rwanda
- Seychelles
- Somalia
- Tanzania
- Uganda

West Africa

- Benin
- Burkina Faso
- Cape Verde
- Côte d'Ivoire
- The Gambia
- Ghana
- Guinea
- Guinea-Bissau
- Liberia
- Mali
- Mauritania
- Niger
- Nigeria
- Saint Helena
- São Tomé and Principe
- Senegal
- Sierra Leone
- Togo

NORTH AFRICA

Access to clean water and sanitary disposal of waste are limited in many areas, so infections related to fecal contamination of food and water remain common and widespread. Vaccine-preventable diseases such as measles, mumps, rubella, and diphtheria persist in the region. More common infections in returned travelers are gastrointestinal: diarrhea (acute and chronic) and occasionally typhoid fever, amebiasis, and brucellosis. Chronic and latent infections in immigrants (and long-term residents) from this region include tuberculosis, schistosomiasis, fascioliasis, hepatitis B and C, intestinal parasites, and echinococcosis.

Vector-borne infections: Many have focal distributions or seasonal patterns. Risk to the usual traveler is low. Vector-borne infections in parts of the region include dengue fever, lymphatic filariasis (especially in the Nile Delta), leishmaniasis (cutaneous and visceral), malaria (risk limited to a few areas), relapsing fever, Rift Valley fever,* sand fly fever, Sindbis virus infection, West Nile fever (especially in Egypt), Crimean-Congo hemorrhagic fever, spotted fever due to *Rickettsia conorii,* and murine typhus.

Food- and water-borne infections: These infections, which are common in travelers to this region, include dysentery and diarrhea caused by bacteria, viruses, and parasites. Risk for hepatitis A is high throughout the region. Hepatitis E and cholera have caused focal outbreaks, and indigenous wild polio was still present in Egypt in 2003. Other risks include typhoid fever, brucellosis, amebiasis, and fascioliasis (rare in visitors to the area). Intestinal helminths are common in some local populations but rare in short-term travelers.

Airborne and person-to-person transmission: The annual incidence of tuberculosis is estimated to be 50–100/100,000. Q fever is widespread in livestock-raising areas.

Sexually transmitted and blood-borne infections: HIV prevalence (in adults 15–49 years) is estimated to be <1%. Chancroid is a common cause of genital ulcers. Prevalence of chronic hepatitis B carriage is estimated to be 2%–7% in the region; hepatitis C prevalence exceeds 15% in Egypt.

Zoonotic infections: Rabies is endemic in the region. Sporadic cases of human plague* are reported, and an outbreak occurred in Algeria in 2003. Sporadic cases and outbreaks of anthrax* occur in the region.

Soil- and water-associated infections: Schistosomiasis is present, especially in the Nile Delta and Valley; it is found focally in other countries. Other risks include leptospirosis.*

Other hazards for travelers include scorpion stings, snake bites, and a high rate of motor-vehicle accidents and violent injuries. Screening of blood before transfusion is inadequate in many hospitals.

CENTRAL, EAST, AND WEST AFRICA

Vector-borne infections are common and widespread and pose a major risk to local residents and travelers. Access to clean water and sanitary disposal of waste are limited in many areas, so infections related to fecal contamination of food and water remain common and widespread. Vaccine-preventable diseases such as measles, mumps, rubella, poliomyelitis, and diphtheria persist in the region.

The most common cause of systemic febrile illness in travelers to this region is malaria caused by *Plasmodium falciparum*. Subacute or chronic infections in immigrants (and long-term residents) from the area include tuberculosis, hepatitis B, HIV, lymphatic filariasis, onchocerciasis, loiasis, schistosomiasis, echinococcosis, leprosy, and intestinal parasites.

Vector-borne infections: Malaria transmission is intense in many parts of the region, including urban areas, where *falciparum* malaria, much of it resistant to chloroquine, predominates. Sporadic cases and outbreaks of yellow fever have occurred in at least 14 of the countries (especially in West Africa) in the past 10 years, with the largest number of cases being reported from Nigeria, Guinea, the Sudan, Côte d'Ivoire, Liberia, Senegal, and Sierra Leone. All countries in the region are considered to be in the endemic zone, and unvaccinated travelers are at risk for infection. Official reports of yellow fever reflect only a small percentage of all infections. African trypanosomiasis has increased in Africa (it is epidemic in Angola, Democratic Republic of Congo, and the Sudan; highly endemic in Cameroon, Central African Republic, Chad, Congo, Côte d'Ivoire, Guinea, Mozambique, Uganda, and Tanzania; and low levels are found in most of the other countries), and an increase in travelers has been noted since 2000. Most had exposures in Tanzania and Kenya, reflecting common tourist routes. *Trypanosoma brucei gambiense* is found in focal areas of western and central Africa; *T. b. rhodesiense,* which causes more acute illness, is found in east Africa. Vector-borne viral infections include dengue fever, Crimean-Congo hemorrhagic fever,* Rift Valley fever,* West Nile fever, and O'nyong nyong fever. Lymphatic

MAP 3-1. REGIONS – AFRICA AND THE MIDDLE EAST

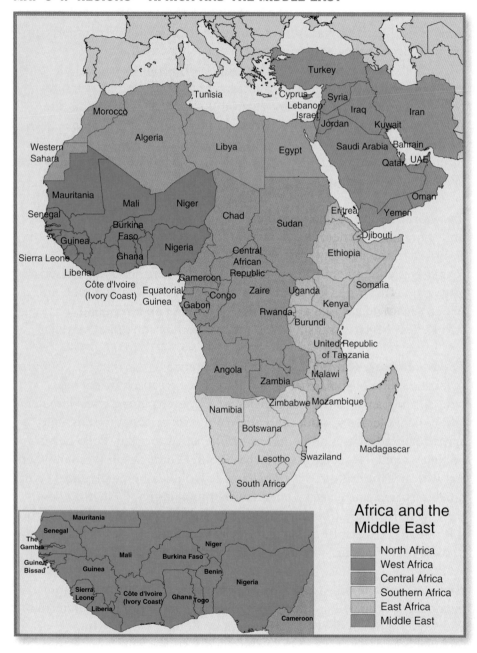

Africa and the Middle East

- North Africa
- West Africa
- Central Africa
- Southern Africa
- East Africa
- Middle East

filariasis is present in many areas; onchocerciasis is widely distributed around river systems, especially in West and Central Africa and as far west as east as Ethiopia. Another filarial infection, loiasis, is widely distributed in the tropical rain forest, especially in Central and West Africa. Filarial infections are rare in short-term travelers. The rickettsial infections murine typhus, louse-borne typhus, and African tick bite fever (due to *Rickettsia africae*) occur in the region. African tick-bite fever has been increasingly recognized in travelers to rural areas. Murine typhus is more common in coastal areas. Tungiasis (penetration of the skin by sand fleas) is widespread in tropical Africa, especially West Africa, including Madagascar.

Tick-borne relapsing fever is widespread in eastern and central Africa and sporadic elsewhere. Epidemics of louse-borne relapsing fever have occurred in the past but pose little risk to usual travelers. Visceral leishmaniasis is endemic in Ethiopia, Kenya, and Sudan (and has caused large epidemics); it is found in the savanna parts of the region. Cutaneous leishmaniasis is also found in the savanna and in Sudan, Ethiopia and Kenya. Myiasis transmitted by the tumbu fly can affect travelers.

Food- and water-borne infections: Dysentery and diarrhea are common in local populations; diarrhea in travelers may be caused by bacteria, viruses, and parasites (especially *Giardia, Cryptosporidium, Entamoeba histolytica*). Cholera is sporadic and epidemic. Risk of hepatitis A is widespread; sporadic cases and outbreaks of hepatitis E occur. Polio persists in Nigeria and has recently spread to 12 other countries in West and Central Africa. Other risks to travelers include typhoid and paratyphoid fever, amebiasis, and brucellosis. Dracunculiasis remains endemic in 12 countries, with the highest number of cases in Sudan, Nigeria, and Ghana, but it is rare in travelers. Intestinal parasites are common in residents in many parts of region but are rare in short-term travelers.

Airborne and person-to-person transmission: The estimated annual incidence rates of tuberculosis (per 100,000) are >100 in all countries and >300 in much of region. Frequent epidemics of serogroup A meningococcal disease occur during the dry season (December through June) in a band of countries from Senegal to Ethiopia. Severe outbreaks have occurred in Burkina Faso, Chad, Mali, Niger, Nigeria, Ethiopia, and the Sudan. Serogroup W135 emerged in Burkina Faso in 2002, causing a large epidemic (13,000 cases). Nosocomial and intrafamilial spread of Ebola* occurs in outbreaks (Sudan, Democratic Republic of the Congo, Côte d'Ivoire, Gabon). Nosocomial spread of Lassa fever virus* has also occurred.

Sexually transmitted and blood-borne infections: Estimated prevalence of HIV in adults (15–49 years) ranges from 1% to 15% in most countries. In most of the region, prevalence of chronic infection with hepatitis B virus exceeds 8%. HTLV-1 is endemic in West Africa. Common causes of genital ulcer disease include chancroid, syphilis, and herpes simplex.

Zoonotic infections: Dogs are the most important source of rabies, which is found throughout the region. A wild rodent is the reservoir host for Lassa fever virus,* which is endemic in West Africa; cases have also been documented in the Central African Republic. Echinococcosis* is widespread in animal breeding areas. Sporadic cases and outbreaks of anthrax* occur in the region (it is hyperendemic in Zambia, Ethiopia, Niger, and Chad and in several countries along the western coast). Monkeypox* is found in West and Central Africa, primarily in remote villages in rain forest areas. Plague* is enzootic, and sporadic cases and outbreaks occur in humans. (Outbreaks have occurred since 2000 in Madagascar, Malawi, Mozambique, Uganda, and Tanzania). Q fever* (airborne spread) is found, especially in West Africa, where stock breeding is common.

Soil- and water-associated infections: Schistosomiasis due to *Schistosoma mansoni* and *S. haematobium* is widespread; *S. intercalatum* has a more limited distribution (West Africa). *Mycobacterium ulcerans* (the cause of Buruli ulcer) is most concentrated in West Africa and is increasing in prevalence. Rare cases have occurred in travelers. Leptospirosis* (both sporadic cases and outbreaks) occurs in tropical areas. Other risks include mycetoma and histoplasmosis.

Other hazards for travelers include motor vehicle accidents and other injuries, including violent injury with assault rifles and other weapons, and sexual assaults. Aflatoxin contamination of grains and snake bites are common, especially in rural areas. Screening of blood before transfusion is inadequate in many hospitals.

SOUTHERN AFRICA

Vector-borne infections are common in parts of the region. Access to clean water and sanitary disposal of waste are highly variable but are poor in some areas (especially some rural areas). Vaccine coverage is high in some populations, but vaccine-preventable diseases, such as measles, mumps, rubella, and diphtheria, persist in parts of the region. Polio reappeared in 2004 in Botswana. More common infections in travelers include gastrointestinal infections, African tick-bite fever, and malaria. Infections in immigrants (and long-term residents from the region) include tuberculosis, HIV, schistosomiasis, and intestinal parasites.

Vector-borne infections: Malaria is present in parts of all countries in the region except Lesotho, although the risk is focal or seasonal in many areas. African tick-bite fever (*Rickettsia africae*) has been common in travelers to the region, especially South Africa, Botswana, Swaziland, Lesotho, and Zimbabwe. Other vector-borne infections include tick-borne relapsing fever, Rift Valley fever,* dengue (focal outbreaks but larger areas infested with *Aedes aegypti*), tick-borne relapsing fever, murine typhus, West Nile fever, and Crimean-Congo hemorrhagic fever.* African trypanosomiasis has been reported from Botswana and Namibia in the past. Tungiasis is reported from South Africa.

Food- and water-borne infections: Risk for hepatitis A is high in parts of region; outbreaks of hepatitis E have been reported. Risk for dysentery and diarrhea is highly variable within the region. Diarrhea in travelers may be caused by bacteria, viruses, and parasites. Other risks for travelers include typhoid and paratyphoid fever and amebiasis. Cholera is sporadic and epidemic (epidemics since 2002 in South Africa, Swaziland, and Zimbabwe). Intestinal helminths, though common in some local populations, are rare in short-term travelers.

Airborne and person-to-person transmission: The estimated incidence rate of tuberculosis is >300 per 100,000 population in the region.

Sexually transmitted and blood-borne infections: HIV prevalence in antenatal clinics exceeds 25% in many countries in region. Prevalence of chronic carriage of hepatitis B virus exceeds 8%.

Zoonotic infections: The mongoose is a source of rabies in addition to domestic dogs and other animals. Plague* is enzootic, and sporadic cases and outbreaks have occurred in Botswana, Namibia, and Zimbabwe since 1990. Anthrax* is hyperendemic in Zimbabwe, with recent outbreaks in animals and also human cases. Sporadic cases of anthrax have been reported elsewhere in the region.

Soil- and water-associated infections: Focal active areas of schistosomiasis persist (caused by *Schistosoma mansoni, S. haematobium,* and *S. mattheei*). Cutaneous larva migrans can occur after exposures on beaches. Leptospirosis* has caused outbreaks. Histoplasmosis has caused an outbreak in South Africa.

Other hazards for travelers include motor vehicle accidents and violent injury, as well as snake bites. Screening of blood before transfusion is inadequate in many hospitals.

THE AMERICAS

Mexico and Central America

- Belize
- Costa Rica
- El Salvador
- Guatemala
- Honduras
- Mexico
- Nicaragua
- Panama

North America

- Canada
- Saint Pierre and Miquelon
- United States

Tropical South America

- Bolivia
- Brazil
- Colombia

Tropical South America—cont'd

- Ecuador
- French Guiana
- Galápagos Islands
- Guyana
- Paraguay
- Peru
- Suriname
- Venezuela

Temperate South America

- Argentina
- Chile
- Easter Island
- Falkland Islands
- South Georgia
- South Sandwich Islands
- Uruguay

The Caribbean

- Anguilla
- Antigua and Barbuda
- Aruba
- The Bahamas
- Barbados
- Bermuda
- Cayman Islands
- Cuba
- Dominica
- Dominican Republic
- Grenada
- Guadaloupe
- Haiti
- Jamaica
- Martinique
- Montserrat
- Netherlands Antilles
- Puerto Rico

- Saint Kitts and Nevis
- Saint Lucia
- Saint Martin
- Saint Vincent and the Grenadines
- Trinidad and Tobago
- Turks and Caicos Islands
- British Virgin Islands
- U.S. Virgin Islands

NORTH AMERICA

Good sanitation and clean water are available in major urban areas and most rural areas. Many vector-borne infections are found in focal areas and can pose a risk to travelers, especially adventure travelers to rural areas. In temperate areas they occur during the summer months. Levels of immunization are high in most areas. Poliomyelitis has been eradicated.

Vector-borne infections: Lyme disease is endemic in northeastern, north central (upper Midwest), and Pacific coastal areas of North America. West Nile fever was first documented in the United States (New York) in 1999 and has since spread throughout continental U.S. and southern Canada. Other vector-borne infections include Rocky Mountain spotted fever, murine typhus, rickettsialpox, St. Louis encephalitis, La Crosse encephalitis, Eastern equine encephalitis, Colorado tick fever, and relapsing fever. Ehrlichiosis (granulocytic and monocytic) has been reported primarily from the central and eastern thirds of the United States. Sporadic local transmission of dengue has occurred since 1995 in Florida and Texas, and the vector mosquito *Aedes aegypti* inhabits the southeastern United States. An outbreak of dengue in Hawaii in 2001-2002 was transmitted by *Aedes albopictus*.

Food- and water-borne infections: Outbreaks of diarrhea caused by enterohemorrhagic *Escherichia coli* O157:H7 have occurred in many areas and have increased in the past decade. *Campylobacter* and *Salmonella* are the most common causes of acute bacterial diarrhea. Giardiasis and cryptosporidiosis occur sporadically and in outbreaks. Outbreaks of diarrhea due to norovirus are increasingly being reported in the United States and Canada.

Airborne and person-to-person transmission: Outbreaks and cases of pertussis have been increasing for more than a decade. The incidence of tuberculosis is low (about 6/100,000 population). Numbers of measles cases have declined in the United States and Canada, and most of these cases are imported or linked to imported cases.

Sexually transmitted and blood-borne infections: The HIV prevalence in adults is estimated to be 0.6%.

Zoonotic infections: Rabies is enzootic in bats, raccoons, foxes, and other wild animals. Human cases are rare. Cases of hantavirus pulmonary syndrome have been widely distributed in North America, with the greatest concentration in the western and southwestern United States. Tularemia* is found in wide areas of the United States, including Alaska, and Canada, with the greatest number of cases in the central states (Missouri and neighboring states). Outbreaks have occurred on Martha's Vineyard (Massachusetts). Q fever* cases occur sporadically, especially in persons having contact with livestock in the western part of region; a number of outbreaks have been documented in the Maritime province, eastern Canada. Plague* is enzootic in the western United States, and rare human cases occur, almost 90% from New Mexico, Colorado, Arizona and California, often associated with prairie dogs.

Soil- and water-associated infections: Coccidioidomycosis is endemic in the southwestern United States and can occur in visitors to the area. Its incidence has increased in Arizona and California in recent years. Histoplasmosis is highly endemic, especially in the Mississippi, Ohio, and St. Lawrence River valleys. Sporadic cases and large outbreaks occur. Hawaii has the highest incidence rate of leptospirosis* in the United States, although sporadic cases and outbreaks have occurred elsewhere, primarily in warmer regions or in summer months. It is often associated with water recreational activities. Nonhuman schistosomes that cause cercarial dermatitis are widely distributed in freshwater and seawater along the Atlantic, Pacific, and Gulf coasts, and inland lakes.

Other hazards for travelers include violent injury and death related to guns; rates are higher in the United States than in most industrialized countries. Nineteen species of venomous snakes inhabit North America; the highest bite rates are found in southern states and southwestern desert states. Tick paralysis is most often reported from western Canada and the northwestern United States.

MEXICO AND CENTRAL AMERICA

Vector-borne infections have focal distributions, and some are seasonal. Access to clean water and sanitary disposal of waste remain limited in many areas, so infections related to fecal contamination of food and water remain common. Levels of vaccine coverage are generally good and improving.

More common infections in travelers to the area include gastrointestinal infections, dengue fever, and myiasis. The risk of malaria is low in most countries; more than half of the cases of malaria in travelers to this region are caused by *P. vivax*. Chronic or latent infections with late sequelae in immigrants (and long-term residents) include cysticercosis, tuberculosis, Chagas' disease, leishmaniasis, and strongyloidiasis.

Vector-borne infections: Malaria is present in focal areas of all these countries; it remains sensitive to chloroquine in all areas except for parts of Panama. Risk for travelers is low in most areas. Dengue epidemics have affected most of these countries in the past 5 years. Other vector-borne infections include rickettsial infections (spotted fever and murine typhus) and relapsing fever (tick borne). Foci of active transmission of leishmaniasis (predominantly cutaneous) are present in all countries. West Nile virus has now been found in Mexico and may spread in Central America. Localized foci of transmission of Chagas disease exist in rural areas. Risk to the usual traveler is low. Onchocerciasis is endemic in focal areas of Mexico and Guatemala; eradication efforts are in progress. Myiasis (primarily botfly) is endemic in Central America.

Food- and water-borne infections: Diarrhea in travelers is common and may be caused by bacteria, viruses, and parasites. Diarrhea caused by enterotoxigenic *E. coli* predominates, but other bacteria and protozoa (including *Giardia, Cryptosporidium,* and *Entamoeba histolytica*) cause diarrhea. Risk of hepatitis A is high in many areas; epidemics of hepatitis E have occurred in Mexico. Other infections include brucellosis, typhoid fever, and amebic liver abscess. Nicaragua and

Guatemala reported cholera in 2002-2003; however, risk for travelers is low. Gnathostomiasis has increased in Mexico, with many cases being reported from the Acapulco area; infection has been reported in travelers. Intestinal helminth infections are common in some local populations but are rare in visitors to the area. Central nervous system cysticercosis is a common cause of seizures in local residents.

Airborne and person-to-person transmission: The estimated annual incidence rate of tuberculosis per 100,000 population is 10–50 in most of the area, but 50–100 in Guatemala, Nicaragua, and Honduras.

Sexually transmitted and blood-borne infections: The estimated prevalence of HIV in adults is 0.1%-1%.

Zoonotic infections: Rabies is found throughout the region. Anthrax* is enzootic throughout the region and can infect humans; this disease is most common in El Salvador, Guatemala, Honduras, and Nicaragua. Cases of hantavirus pulmonary syndrome have been reported from Panama.

Soil- and water-associated infections: Outbreaks of leptospirosis have occurred in travelers to the area (including whitewater rafters in Costa Rica and U.S. troops training in Panama); hemorrhagic pulmonary leptospirosis* has occurred in Nicaragua. Sporadic cases and outbreaks of coccidioidomycosis and histoplasmosis have occurred in travelers to area. Risky activities include disturbing soil and entering caves and abandoned mines. Paracoccidioidomycosis is endemic in parts of Mexico and Central America. Hookworm infections are common in some local populations but rare in travelers. Cutaneous larva migrans occurs in visitors, especially those visiting beaches.

Other risks for travelers include scorpion and snake bites and motor vehicle accidents. Screening of blood before transfusion is inadequate in many hospitals.

THE CARIBBEAN

Access to clean water and levels of sanitation are highly variable in the region.

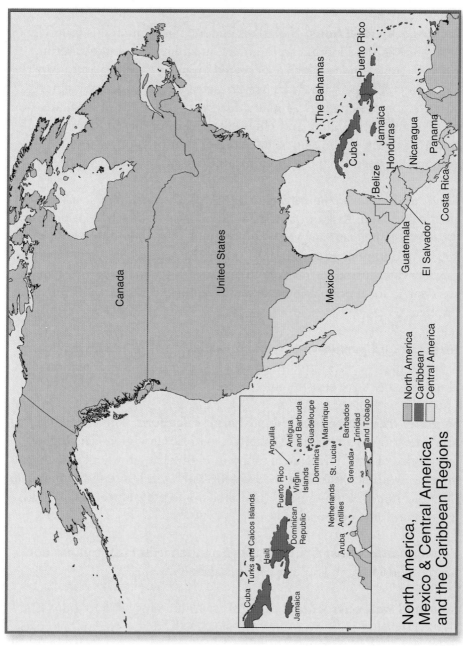

North America, Mexico & Central America, and the Caribbean Regions

North America
Caribbean
Central America

More common infections in travelers include gastrointestinal infections; dengue fever is reported during periods of epidemic activity.

Vector-borne infections: Malaria is endemic in Haiti and is found in focal areas in the Dominican Republic, including a recent cluster in 2004. Dengue epidemics have occurred on many of the islands. Most islands are infested with *Aedes aegypti,* so these places are at risk for introduction of dengue. Lymphatic filariasis is endemic in focal areas of the Dominican Republic and Haiti. Spotted fever due to *Rickettsia africae* has been acquired in Guadeloupe. Transmission of cutaneous leishmaniasis occurs in the Dominican Republic.

Food- and waterborne infections: Risk of diarrheal illness varies greatly by island. Risk of diarrhea and hepatitis A is high, especially on the island of Hispaniola, where an outbreak of typhoid fever occurred in 2003. An outbreak of eosinophilic meningitis caused by *Angiostrongylus cantonensis* occurred in travelers to Jamaica. Intestinal helminths are common in local populations on some islands but are rare in short-term travelers.

Airborne and person-to-person transmission: The annual incidence of tuberculosis is estimated to exceed 300 per 100,000 population in Haiti. The rates are substantially lower on other islands.

Sexually transmitted and blood-borne infections: The prevalence of HIV infection in adults is estimated to be 2.3% in region. The highest prevalence of HIV infection is found in Haiti. The prevalence of chronic infection with hepatitis B is moderate (2%–7%) in Haiti and Dominican Republic but >2% on most of the islands. The prevalence of HTLV-I is 2%–4% on some of the islands.

Zoonotic infections: Anthrax* is hyperendemic in Haiti but has not been reported on most of the other islands.

Soil- and water-associated infections: Cutaneous larva migrans is a risk for travelers with exposures on beaches. Endemic foci of histoplasmosis are found on many islands, and outbreaks have occurred in travelers. Leptospirosis* is common in many areas and poses a risk to travelers engaged in recreational freshwater activities. Foci of schistoso-

MAP 3-3. REGIONS - SOUTH AMERICA

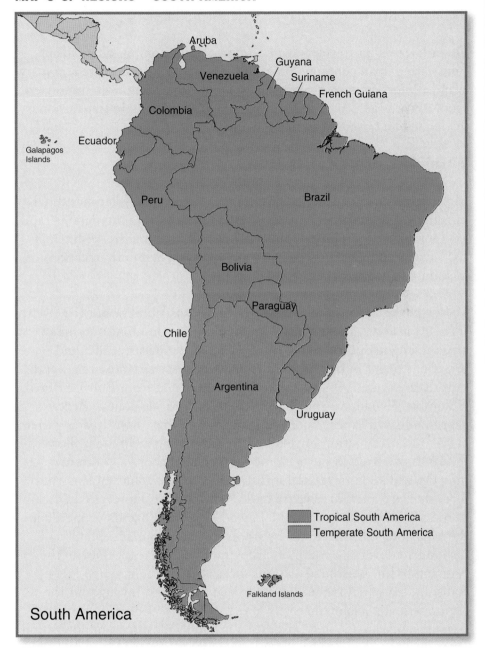

South America

Tropical South America
Temperate South America

miasis have been active in the past in the Dominican Republic, Puerto Rico, and other islands, but pose little risk to travelers.

Other hazards for travelers include ciguatera poisoning, which results from eating toxin-containing reef fish; outbreaks have occurred on many islands. Injury from motor vehicle accidents (including from motorized scooters) is a risk for travelers. Screening of blood before transfusion is inadequate in hospitals on many islands.

TROPICAL SOUTH AMERICA

More common infections in travelers include dengue, gastrointestinal infections, and malaria. Chronic or latent infections in immigrants (and long-term residents) include tuberculosis, schistosomiasis, leishmaniasis, Chagas' disease, cysticercosis, and intestinal helminth infections, including strongyloidiasis.

Vector-borne infections: Malaria is widely distributed, but the risk to travelers is low in most areas. *Vivax* malaria predominates in many areas. Dengue outbreaks have increased in the past decade, and infections occur in travelers. Yellow fever causes sporadic cases and outbreaks. Since 1993, cases have been reported from Bolivia, Brazil, Colombia, Ecuador, French Guiana, Peru, and Venezuela. *Aedes aegypti* infests all these countries, including urban areas, placing them at risk for introduction of yellow fever (and dengue). Fatal yellow fever has occurred in unvaccinated travelers. Other vector-borne infections include rickettsial infections (murine typhus and spotted fever due to *Rickettsia rickettsii* and *R. felis*), relapsing fever (the tick-borne is widely distributed; the louse-borne form occurs primarily in the highlands of Bolivia and Peru), and Venezuelan encephalitis. Oropouche fever is a common arboviral infection, especially in the Amazon basin. Leishmaniasis has increased in recent years; foci of transmission of cutaneous leishmaniasis are found throughout the region; visceral leishmaniasis is found primarily in Brazil. American trypanosomiasis (Chagas' disease) has been widespread in poor, rural areas, but transmission has been interrupted or slowed in many areas (e.g., Brazil) through eradication programs. Onchocerciasis is endemic in focal areas of Brazil, Colombia, Ecuador, and Venezuela; eradication efforts are in progress. Bartonellosis is found in the mountain valleys of Peru (largest endemic focus), Ecuador, and southwestern Colombia (at altitudes between 600 and 2800 meters). Lymphatic filariasis is endemic in Guyana and in focal areas of Brazil and has been found in other countries of the region in the past. Myiasis occasionally occurs in travelers.

Food- and waterborne infections: Gastrointestinal infections in travelers are caused by bacteria, viruses, and parasites. Hepatitis A risk is widespread. Cholera was widespread in South America in the 1990s; only Peru reported infections in 2003. Typhoid fever, brucellosis, and amebic liver abscess are occasionally seen in travelers. Fascioliasis is highly endemic in some areas, especially in Bolivia, Peru, and Venezuela, but risk is low for the usual traveler. Paragonimiasis is endemic in Ecuador and Peru and occurs sporadically in other countries; infections are rare in the usual traveler.

Airborne and person-to-person transmission: The annual incidence rate of tuberculosis per 100,000 is estimated to be 100–300 in Peru, Ecuador, Bolivia, and Guyana and 50–100 or less in the rest of the region. Multidrug resistance has been a problem, especially in Peru. Leprosy is highly endemic in some focal areas (e.g., high prevalence in the Amazon and parts of the Andes).

Sexually transmitted and blood-borne infections: Prevalence of HIV in adults is estimated to be 0.1%-1% in most of the region, but the prevalence is higher in Guyana and Suriname. The prevalence of chronic infection with hepatitis B exceeds 8% in Peru, northern Brazil, and southern Colombia and Venezuela and is 2%-7% in the rest of the region. Hepatitis D has caused epidemics of fulminant hepatitis in the Amazon Basin. HTLV-I is found especially in areas adjacent to the Caribbean and in Colombia, Venezuela, Surinam, Guyana, and Brazil.

Zoonotic infections: Rabies is found throughout the region; vampire bats transmit infection in some areas. Hantavirus pulmonary syndrome caused by hantaviruses with rodent reservoirs has been documented in Bolivia, Brazil, and Paraguay; these viruses may be more widely distributed. Other rodent-associated viruses include Machupo virus,* which causes sporadic infections in rural northeastern Bolivia, and Guaranito virus in Venezuela. Plague* has been reported from Bolivia, Brazil, Ecuador, and Peru since 1990 (most cases are from Peru). Echinococcosis* is found in some rural areas; the risk to travelers is low.

Soil- and water-associated infections: Endemic foci of schistosomiasis (*Schistosoma mansoni*) are found in Brazil, Venezuela, and Suriname. Buruli ulcer (*Mycobacterium ulcerans*) is endemic in French Guyana; a few cases have been reported from other countries (e.g., Peru and Suriname). Risk of leptospirosis* is widespread in tropical areas; outbreaks have followed flooding. Histoplasmosis has been reported from all countries in the region, and paracoccidioidomycosis is endemic throughout the area, with the highest transmission in Peru, Ecuador, Colombia, and Brazil. Coccidioidomycosis is more focal in distribution, with endemic areas in Brazil, Colombia, Paraguay, and Venezuela.

Other risks for travelers include venomous snake bites, injury from motor vehicle accidents, and high altitude-related illness in the Andes. Screening of blood before transfusion is inadequate in many hospitals.

TEMPERATE SOUTH AMERICA

The overall risk for infections is low for most travelers to area. Gastrointestinal infections are a risk, especially in rural areas. Chronic and latent infections in immigrants (and long-term residents) include cysticercosis, Chagas' (from remote acquisition), echinococcosis, soil-associated fungal infections (see below), and intestinal helminth infections.

Vector-borne infections: Limited areas of malaria risk are found in Argentina. Dengue outbreaks have occurred in Argentina since 1997, and *Aedes aegypti* infests the country as far south as Buenos Aires. An outbreak occurred on Easter Island (Chile) in 2002. Other vector-borne infections include bartonellosis (limited to the slopes of the Andes in Chile), tick-borne relapsing fever (reported from northern Argentina and Chile), murine typhus, and spotted fever due to *R. rickettsii* (reported from Argentina). Leishmaniasis (both cutaneous and mucocutaneous) is endemic in northern Argentina and may be present in Uruguay. Programs to eradicate American trypanosomiasis (Chagas' disease) have reduced or interrupted active transmission in many areas.

Food- and water-borne infections: Risk of hepatitis A is moderate to high in parts of the region. Diarrhea in travelers is caused by bacteria, viruses, and parasites. Typhoid fever outbreaks have occurred in Chile in the past, and sporadic infections occur in the region. Typhoid fever, amebic abscesses, and brucellosis can be acquired by travelers. Fascioliasis occurs sporadically, but travelers are at low risk.

Airborne and person-to-person transmission: The annual incidence of tuberculosis is estimated to be 10–50 per 100,000 population. Influenza outbreaks peak in May–August.

Sexually transmitted and blood-borne infections: The estimated prevalence of HIV infection in adults is low (0.1%–1%).

Zoonotic infections: Q fever* (airborne spread) is common in areas where livestock are raised; frequent outbreaks have been noted in Uruguay. Rabies is present in the region. Anthrax* is enzootic in Argentina. Sporadic cases of hantavirus pulmonary syndrome (Andes virus; rodent reservoir host) have been reported from Argentina and Chile. Argentine hemorrhagic fever caused by Junin virus (rodent reservoir) is found in an agricultural area of Argentina. Risk to travelers is low.

Soil- and water-associated infections: Histoplasmosis is endemic in Uruguay and parts of Venezuela. Coccidioidomycosis is found in focal areas of Argentina and Chile; paracoccidioidomycosis is highly endemic in Uruguay and in parts of Argentina and sporadic elsewhere. Sporotrichosis is highly endemic in Uruguay and sporadic elsewhere. Hookworm infections are endemic in warm, wet areas but are rare in travelers. Leptospirosis* is a risk in warmer months.

Other hazards for travelers: Screening of blood prior to transfusion is inadequate in many hospitals.

ASIA

South Asia

- Afghanistan
- Bangladesh
- Bhutan
- British Indian Ocean Territory
- India
- Maldives
- Nepal

South Asia—cont'd

- Pakistan
- Sri Lanka

East Asia

- China
- Hong Kong SAR[1]
- Japan
- Macau SAR[1]
- Mongolia
- North Korea
- South Korea
- Taiwan

Southeast Asia

- Brunei
- Burma (Myanmar)
- Cambodia
- East Timor
- Indonesia
- Laos
- Malaysia
- Philippines
- Singapore
- Thailand
- Vietnam

EAST ASIA

Risk of infection is highly variable in the region. Access to clean water and good sanitary facilities are limited in many rural areas, especially in China and Mongolia. Respiratory infections (etiology often undefined) are common in travelers to the region. Chronic and latent infections in immigrants (and long-term residents) include tuberculosis, complications from chronic hepatitis B (and also hepatitis C) infection, schistosomiasis, paragonimiasis, and strongyloidiasis.

[1]Special Administrative Region

MAP 3-4. REGIONS - ASIA

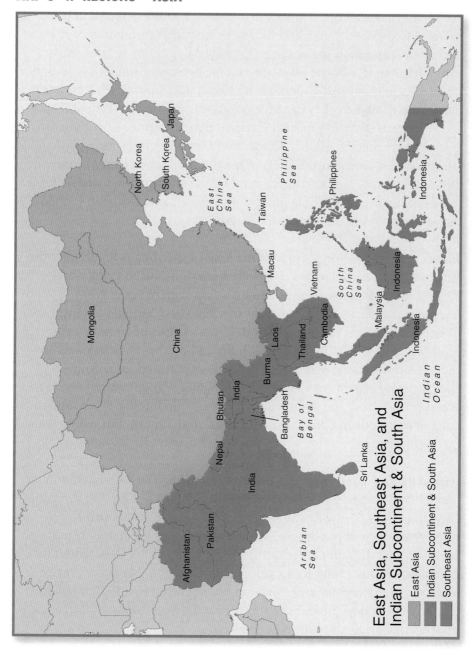

East Asia, Southeast Asia, and
Indian Subcontinent & South Asia

East Asia
Indian Subcontinent & South Asia
Southeast Asia

Vector-borne infections: Malaria is found in focal areas of China and North and South Korea. Japanese encephalitis (JE) is found in wide areas of China and Japan and focally in Korea. Transmission of malaria and JE is seasonal in many areas. Reported infections in travelers are rare. Other vector-borne infections include dengue, which has caused outbreaks in mainland China, Hong Kong, and Taiwan; spotted fever caused by *R. sibirica* (China, Mongolia); murine typhus; Oriental spotted fever caused by *R. japonica* (Japan); rickettsialpox (Korea); scrub typhus (especially in China, Korea, and Japan); tick-borne encephalitis (in forested regions northeastern China and in South Korea); visceral and cutaneous leishmaniasis (in rural China); lymphatic filariasis (in focal coastal areas of China and South Korea); and Crimean-Congo hemorrhagic fever* (in western China).

Food- and water-borne infections: Risk of diarrhea is highly variable within the region. Diarrhea in travelers may be caused by bacteria, viruses, and parasites. Risk of hepatitis A is high in some areas (excluding Japan), especially in rural areas of China and Mongolia. Outbreaks of hepatitis E have been reported in China. Cases of cholera were reported from China in 2002–2003. Sporadic cases of anisakiasis are reported from Korea and Japan. Brucellosis is found, especially in sheep-raising regions of China and Mongolia. Paragonimiasis is endemic in China and still occurs in Korea. Clonorchiasis is found in local populations in China, Japan, Korea, and Taiwan, but risk to usual traveler is low.

Airborne and person-to-person transmission: The estimated annual incidence of tuberculosis per 100,000 population is 100–300 in China, Mongolia, and North Korea and 50–100 in Japan and South Korea. High rates of multiple drug-resistant tuberculosis are found in parts of China (about 10% in new patients). Outbreaks of SARS occurred in mainland China, Hong Kong, and Taiwan in 2003. Measles remains endemic in the region, and infection has occurred in adopted children from China and in travelers to the region. In tropical areas, influenza may occur during all months of the year.

Sexually transmitted and blood-borne infections: The prevalence of HIV in adults is low (0.1%–1%) in most of the region, but a much higher prevalence is found in focal areas in southern China. Hepatitis B is highly endemic among adults in region, excluding Japan. Prevalence of chronic infection exceeds 8% in many areas. Prevalence of hepatitis C is 10% or higher in Mongolia; 2.5%–9.9% in mainland China and Taiwan, and 1%–2.4% in the rest of the region. A high prevalence of HTLV-I is found focally in the southern islands of Japan.

Zoonotic infections: Rabies is widespread in China (not Hong Kong) and Mongolia. Avian influenza has been transmitted to humans in Hong Kong and China. To date, the virus has caused high mortality in humans but has not been readily transmissible from person to person. Highly pathogenic H5N1 has also been found in bird populations in Japan, and South Korea. Cases of human plague* are reported most years from China and Mongolia. Hantaviruses causing hemorrhagic fever with renal syndrome are a major health threat in China and the Republic of Korea, primarily affecting residents of rural areas in late fall and early winter. Risk to the usual traveler is low. Anthrax* is enzootic in China and Mongolia, and sporadic infection is reported in the rest of the region. Tularemia* occurs in China and Japan and is found especially in northern parts of region. Echinococcosis* is endemic in rural areas of China and Mongolia.

Schistosomiasis (*S. japonicum*) is present in focal areas in China, especially in the Yangtze River basin. Leptospirosis* is a risk, especially in tropical areas of China and South Korea. Cutaneous larva migrans is common in warm coastal areas. Cases of histoplasmosis have been reported.

Other risks for travelers include injury from motor vehicle accidents and venomous snake bites. Screening of blood before transfusion is inadequate in many hospitals in the region.

SOUTHEAST ASIA

More common infections in travelers to the area include dengue fever, respiratory infections, and diarrheal infections. Chronic and latent infections in immigrants (and long-term residents) include tuberculosis, late complications of hepatitis B infection, intestinal helminth infections (including strongyloidiasis), and other helminth infections, such as paragonimiasis, opisthorchiasis, and clonorchiasis.

Vector-borne infections: Dengue fever is hyperendemic in the region, and epidemics are common; cases occur in travelers to the region. Malaria is found in focal areas (primarily rural) in all these countries (except Brunei and Singapore), especially in rural areas. Japanese encephalitis is widely distributed in the region and is hyperendemic in some areas; risk is seasonal in some countries. Scrub typhus is a common cause of fever in the region. Other vector-borne infections include murine typhus, Chikungunya virus, and relapsing fever. Foci of transmission of lymphatic filariasis are found throughout the area, with the exception of some of the Indonesian islands.

Food- and water-borne infections: Risk of hepatitis A is widespread in the region. Risk of diarrhea caused by bacteria, viruses, and parasites is high in parts of the area. Campylobacter infections are especially common in Thailand and are often resistant to fluoroquinolones. Amebic liver abscesses, typhoid fever, and brucellosis occur. Isolates of *Salmonella* causing typhoid fever may be resistant to multiple drugs, including the fluoroquinolones. Cholera epidemics have been common in the past. Outbreaks of hepatitis E have been reported from the region (Indonesia and Burma). Cysticercosis is especially common in Indonesia. Gnathostomiasis is endemic in region and especially common in Thailand. Intestinal helminth infections are common in some rural areas; risk to the usual traveler is low. Opisthorchiasis, clonorchiasis, fasciolopsiasis, and paragonimiasis are endemic in parts of the region (especially Laos and Burma).

Airborne and person-to-person transmission: The annual incidence rate of tuberculosis per 100,000 population is estimated to be >300 in Cambodia and 100–300 in the rest of the region. Measles transmission persists in region, although vaccination coverage is improving in some countries. SARS outbreaks occurred in the region (especially in Singapore and Vietnam) in 2003. Influenza infections can occur throughout the year in tropical areas.

Sexually transmitted and blood-borne infections: The prevalence of HIV is 1%–5% in Thailand and Cambodia in adults and <1% in the rest of the region. Higher prevalence may be found in specific populations. The prevalence of hepatitis B chronic carriage exceeds 8% in many parts of region. The prevalence of chronic hepatitis C is 1%–2.4%. Chancroid is a common cause of genital ulcer disease.

Zoonotic infections: Rabies is common in the region, and travelers are at risk for exposure to rabid animals, especially dogs. Outbreaks of avian influenza occurred in 2003–2005 in Thailand, Vietnam, Indonesia, Malaysia, and Cambodia. Human cases (with high mortality rates) occurred in Vietnam and Thailand. Anthrax* is hyperendemic in Burma; sporadic cases occur in much of the rest of the region. An outbreak of Nipah virus, with a probable reservoir in fruit bats and documented transmission to humans from pigs, occurred in Malaysia (1998–1999) and in Singapore (after contact with pigs imported from Malaysia). Cases of human plague* have been reported since 1990 from Indonesia, Laos, Burma, and Vietnam.

Soil- and water-associated infections: Schistosomiasis caused by *S. japonicum* is found in the Philippines and Indonesia (Sulawesi [Celebes]); caused by *S. mekongi* in Cambodia and Laos; and caused by *S. malayensis* in peninsular Malaysia. Leptospirosis* is common in tropical areas and has been reported in travelers to the area. Melioidosis is a common cause of community-acquired sepsis, especially in rural areas of Thailand; it is also common in Cambodia, Laos, and Vietnam. Cases have increased in 2004 in Singapore. Infection in travelers is rare. *Penicilliosis marneffei* is found in southeast Asia and is a common opportunistic infection in HIV-infected patients, especially in Thailand. Rare cases have been reported in travelers to the region. Cutaneous larva migrans is common on warm coastal areas.

Other risks for travelers include injury from motor vehicle accidents and venomous snake bites. Screening of blood before transfusion is inadequate in many hospitals in the region.

SOUTH ASIA

More common infections in travelers are gastrointestinal infections (including acute bacterial diarrhea and amebic disease), typhoid fever, and malaria. Chronic and latent infections in immigrants (or long-term residents) include tuberculosis, cysticercosis, visceral leishmaniasis, lymphatic filariasis, echinococcosis, and intestinal helminths. Primary varicella may be seen in adults, as childhood infection is less common in tropical areas.

Vector-borne infections: Malaria is widespread in areas at altitudes <2000 meters and is found in the Terai and Hill districts of Nepal at altitudes <1200 meters. Dengue fever has caused epidemics in all these countries except Nepal. Japanese encephalitis transmission occurs widely in lowland areas of the region (except for Afghanistan). Transmission is seasonal. Focal areas of transmission of visceral leishmaniasis are present in rural India, Pakistan, Nepal, and Bangladesh. Cutaneous leishmaniasis is present in Afghanistan, where it has infected US troops; India; and Pakistan. Lymphatic filariasis is endemic in large areas of India, Sri Lanka, and Bangladesh. Other vector-borne infections include scrub typhus, murine typhus, epidemic typhus (in remote, cooler areas), relapsing fever, sandfly fever, spotted fever due to *R. conorii* (especially in India), Kyasanur Forest disease (tick-borne; Karnataka State, India, and Pakistan), and Crimean-Congo hemorrhagic fever* (in Pakistan and Afghanistan).

Food- and water-borne infections: Hepatitis A is widespread, and risk to travelers is high. Large outbreaks of hepatitis E have occurred in Bangladesh, India, Nepal, and Pakistan. Typhoid and paratyphoid fever (increasingly resistant to multiple antimicrobial agents) occur sporadically and in outbreaks and can affect travelers to region. Amebic infections are common and can cause liver abscesses. Indigenous wild polio was present in 2003 in India, Pakistan, and Afghanistan. *Cyclospora* infections have been reported, especially from Nepal. Cholera outbreaks have occurred frequently in the region, especially in Bangladesh. Cysticercosis is found, especially in India. Paragonimiasis is endemic in India (Manipur Province). Gnathostomiasis has caused sporadic cases and outbreaks.

Airborne and person-to-person: The annual incidence rates of tuberculosis per 100,000 population are estimated to be >300 in Afghanistan and 100–300 in most of the rest of the region. Measles occurs in the region and can be a source of infection for unvaccinated travelers.

Sexually transmitted and blood-borne infections: The prevalence of HIV is <1% in most of the region but is rising rapidly in some populations in India. The prevalence of chronic infection with hepatitis B is 2%–7% in most of the region.

Zoonotic infections: Rabies is common in the region and poses a risk to travelers. Q fever* is widespread. Anthrax* is endemic in much of the region, and cases occur sporadically. Plague* is endemic in India, and outbreaks have occurred. Echinococcosis* is highly endemic in focal rural areas. An outbreak of Nipah virus (encephalitis) occurred in Bangladesh in early 2004, and person-to-person spread may have occurred. Macaques throughout the region are infected with B virus (Herpes).

Soil- and water-associated infections: Leptospirosis* is common, especially in tropical areas.

Other risks for travelers include snake bites, injury from motor vehicle accidents, and injury related to ongoing conflicts. Screening of blood before transfusion is inadequate in many hospitals.

MIDDLE EAST

- Bahrain
- Cyprus
- Iran
- Iraq
- Israel
- Jordan
- Kuwait
- Lebanon
- Oman
- Qatar
- Saudi Arabia
- Syria
- Turkey
- United Arab Emirates
- Yemen

MIDDLE EAST

Common infections in travelers are gastrointestinal infections. Chronic and latent infections in immigrants (and long-term residents) include tuberculosis, echinococcosis, cutaneous leishmaniasis, brucellosis.

Vector-borne infections: Malaria is present in focal areas of Iran, Iraq, Oman, Saudi Arabia, Syria, Turkey, and Yemen. Epidemic dengue activity occurred in Saudi Arabia and Yemen in 2002. Cutaneous leishmaniasis is widespread and common, especially in countries bordering the

Mediterranean. Transmission of visceral leishmaniasis occurs focally in Turkey, Iraq, Saudi Arabia, and Syria. Other vector-borne infections include murine typhus, spotted fever due to *R. conorii*, tick-borne encephalitis (in Turkey), Crimean-Congo hemorrhagic fever* (in Iran, Iraq, and the Arabian peninsula), tick-borne relapsing fever, sandfly fever, and West Nile fever. Lymphatic filariasis and onchocerciasis are endemic in focal areas of Yemen.

Food- and water-borne infections: Risk of hepatitis A is high in many parts of the area; typhoid fever occurs sporadically and in outbreaks. Outbreaks of hepatitis E have been reported in Iran and Jordan. Cholera was reported from Saudi Arabia, Iraq, and Iran in 2002–2003. Brucellosis is widespread and common in parts of the region.

Airborne and person-to-person transmission: Pilgrims to the Hajj (Saudi Arabia) have acquired meningococcal infections caused by serotypes A and W-135, as well as influenza infections. The annual incidence of tuberculosis per 100,000 population is estimated to be 100–300 in Yemen and Iraq and 50–100 or less in the rest of the region. Measles continues to be reported from the region.

Sexually transmitted and blood-borne infections: The prevalence of hepatitis B chronic infection is >8% in Saudi Arabia and 2%–7% in much of the rest of the region. The prevalence of HIV is estimated to be <1% throughout the region.

Zoonotic infections: Anthrax* is enzootic in Turkey, and sporadic cases occur in most of the region except for Oman. Rabies is widespread in the region. Endemic foci of plague* have been identified in the region in the past. Q fever* is common in most countries in the region. Echinococcosis* is endemic in many rural areas. Outbreaks of oropharyngeal tularemia* have been reported from Turkey.

Soil- and water-associated infections: Schistosomiasis has been found in focal areas in Saudi Arabia, Yemen, Iraq, and Syria.

Other risks for travelers include motor vehicle accidents, intentional injuries, and injuries related to ongoing conflicts. Snake and scorpion bites are an additional hazard. Screening of blood before transfusion is inadequate in many hospitals.

EUROPE

Eastern Europe & Northern Asia

- Albania
- Armenia
- Azerbaijan
- Belarus
- Bosnia and Herzegovina
- Bulgaria
- Croatia
- Czech Republic
- Estonia
- Georgia
- Hungary
- Kazakhstan
- Kyrgyzstan
- Latvia
- Lithuania
- Macedonia
- Moldova
- Poland
- Romania
- Russia
- Serbia and Montenegro
- Slovakia
- Slovenia
- Tajikistan
- Turkmenistan
- Ukraine
- Uzbekistan

Western Europe

- Andorra
- Austria
- Azores
- Belgium
- Denmark
- Faroe Islands
- Finland

Western Europe—cont'd

- France
- Germany
- Gibraltar
- Greece
- Greenland
- Holy See
- Iceland
- Ireland
- Italy
- Liechtenstein
- Luxembourg
- Malta
- Monaco
- Netherlands
- Norway
- Portugal
- San Marino
- Spain
- Sweden
- Switzerland
- United Kingdom

WESTERN EUROPE

The area is characterized by a low risk for most infectious diseases.

Vector-borne infections: The only malaria cases are "airport" malaria and imported cases. Lyme disease is found in broad areas of Europe in temperate forested areas. Tick-borne encephalitis is found in Austria, Germany, Finland, Sweden, Switzerland, and Denmark (only on island of Bornholm); a few cases have also been reported from Italy, Norway, and France. Leishmaniasis (cutaneous and visceral) is found, especially in countries bordering the Mediterranean, with the highest numbers of cases from Spain, where it is an important opportunistic infection in HIV-infected persons. Relapsing fever (tick-borne) is found in focal areas in Greece, Italy, Portugal, and Spain; sporadic cases may occur elsewhere in region. Murine typhus is more common in warmer areas, especially Mediterranean port cities. Sandfly fever occurs in warmer months in southern Europe, especially in Italy, Spain, Portugal, and

MAP 3-5. REGIONS - WESTERN EUROPE

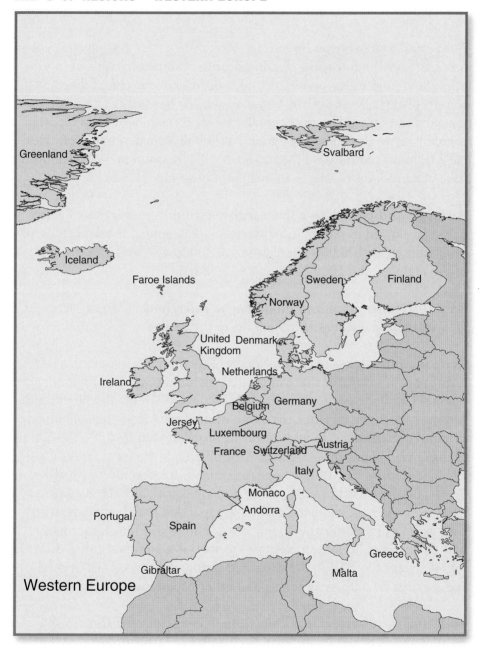

Greece. Small numbers of cases of babesiosis have been reported from the region.

Food- and water-borne infections: Risk of hepatitis A is low (except for Greenland). Outbreaks of salmonellosis, campylobacteriosis, and other food- and water-borne infections occur, but the risk of diarrhea in travelers is low. Brucellosis is found, especially in southern countries on the Mediterranean. Variant Creutzfeldt-Jakob cases have been reported primarily from the United Kingdom, although a small number of cases have been reported from other countries. Large outbreaks of trichinosis have occurred; outbreaks in France have been linked to horse meat.

Airborne and person-to-person transmission: Measles transmission has been slowed by vaccination programs. The annual incidence rate of tuberculosis per 100,000 population is estimated to be 10–50 for most of the region and <10 in Norway and Sweden.

Sexually transmitted and blood-borne infections: The prevalence of HIV in adults is estimated to be 0.3% in this region.

Zoonotic infections: Large outbreaks of tularemia* have occurred in rural areas in several of these countries, including Sweden, Finland, and Spain. Hantaviruses causing hemorrhagic fever with renal syndrome are widespread; Puumala virus, the cause of mild nephropathia epidemica, is found in Scandinavian and western European countries. Rabies is present in many countries in western Europe; human cases are rare. Echinococcosis* due to *Echinococcus granulosus* is found, especially in Spain and the Mediterranean countries; areas with alveolar echinococcosis (caused by *E. multilocularis*) have expanded in recent years, with the largest number of cases found in focal areas of France, Germany, and Switzerland. Q fever* (airborne spread) is a common cause of febrile illness (both sporadic cases and outbreaks), especially in rural areas of Spain, southern France, and other Mediterranean countries.

Soil- and water-associated infections: Legionnaires' disease is sporadic; some outbreaks have involved tourists at resort hotels.

Other risks for travelers include motor vehicle accidents and injuries related to ongoing conflicts and alcohol abuse. Nosocomial transmission of infections is a problem in many areas because of inadequate

MAP 3-6. REGIONS – EASTERN EUROPE AND NORTHERN ASIA

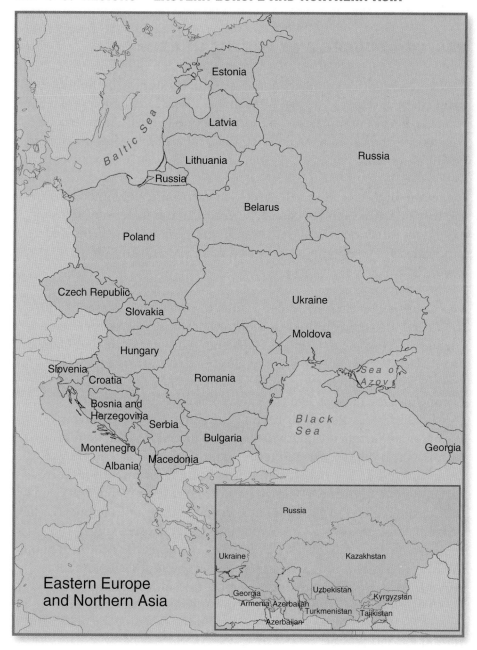

infection control procedures. Screening of blood before transfusion is inadequate in many hospitals.

EASTERN EUROPE AND NORTHERN ASIA

Access to clean water and adequate levels of sanitation are limited in many parts of region. Vaccine-preventable diseases remain a problem where levels of immunization are low. The public health infrastructure has deteriorated in areas of conflict; political instability has threatened health in some areas.

Common infections in travelers include gastrointestinal infections, respiratory infections, and occasionally vector-borne infections. Chronic and latent infections immigrants (and long-term residents) include tuberculosis (including multidrug-resistant TB) and late sequelae of hepatitis B.

Vector-borne infections: Malaria transmission occurs seasonally in focal rural areas of countries in the southernmost part of the region (Armenia, Azerbaijan, Georgia, Tajikistan, Turkmenistan, and Uzbekistan). Tick-borne encephalitis is widespread, occurring in warmer months in the southern part of the nontropical forested region of Europe and Asia. Most intense transmission has been reported in Russia, the Czech Republic, Latvia, Lithuania, Estonia, Hungary, Poland, and Slovenia. Other vector-borne infections include murine typhus, scrub typhus, spotted fever due to *Rickettsia sibirica* (North Asian spotted fever), rickettsialpox, relapsing fever (more southern parts of region), Crimean-Congo hemorrhagic fever* (in many countries of the region but primarily in persons working with animals or in hospitals), leishmaniasis (cutaneous and visceral; especially in the southern areas of the former Soviet Union), Lyme disease (throughout the former Soviet Union), sandfly fever (in the southern parts of region), West Nile (a large outbreak occurred in Romania in late 1990s), and Japanese encephalitis (transmission occurs in a limited area of far eastern Russia).

Food- and water-borne infections: A high risk of hepatitis A is present in many parts of the region. Sporadic cases of typhoid fever are reported, and outbreaks occur. Outbreaks of hepatitis E have been reported from the southern areas of Russia. Brucellosis is a risk in many areas. Outbreaks of botulism are usually linked to home-canned foods. Sporadic cases of fascioliasis occur.

Airborne and person-to-person transmission: The annual incidence rate of tuberculosis per 100,000 population is estimated to be 100–300 in many parts of the region. High rates of drug-resistant TB are found in Estonia, Kazakhstan, Latvia, Lithuania, parts of Russia, and Uzbekistan, where rates of drug resistance in newly diagnosed TB patients are as high as 14%. Cases of diphtheria have declined (after the massive outbreak of the 1990s) with improved rates of immunization. Transmission of measles is declining.

Sexually transmitted and blood-borne infections: The prevalence of HIV in adults is estimated to be 0.6% in the region. The prevalence of hepatitis B is intermediate (2%–7%) or high (> 8%) in most of the region. The prevalence of hepatitis C is 1%–2.4% in much of the area (2.5%–9.9% in Romania).

Zoonotic infections: Rabies is widespread in the region and is increasing in some countries. Tularemia* is widespread and occurs in focal outbreaks. Wild rodent plague* is broadly distributed in southern areas of the former Soviet Union; human cases are rare. Sporadic cases and occasional outbreaks of anthrax* are reported. Q fever* is found, especially in cattle-raising areas. Hantaviruses causing hemorrhagic fever with renal syndrome are found in many countries in the region; infection is sporadic and epidemic. Echinococcosis* occurs sporadically in the area.

Soil- and water-associated infections: Cases of cholera have been reported from Russia in 2002–2003.

Other risks for travelers include motor vehicle accidents and injuries related to ongoing conflicts and alcohol abuse. Nosocomial transmission of infections is a problem in many areas because of inadequate infection control procedures. Screening of blood before transfusion is inadequate in many hospitals.

AUSTRALIA AND THE SOUTH PACIFIC

- American Samoa
- Australia

- Christmas Island
- Cocos (Keeling) Islands
- Cook Islands
- Fiji
- French Polynesia
- Guam
- Kiribati
- Marshall Islands
- Micronesia
- Nauru
- New Caledonia
- New Zealand
- Niue
- Norfolk Island
- Northern Mariana Islands
- Palau
- Papua New Guinea
- Pitcairn Islands
- Samoa
- Solomon Islands
- Tahiti
- Tokelau
- Tonga
- Tuvalu
- Vanuatu
- Wake Island

AUSTRALIA AND THE SOUTH PACIFIC

Risk of infection is highly variable within the region. The risk of food and water-borne infections is low in most of Australia and New Zealand; immunization coverage is also generally high in those countries. Vector-borne infections and gastrointestinal infections are common in travelers to other islands.

Vector-borne infections: Malaria is transmitted on Papua New Guinea, Vanuatu, and the Solomon Islands. Dengue has caused recurring epidemics on many of the islands and in northern Australia. Japanese encephalitis (JE) is found in Papua New Guinea and the Torres Strait

MAP 3-7. REGIONS – AUSTRALIA AND THE SOUTH PACIFIC ISLANDS

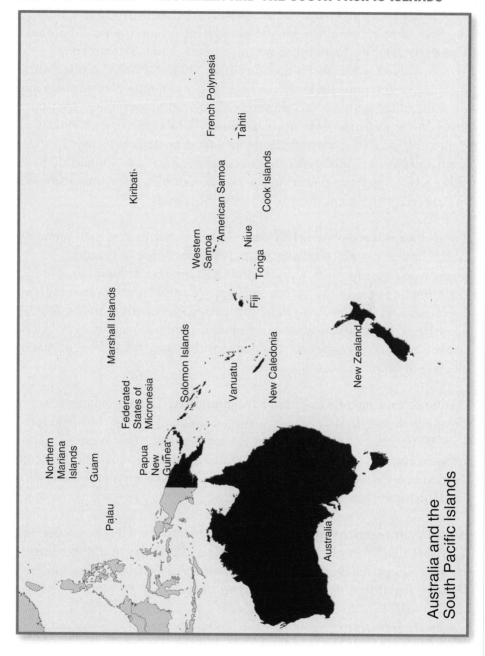

Australia and the
South Pacific Islands

and far northern Australia. JE infections have occurred in the western Pacific islands (e.g., Guam) in the past. Lymphatic filariasis is widely distributed on many of the Pacific islands, including American Samoa, Cook Islands, Fiji, French Polynesia, Kiribati, Niue, Samoa, Tonga, Tuvalu, Vanuatu, and Wallis and Futuna. Other vector-borne infections include scrub typhus (in northern Australia and Papua New Guinea and on some of the western and southern islands), murine typhus, spotted fever due to *Rickettsia australis* (Queensland tick typhus), and Murray Valley encephalitis (recurring epidemics are reported, especially in southeastern Australia; rare cases occur in Papua New Guinea). Ross River fever (epidemic polyarthritis) causes sporadic cases and outbreaks in Australia and on a number of the Pacific islands.

Food- and water-borne infections: Risk of hepatitis A is high on many of the Pacific islands. Gastrointestinal infections due to bacteria, viruses, and parasites (including *Entamoeba histolytica*) have been common on some of the islands, including Papua New Guinea. Typhoid fever is uncommon in Australia; outbreaks have occurred on some of the islands. Cases of eosinophilic meningitis due to *Angiostrongylus cantonensis* have been reported from many of the islands. Occasional cases of cholera occur in Australia.

Airborne and person-to-person transmission: The annual incidence of tuberculosis per 100,000 population is estimated to be 100–300 for the Pacific islands, 10–50 for New Zealand, and <10 for Australia. The influenza transmission season in Australia typically occurs April through September. Periodic outbreaks of measles have occurred on islands with inadequate immunization coverage.

Sexually transmitted and blood-borne infections: The prevalence of HIV is 0.1%–1% in most of the region. The prevalence of chronic infection with hepatitis B is ≥8% on many of the Pacific islands. The prevalence of hepatitis C is 1%–2.4% in most of the area.

Zoonotic infections: Sporadic cases and outbreaks of Q fever* occur in Australia (rarely in New Zealand). Most of the islands are reported to be rabies free, although bat rabies exists in some of these areas. Fatal cases of Hendra virus (closely related to Nipah virus) infection occurred in Australia in 1994. Fruit bats, widely distributed in Australia and the South Pacific, may be the natural host.

Soil- and water-associated infections: Buruli ulcer (caused by *Mycobacterium ulcerans*) increased in incidence in Australia in the 1990s, with the development of new foci on Phillip Island and in a district southwest of Melbourne. Most cases are in Victoria and Queensland. Cases of melioidosis have been reported from Papua New Guinea, Guam, and Australia; risk may exist on other islands. Leptospirosis is common on some of the islands. Sporadic cases of histoplasmosis have been documented. Hookworm infections and strongyloidiasis are common on some of the Pacific Islands.

Other hazards for travelers include ciguatera poisoning from eating large reef-dwelling fish; high attack rates have been reported on some of the islands. Venomous snakes and spiders are a risk in many areas. Screening of blood before transfusion is inadequate in hospitals on many of the islands.

Bibliography

Heymann DL, editor. *Control of communicable diseases manual.* 18th ed. Washington DC: American Public Health Association; 2004.

Promedmail.org [database on the Internet]. Boston: International Society for Infectious Diseases. ©2001 [cited 2004 Oct 17]. Available from: http://www.promedmail.org.

Ryan ET, Wilson ME, Kain KC. Illness after international travel. *N Engl J Med.* 2002;347:505-16.

Wilson ME. *A world guide to infections: diseases, distribution, diagnosis.* New York: Oxford; 1991.

World Health Organization. International travel and health [monograph on the Internet]. Geneva, Switzerland: World Health Organization; 2004 [cited 2004 Oct 17]. Available from: http://www.who.int/ith/.

World Health Organization [homepage on the Internet]. Geneva, Switzerland: World Health Organization; ©2004 [updated 2004 Oct 15; cited 2004 Oct 17]. Weekly Epidemiological Record. Available from: http://www.who.int/wer/.

—MARY E. WILSON

CHAPTER 4

Prevention of Specific Infectious Diseases

>>Acquired Immunodeficiency Syndrome (AIDS)

DESCRIPTION

AIDS is a serious disease, first recognized as a distinct syndrome in 1981. AIDS represents the late clinical stage of infection with human immunodeficiency virus (HIV), which progressively damages the immune system. Without an effective immune system, life-threatening infections and other noninfectious conditions related to failing immunity (such as certain cancers) eventually develop.

OCCURRENCE

AIDS and HIV infection occur worldwide. Many countries lack comprehensive surveillance systems, so the true number of cases is likely far greater than officially reported, particularly in developing countries. The Joint United Nations Programme on HIV/AIDS estimates that, as of the end of 2003, 40 million persons were living with HIV/AIDS worldwide and that there were 14,000 new infections daily. Because HIV infection and AIDS are distributed globally, the risk for international travelers is determined less by geographic destination and more by behaviors that put them at risk of becoming infected, such as sexual and drug-using behaviors.

RISK FOR TRAVELERS

The risk of HIV infection for international travelers is generally low. Factors to consider in assessing risk include the extent of direct contact with blood or other potentially infectious secretions and the extent of sexual contact with potentially infected persons. In addition, the blood supply in developing countries might not be adequately screened.

PREVENTION

No vaccine is available to prevent infection with HIV. For information on the safety of vaccines for HIV-infected persons, see section on *The Immunocompromised Traveler.*

Travelers should be advised that HIV infection is preventable. HIV can be transmitted through sexual intercourse and needle- or syringe-sharing; by medical use of blood, blood components, or organ or tissue transplantation; through artificial insemination; and perinatally from an infected woman to her infant. HIV is not transmitted through casual contact; air, food, or water routes; contact with inanimate objects; or by mosquitoes or other arthropod vectors. The use of any public conveyance (e.g., an airplane, an automobile, a boat, a bus, or a train) by persons with AIDS or HIV infection does not pose a risk of infection for the crew members or other travelers.

Travelers should be advised that they are at risk if they—

- Have sexual contact (heterosexual or homosexual) with an infected person.
- Use or allow the use of contaminated, unsterilized syringes or needles for any injections or other procedures that pierce the skin, including acupuncture, use of illicit drugs, steroid or vitamin injections, medical or dental procedures, ear or body piercing, or tattooing.
- Use infected blood, blood components, or clotting factor concentrates. HIV infection by this route is rare in countries or cities where donated blood and plasma are screened for antibodies to HIV.

Travelers should be advised to avoid sexual encounters with persons who are infected with HIV or whose HIV infection status is unknown. Travelers should also be advised to avoid sexual activity with persons who are at high risk for HIV infection, such as intravenous drug users, commercial sex workers (both male and female), and other persons with multiple sexual partners. In countries with high rates of HIV infection, many persons without these risk factors may be infected and be unaware of their status. Condoms, when used consistently and correctly, prevent transmission of HIV. Travelers who engage in vaginal, anal, or oral-genital sexual contact with a person who is HIV-infected or whose HIV status is unknown should use a latex condom. Persons who are sensitive to latex should use condoms made of polyurethane or other synthetic materials. Some areas may have a limited supply and selection of condoms, or available condoms may be of inferior quality. Persons traveling to these areas who engage in sexual contact with persons who are HIV-infected or whose HIV status is unknown should carry their own supply of condoms. When a male condom cannot be used properly, a female condom should be considered. When no condom is available, travelers should abstain from anal, vaginal, and oral-genital sexual contact with persons who are HIV-infected or whose HIV status is unknown. Barrier methods other than condoms have not been shown to be effective in the prevention of HIV transmission. Spermicides alone have also not been shown to be effective, and the widely used spermicide nonoxynol-9 can increase the risk of HIV transmission in some cases. In many countries, needle-sharing by intravenous drug users is a major means of HIV transmission and transmission of other infections, such as hepatitis B and hepatitis C. Travelers should be advised not to use drugs intravenously or share needles for any purpose. Travelers should also be advised to avoid, if at all possible, receiving medications from multidose vials, which may have become contaminated by used needles.

In many developed countries (e.g., Australia, Canada, Japan, New Zealand, western European nations, United States), the risk of transfusion-associated HIV infection has been virtually eliminated through required testing of all donated blood for antibody to HIV. In the United States, donations of blood and plasma must be screened for HIV-1 and HIV-2 antibodies, the HIV-1 p24 antigen, and traces of HIV genetic material that may indicate infection.

If produced in the United States according to U.S. Food and Drug Administration-approved procedures, immune globulin preparations (such as those used for the prevention of hepatitis A and B) and hepatitis B virus vaccines undergo processes that inactivate HIV; therefore, these products should be used as indicated. Developing countries may have no formal program for testing blood or biological products for contamination with HIV. In those countries, travelers should (when medically prudent) avoid use of unscreened blood-clotting factor concentrates or concentrates of uncertain purity. If transfusion is necessary, the blood should be tested, if at all possible, for HIV antibody by appropriately trained laboratory technicians using a reliable test. See *Seeking Health Care Abroad* for additional information.

Needles used to draw blood or administer injections should be sterile, single use, disposable, and prepackaged in a sealed container. Travelers with insulin-dependent diabetes, hemophilia, or other conditions that necessitate routine or frequent injections should be advised to carry a supply of syringes, needles, and disinfectant swabs (e.g., alcohol wipes) sufficient to last their entire stay abroad. Before traveling, such persons should consider requesting documentation of the medical necessity for traveling with these items (e.g., a doctor's letter) in case their need is questioned by inspection personnel at ports of entry.

International travelers should be advised that some countries screen incoming travelers for HIV infection and may deny entry to persons with AIDS and evidence of HIV infection. These countries usually screen only persons planning extended visits, such as for work or study. Persons intending to visit a country for an extended stay should be informed of that country's policies and requirements. This information is usually available from the consular officials of the individual nations. An unofficial list compiled by the U.S. Department of State can be found at the following URL: http://travel.state.gov/HIVtestingreqs.html.

Further information is available from 1-800-342-AIDS, toll free from the United States or its territories (for Spanish-speaking callers, 1-800-344-SIDA; for hearing-impaired callers with teletype equipment, 1-800-AIDS-TTY).

Bibliography

CDC. HIV Prevention Bulletin: Medical Advice for Persons who Inject Illicit Drugs. Available at: http://www.cdc.gov/idu/pubs/hiv_prev.htm. Last accessed July 6, 2004.

CDC. Management of possible sexual, injecting-drug-use, or other nonoccupational exposure to HIV, including considerations related to antiretroviral therapy. MMWR Recommendations and Reports 47(RR-17): 1–19, 1998. http://www.cdc.gov/mmwr/preview/mmwrhtml/00054952.htm. Last accessed July 6, 2004.

Memish ZA, Osoba AO. Sexually transmitted diseases and travel. Int J Antimicrob Agents 2003;21: 131–4.

Perrin L, Kaiser L, Yerly S. Travel and the spread of HIV-1 genetic variants. Lancet Infect Dis 2003;3:22–27.

Wright ER. Travel, tourism, and HIV risk among older adults. J AIDS 2003; 33(suppl. 2): S233–7.

–JOHN T. BROOKS

>>African Trypanosomiasis (African Sleeping Sickness)

DESCRIPTION

Trypanosomiasis is a systemic disease caused by the parasite *Trypanosoma brucei*. East African trypanosomiasis is caused by *T. b. rhodesiense* and West African trypanosomiasis by *T. b. gambiense*. Both forms are transmitted by the bite of the tsetse fly, a gray-brown insect about the size of a honeybee.

OCCURRENCE

African trypanosomiasis is confined to tropical Africa between 15° north latitude and 20° south latitude, or from north of South Africa to south of Algeria, Libya, and Egypt. According to WHO, 25,000–45,000 cases of trypanosomiasis are reported annually; however, the actual prevalence of cases is estimated to be 300,000 to 500,000.

RISK FOR TRAVELERS

Tsetse flies inhabit rural areas, living in the woodland and thickets of the savannah and the dense vegetation along streams. Infection of international travelers is rare. Approximately 1 case per year is reported among U.S. travelers. Most of these infections are caused by *T. b. rhodesiense* and they are acquired in East African game parks. Travelers visiting game parks and remote areas should be advised to take precautions. Travelers to urban areas are not at risk.

CLINICAL PRESENTATION

Signs and symptoms are initially nonspecific (fever, skin lesions, rash, edema, or lymphadenopathy); however, the infection progresses to meningoencephalitis. Symptoms generally appear within 1 to 3 weeks of infection. East African trypanosomiasis is more acute clinically, with earlier central nervous system involvement than in the West African form of the disease. Untreated cases are eventually fatal.

PREVENTION

No vaccine is available to prevent this disease. Tsetse flies are attracted to moving vehicles and dark, contrasting colors. They are not affected by insect repellents and can bite through lightweight clothing. Areas of heavy infestation tend to be sporadically distributed and are usually well known to local residents. Avoidance of such areas is the best means of protection. Travelers at risk should be advised to wear clothing of wrist and ankle length that is made of medium-weight fabric in neutral colors that blend with the background environment.

TREATMENT

Travelers who sustain tsetse fly bites and become ill with high fever or other manifestations of African trypanosomiasis should be advised to seek early medical attention. The infection can usually be cured by an appropriate course of anti-trypanosomal therapy. The drug of choice for treatment of East African trypanosomiasis is suramin (for the hemolymphatic stage) or melarsoprol (for late disease with central nervous system involvement). These drugs are available under an Investigational New Drug protocol from the CDC Drug Service. West African trypanosomiasis is best treated with pentamidine isethionate (for the hemolymphatic stage) or eflornithine. Travelers should be advised to consult an infectious disease or tropical medicine specialist.

Bibliography

Lejon V, Boelaert M, Jannin J, et al. Diagnosis of imported sleeping sickness. Lancet Infect Dis. 2003;3:804–8.

Moore A. Human African trypanosomiasis: a reemerging public health threat. In: Scheld WM, Murray BE, Hughes J, editors. Emerging Infections VI. Washington, DC: ASM Press; 2004. p. 143–57.

Moore A, Ryan ET, Waldron MA. A 37-year-old man with fever, hepatosplenomegaly, and a cutaneous foot lesion after a trip to Africa. N Engl J Med. 2002;346:2069–6.

Moore DAJ, Edwards M, Escombe R, et al. African trypanosomiasis in travelers returning to the United Kingdom. Emerg Infect Dis. 2002;8:74–6.

Sinha A, Grace C, Alston WK, et al. African trypanosomiasis in two travelers from the United States. Clin Infect Dis. 1999;29:840–4.

Van Nieuwenhove S. Present strategies in the treatment of human African trypanosomiasis. In: Dumas M, Bouteille B, Buguet A, editors. Progress in human African trypanosomiasis, sleeping sickness. Paris: Springer Verlag; 1999. p. 253–80.

–ANNE MOORE

>>Amebiasis

DESCRIPTION

Amebiasis is caused by the protozoan parasite *Entamoeba histolytica*. Infection is acquired by the fecal-oral route, either by person-to-person contact or indirectly by eating or drinking fecally contaminated food or water.

OCCURRENCE

Amebiasis occurs worldwide, especially in regions with poor sanitation. *E. histolytica* antibody prevalence rates (reflecting past or recent infection), commonly range from 6% to 25% in developing countries, but may exceed 50% in some communities.

RISK FOR TRAVELERS

For travelers to developing countries, risk for infection is highest for those who live in or visit rural areas, spend time in backcountry areas, or eat or drink in settings of poor sanitation.

CLINICAL PRESENTATION

The incubation period is commonly 2–4 weeks but ranges from a few days to years. The clinical spectrum of intestinal amebiasis ranges from asymptomatic infection to fulminant colitis and peritonitis. The parasite initially infects the colon, but it occasionally may spread to other organs, most commonly the liver (amebic liver abscess). In persons infected with *E. histolytica* who are symptomatic, the most common symptom is diarrhea. The diarrhea can worsen to painful, bloody bowel movements, with or without fever (amebic dysentery). *Entamoeba dispar,* a nonpathogenic amoeba that also inhabits the colon, cannot be distinguished from the pathogen *E. histolytica* by routine microscopy; however, an enzyme immunoassay kit for distinguishing the two organisms in fresh stool specimens is commercially but not widely available. Similarly, polymerase chain reaction (PCR)-based diagnostic tests have been developed but are not widely available.

PREVENTION

No vaccine is available. Travelers to developing countries should be advised to follow the precautions detailed in the section *Risks from Food and Water* in Chapter 2 and avoid sexual practices that may lead to fecal-oral transmission.

TREATMENT

Travelers may be advised to consult with an infectious disease specialist to ensure proper diagnosis and treatment. Iodoquinol or paromomycin are the drugs of choice for asymptomatic but proven *E. histolytica* infections. For mild or moderate to severe intestinal disease and extraintestinal disease (e.g., hepatic abscess), treatment with metronidazole or tinidazole should be immediately followed by treatment with paromomycin or iodoquinol. *E. dispar* infection does not require treatment.

Bibliography

Ravdin JI, editor. Amebiasis. Human infection by *Entamoeba histolytica.* New York: John Wiley & Sons; 1988.

Ravdin JI. *Entamoeba histolytica* (amebiasis). In: Mandell GL, Bennett JE, Dolin R, editors. Mandell, Douglas and Bennett's principles and practice of infectious diseases. 5th ed. Philadelphia, PA: Churchill Livingstone; 2000. p. 2798–810.

Sanuki JT, Asai E, Okuzawa S, et al. Identification of *Entamoeba histolytica* and *E. dispar* cysts in stool by polymerase chain reaction. Parasitol Res. 1997;83:96–8.

Tanyuksel M, Petri WA Jr. Laboratory diagnosis of amebiasis. Clin Microbiol Rev. 2003;16:713–29.

Verweij JJ, Blotkamp J, Brienen A, et al. Differentiation of *Entamoeba histolytica* and *Entamoeba dispar* cysts using polymerase chain reaction on DNA isolated from faeces with spin columns. Eur J Clin Microbiol Infect Dis. 2000;19:358–61.

—DENNIS JURANEK

>>American Trypanosomiasis (Chagas' Disease)

DESCRIPTION

Chagas' disease is caused by the protozoan parasite *Trypanosoma cruzi*. Chagas' disease is usually transmitted by contact with the feces of an infected triatomine ("cone nose" or "kissing") bug. Transmission can also occur through blood transfusion and organ transplantation and congenitally through passage of parasites across the placenta.

OCCURRENCE

Chagas' disease occurs in Mexico, Central America, and South America; acquisition of infection in the United States is rare. An estimated 11 million people are infected worldwide; of these, 15%–30% have clinical symptoms.

RISK FOR TRAVELERS

Travelers rarely acquire Chagas' disease. Triatomine bugs typically infest poor-quality buildings constructed of mud, adobe brick, or palm thatch, particularly those with cracks or crevices in the walls and roof. Because the bugs primarily feed at night, travelers can greatly reduce their risk for acquiring infection by avoiding overnight stays in such dwellings and by not camping or sleeping outdoors in endemic areas. Travelers should be aware that blood products might not be routinely or adequately tested for *T. cruzi* prior to transfusion.

CLINICAL PRESENTATION

Acute infection is usually asymptomatic but may be accompanied by local swelling at the site of inoculation, fever, and in 5%–10% of cases, meningoencephalitis, myocarditis or both. An asymptomatic phase follows the acute infection and lasts for life in 70%-80% of cases. Cardiomyopathy and/or intestinal "mega" syndromes (e.g., megaesophagus and megacolon) develop in the rest of infected persons 10-40 years after infection.

PREVENTION

No vaccine is available. Preventive measures include insecticide spraying of infested houses. Insecticide-impregnated bed nets may reduce the risk of infection for travelers who cannot avoid camping or sleeping outdoors or in poorly constructed houses in endemic areas.

TREATMENT

Treatment is recommended for all cases of acute infection, congenital infection, and reactivated infection in immunocompromised patients. Treatment of chronically infected persons (especially children) may eliminate parasites in up to 60% of cases. The drugs of choice are nifurtimox (under an Investigational New Drug protocol from the CDC Drug Service) or benznidazole (not available in the United States). Travelers should be advised to consult an infectious disease or tropical medicine specialist. Persons with chronic cardiac or gastrointestinal disease may benefit from symptomatic therapy.

Bibliography

Barrett MP, Burchmore RJS, Stich A, et al. The trypanosomiases. Lancet. 2003;362:1469–80.

Dias JCP, Silveira AC, Schofield CJ. The impact of Chagas' disease control in Latin America: a review. Mem Inst Oswaldo Cruz. 2002;97:603–12.

Miles, M. American trypanosomiasis (Chagas' disease). In: Cook GC, Zumla A, editors. Manson's tropical disease. 21st ed. London: Elsevier Science; 2003. p. 1325–37.

Miles MA, Feliciangeli MD, de Arias AR. American trypanosomiasis (Chagas' disease) and the role of molecular epidemiology in guiding control strategies. BMJ. 2003;326:1444–8.

Prata A. Clinical and epidemiological aspects of Chagas' disease. Lancet Infect Dis. 2001;1:92–100.

Tyler KM, Miles MA, editors. World class parasites. Volume 7: American trypanosomiasis. Boston: Kluwer Academics; 2003.

WHO Expert Committee. Control of Chagas' disease. World Health Organ Tech Rep Ser. 2002;905:1–109.

–JAMES H. MAGUIRE, BARBARA HERWALDT, AND NATASHA HOCHBERG

>>Bovine Spongiform Encephalopathy and Variant Creutzfeldt-Jakob Disease

DESCRIPTION

Since 1996, strong evidence has accumulated for a causal relationship between ongoing outbreaks in Europe of a disease in cattle called bovine spongiform encephalopathy (BSE, or "mad cow disease") and a disease in humans called variant Creutzfeldt-Jakob disease (vCJD). Both disorders, which are caused by an unconventional transmissible agent, are invariably fatal brain diseases with incubation periods typically measured in years. Transmission of the BSE agent to humans, leading to vCJD, is believed to occur via ingestion of cattle products contaminated with the BSE agent; however, the specific foods associated with this transmission are unknown. Bioassays have identified the BSE agent in the brain, spinal cord, retina, dorsal root ganglia, distal ileum, and bone marrow of cattle experimentally infected by the oral route, suggesting that these tissues represent the highest risk of transmission.

OCCURRENCE

From 1995 through August 2004, 147 human cases of vCJD were reported in the United Kingdom (UK), 7 in France, and 1 each in

Canada, Ireland, Italy, and the United States. The patients from Canada, Ireland, and the United States had lived in the UK during a key exposure period of the UK population to the BSE agent. By year of onset, the incidence of vCJD in the UK appears to have peaked in 1999 and to have been declining thereafter. However, the future pattern of this epidemic remains uncertain.

From 1986 through 2001, >98% of BSE cases worldwide were reported from the UK, where the disease was first described. During this same period, the number of European countries reporting at least one indigenous BSE case increased from 4 to18 through 2001. During 2001–2003, three countries outside Europe (Canada, Japan, and Israel) reported their first indigenous BSE cases, and others followed.

The reported BSE incidence rates, by country and year, are available on the Internet website of the Office International des Epizooties and new information is being generated on a regular basis. (http://www.oie.int/ eng/info/en_esbincidence.htm.).

The identification in 2003 of a BSE case in Canada, and the subsequent identification later that year of a BSE case in the United States that had been imported from Canada led to the concern that indigenous transmission of BSE may be occurring in North America. Safeguards to minimize the risk for human exposure to BSE have been implemented in the United States by the Department of Agriculture (http://aphis.usda. gov/lpa/issues/bse_testing/plan.html). Transfusion of blood contaminated with the vCJD agent is believed responsible for a few cases of disease in the UK. This prompted the US Food and Drug Administration to publish guidance outlining a geography-based donor deferral policy to reduce the risk of bloodborne transmission of vCJD in the United States. This guidance document included an appendix that listed European countries with BSE or a possible increased risk of BSE for use in determining blood donor deferrals. One deferral criterion was living cumulatively for 5 or more years in continental Europe from 1980 to the present (http://www.aphis.usda.gov/NCIE/country.html#BSE).

RISK FOR TRAVELERS

The current risk of acquiring vCJD from eating beef (muscle meat) and beef products produced from cattle in countries with at least a possibly increased risk of BSE cannot be determined precisely. Nevertheless, in the UK, the current risk of acquiring vCJD from eating beef and beef products appears to be extremely small, perhaps about 1 case per 10 billion servings. In the other countries of the world, this current risk, if it exists at all, would not likely be any higher than that in the UK if BSE-related, public health control measures are being well implemented. Among many uncertainties affecting this determination are the incubation period between exposure to the infective agent and onset of illness, the sensitivities of each country's surveillance for BSE and vCJD, the compliance with and effectiveness of public health measures instituted in each country to prevent BSE contamination of human food, and details about cattle products from one country distributed and consumed elsewhere. Despite the exceedingly low risk, the US blood donor deferral criteria in effect as of September 2004 focus on the time (cumulatively 3 months or more) that a person lived in the UK from 1980 through 1996, whereas for the rest of Europe the criteria focus on the time (cumulatively 5 years or more) that a person lived in these countries from 1980 through the present.

PREVENTION

Public health control measures, such as surveillance, culling sick animals, or banning specified risk materials, have been instituted in many countries, particularly in those with indigenous cases of confirmed BSE, in order to prevent potentially BSE-infected tissues from entering the human food supply. The most stringent of these control measures, including a program that excludes all animals >30 months of age from the human food and animal feed supplies, have been applied in the UK and appear to be highly effective. In June 2000, the European Union Commission on Food Safety and Animal Welfare strengthened the European Union's BSE control measures by requiring all member states to remove specified risk materials from animal feed and human food chains as of October 1, 2000; such bans had already been instituted in most member states.

To reduce any risk of acquiring vCJD from food, travelers to Europe or other areas with indigenous cases of BSE may consider either avoiding beef and beef products altogether or selecting beef or beef products, such as solid pieces of muscle meat (rather than brains or beef products like burgers and sausages), that might have a reduced opportunity for contamination with tissues that may harbor the BSE agent. These measures, however, should be taken with the knowledge of the very low risk of transmission as defined above. Milk and milk products from cows are not believed to pose any risk for transmitting the BSE agent.

TREATMENT

As of September 2004, treatment of prion diseases remains supportive; no specific therapy has been shown to stop the progression of these diseases.

Bibliography

Belay ED, Schonberger LB. The public health impact of prion diseases. Annu Rev Public Health 2005; 26:in press.

Centers for Disease Control and Prevention. Bovine spongiform encephalopathy in a dairy cow — Washington State, 2003. MMWR 2003;52:1280–1285.

Llewelyn CA, Hewitt PE, Knight RSG, et al. Possible transmission of variant Creutzfeldt-Jakob disease by blood transfusion. Lancet 2004;363:417–421.

Peden AH, Head MW, Ritchie DL, et al. Preclinical vCJD after blood transfusion in a PRNP codon 129 heterozygous patient. Lancet 2004;264:527–529.

Will RG, Alpers MP, Dormont D, Schonberger LB. Infectious and sporadic prion diseases. In: Prusiner SB, ed. Prion Biology and Diseases, 2nd Ed., Cold Spring Harbor Laboratory Press, Cold Spring Harbor, New York, 2004: 629–671.

–LAWRENCE B. SCHONBERGER, ERMIAS D. BELAY, AND JAMES J. SEJVAR

>>Cholera

DESCRIPTION

Cholera is an acute intestinal infection caused by toxigenic *Vibrio cholerae* O-group 1 or O-group 139. The infection is often mild and self limited or subclinical. Patients with severe cases respond dramatically to simple fluid- and electrolyte-replacement therapy. Infection is acquired primarily by ingesting contaminated water or food; person-to-person transmission is rare.

OCCURRENCE

Since 1961, *V. cholerae* has spread from Indonesia through most of Asia into Eastern Europe and Africa, and from North Africa to the Iberian Peninsula. In 1991, an extensive epidemic began in Peru and spread to neighboring countries in the Western Hemisphere. In 2003, 111,575 cases from 45 countries were reported to the WHO.

RISK FOR TRAVELERS

Travelers who follow usual tourist itineraries and who observe food safety recommendations while in countries reporting cholera have virtually no risk. Risk increases for those who drink untreated water or eat poorly cooked or raw seafood in disease-endemic areas.

PREVENTION

Vaccine

The risk of cholera to U.S. travelers is so low that vaccination is of questionable benefit. The manufacture and sale of the only cholera vaccine licensed in the United States (by Wyeth Ayerst) have been discontinued. The vaccine is not recommended for travelers because of the brief and incomplete immunity it confers.

Two recently developed oral vaccines for cholera are licensed and available in other countries (Dukoral from Biotec AB and Mutacol from Berna). Both vaccines appear to provide somewhat better immunity and have fewer adverse effects than the previously available vaccine. However, CDC does not recommend either of these two vaccines for most travelers, nor are they available in the United States. Further information on these vaccines can be obtained from the manufacturers: Dukoral, Active Biotec AB, P.O. Box 724, SE-220 07, Lund, Sweden; telephone: 46 46 19 20 00; fax: 46 46 19 20 50; e-mail: info@activebiotech.com; and website: http://www.activebiotech.com; and Mutacol, Berna, Switzerland Division, P.O. Box CH-3001, Bern, Switzerland; telephone: 41 31 981 22 11; fax: 41 31 981 20 66. E-mail information is available at http://www.bernaproducts.com/contact.cfm and from the website http://www.bernaproducts.com.

Currently, no country or territory requires vaccination against cholera as a condition for entry. Local authorities, however, may continue to require documentation of this vaccination. In such cases, a single dose of either oral vaccine is sufficient to satisfy local requirements, or the traveler may request a medical waiver from a physician.

Other

Travelers to cholera-affected areas should be advised to avoid eating high-risk foods, especially fish and shellfish. Food that is cooked and served hot, fruits and vegetables peeled by the traveler personally, beverages and ice that are made from boiled or chlorinated water, or carbonated beverages are usually safe. (See *Risks from Food and Water*, for additional information.) Chemoprophylaxis is almost never indicated.

TREATMENT

Rehydration is the cornerstone of therapy for cholera; antibiotics are an adjunct useful in severe cases only. Oral rehydration salts, and when necessary intravenous fluids and electrolytes, if administered in a timely manner and in adequate volumes, will reduce case-fatality rates to well under 1%.

Bibliography

Cholera, 2003. Weekly Epidemiologic Record. 2004;31:281-8.

Steinberg EB, Greene KD, Bopp CA, Cameron DN, Wells JG, Mintz ED. Cholera in the United States, 1995-2000: trends at the end of the milennium. J Infect Dis. 2001;184:799–802.

World Health Organization. Guidelines for cholera control. Geneva, Switzerland: World Health Organization; 1993.

–ERIC MINTZ

>>Coccidioidomycosis

DESCRIPTION

Coccidioidomycosis or "Valley fever," is a disease caused by the fungus *Coccidioides immitis,* found in the soil of disease-endemic areas. The disease is acquired by inhalation of fungal spores from dust, usually generated by human activities or natural disasters.

OCCURRENCE

Coccidioides immitis is endemic in regions in the Americas characterized by an arid climate, yearly rainfall 5–20 inches, hot summers, winters with few freezes, and alkaline soils. In the United States, this fungus is found in Arizona, Southern California, New Mexico, western Texas, and parts of Utah. Outside the United States, coccidioidomycosis is endemic in parts of Argentina, Brazil, Colombia, Guatemala, Honduras, Mexico, Nicaragua, Paraguay, and Venezuela.

RISK FOR TRAVELERS

In disease-endemic areas, persons can be at increased risk for disease if they participate in or are present during activities that disturb the ground, resulting in exposure to dust. These outdoor activities include construction, landscaping, mining, agriculture, archaeologic excavation, military maneuvers, and recreational pursuits such as dirt biking. Natural events such as earthquakes or windstorms that result in generation of dust clouds in disease-endemic areas increase the risk of infection among exposed persons. Coccidioidomycosis is not transmitted from person to person.

CLINICAL PRESENTATION

The incubation period ranges from 7 to 21 days. Most infections (60%) are asymptomatic. Persons who have symptoms usually have a self-limited influenza-like illness characterized by fever, headache, rash, muscle aches, dry cough, weight loss, and malaise. In rare instances, severe lung disease (e.g., cavitary pneumonia) or dissemination to the central nervous system (e.g., meninges), joints, bones, and skin may develop. Persons at increased risk for severe pulmonary disease are the elderly and those with chronic medical conditions such as congestive heart failure, diabetes, chronic obstructive pulmonary disease, cancer, and corticosteroid use. Persons at increased risk for disseminated disease include African-Americans and Filipinos, those with immunocompromising conditions (e.g., HIV), and pregnant women. Once infected with *C. immitis,* a person is immune to reinfection.

PREVENTION

Although complete prevention of infection is not possible, travelers, especially those at increased risk for severe and disseminated disease, can decrease their risk by limiting their exposure to outdoor dust in disease-endemic areas. Dust-control measures include wetting soil before disturbing the earth or using outdoor vehicles with enclosed, air-conditioned cabs. Persons should also be advised to avoid transporting items contaminated with soil (e.g., cotton or straw) from disease-endemic areas, because infections have been reported among persons who had never visited the areas but were exposed to such fomites. Wearing well-fitted dust masks capable of filtering particles as small as 0.4 µm can provide added protection for those at high risk for exposure to dust from disease-endemic areas or those at high risk for severe or disseminated disease. No effective vaccine for coccidioidomycosis is currently available.

TREATMENT

Most persons with acute symptomatic coccidioidomycosis do not require treatment because the illness is self-limited. Persons at increased risk for dissemination may need to receive antifungal therapy when diagnosed with acute coccidioidomycosis. All persons with disseminated disease should receive antifungal treatment. Amphotericin B should be used for severe disease and pregnant women, and the family of drugs that includes ketoconazole, fluconazole or itraconazole should be used for milder disease or for prolonged treatments. Recommended duration of therapy ranges from 3 to 6 months in those with uncomplicated respiratory infection to lifelong treatment in those with meningitis. An infectious diseases specialist should manage these patients.

Bibliography

Chiller TM, Galgiani JN, Stevens DA. Coccidioidomycosis. Infect Dis Clin North Am. 2003;17:41–57.

Fisher FS, Bultman MW, Pappagianis D. Operational guidelines for geological fieldwork in areas endemic for coccidioidomycosis (Valley fever). Reston, VA: US Geological Survey Open-File Report. 2000:1–16.

Galgiani JN, Ampel NM, Catanzaro A, et al. Practice guideline for the treatment of coccidioidomycosis. Infectious Diseases Society of America. Clin Infect Dis. 2000;30:658–61.

Panackal AA, Hajjeh RA, Cetron MS, et al. Fungal infections among returning travelers. Clin Infect Dis. 2002;35:1088–95.

–JULIETTE MORGAN

>>Cryptosporidiosis

DESCRIPTION

Cryptosporidiosis is a parasitic infection caused by *Cryptosporidium parvum* and occasionally other species of *Cryptosporidium*. It is transmitted by ingestion of fecally contaminated food or water, including water swallowed while swimming; by exposure to fecally contaminated environmental surfaces; and by the fecal-oral route from person to person (e.g., while changing diapers, caring for an infected person, or engaging in certain sexual behaviors).

OCCURRENCE

Cryptosporidiosis occurs worldwide.

RISK FOR TRAVELERS

For travelers to developing countries, risk of infection is highest for those with the greatest exposure to potentially contaminated food or water.

CLINICAL PRESENTATION

Symptoms include watery diarrhea, abdominal cramps, vomiting, and fever. In immune competent persons, symptoms last an average of 6–10 days but can last up to several weeks. In persons with severely weakened immune systems, cryptosporidiosis can become chronic and can be fatal.

PREVENTION

No vaccine is available. To avoid contracting cryptosporidiosis, travelers should be advised to follow the precautions described in the section *Risks from Food and Drink*. Cryptosporidiosis is poorly inactivated by chlorine or iodine disinfection. Water can be treated effectively by boiling or filtration with an absolute 1-micron filter. Specific information on preventing cryptosporidiosis through filtration can be found in "Preventing Cryptosporidiosis: A Guide to Water Filters and Bottled Water" at http://www.cdc.gov/ncidod/dpd/parasites/cryptosporidiosis/factsht_crypto_prevent_water.htm.

TREATMENT

The FDA has approved nitaxozanide suspension (Alinia, Romark Laboratories) for treatment of cryptosporidiosis and giardiasis in children and nitaxozanide tablets for treatment of giardiasis in adults. Nitazoxanide tablets are a potentially useful treatment for immunocompetent adults with cryptosporidiosis.

Bibliography

Bailey JM, Erramouspe J. Nitazoxanide treatment for giardiasis and cryptosporidiosis in children. Ann Pharmacother. 2004;38:634–40.

Guerrant RL. Cryptosporidiosis: an emerging, highly infectious threat. Emerg Infect Dis. 1997;3:51–7.

Kosek M, Alcantara C, Lima AA, et al. Cryptosporidiosis: an update. Lancet Infect Dis. 2001;1:262–9.

Roy SL, DeLong SM, Stenzel SA, et al. Risk factors for sporadic cryptosporidiosis among immunocompetent persons in the United States from 1999 to 2001. J Clin Microbiol. 2004;42:2944–51.

Taylor DN, Connor BA, Shlim DR. Chronic diarrhea in the returned traveler. Med Clin North Am. 1999;83:1033–52.

Thielman NM, Guerrant RL. Persistent diarrhea in the returned traveler. Infect Dis Clin North Am. 1998;12:489–501.

Nitazoxanide (Alinia)—a new anti-protozoal agent. Med Lett Drugs Ther. 2003;45:29–31.

—CARYN BERN

>>Cyclosporiasis

DESCRIPTION

Cyclospora cayetanensis, previously known as cyanobacterium-like, coccidia-like, and cyclospora-like bodies, is a protozoan parasite that causes gastrointestinal infection.

OCCURRENCE

Infection can be acquired worldwide by persons of all ages by ingestion of water or food contaminated with the parasite. Outbreaks in North America have been linked to various types of imported fresh produce. Usually the symptoms of infection begin about 1 week after the exposure.

RISK FOR TRAVELERS

Travelers to developing countries can be at increased risk for this infection, and the risk can vary with the season. Which season is of greatest risk varies by country; for example, in Nepal, risk of infection is greater in the summer and the rainy season.

CLINICAL PRESENTATION

Infection can be asymptomatic or manifested by such symptoms as watery diarrhea, loss of appetite, substantial weight loss, bloating, increased gas, stomach cramps, nausea, vomiting, prolonged fatigue, muscle aches, and low-grade fever. Some travelers first notice influenza-like symptoms. If untreated, the illness can last for weeks to months, and the symptoms can come and go.

PREVENTION

No vaccine is available. Travelers to resource-poor countries should be advised to follow the precautions in the *Risks from Food and Drink* section. Direct, person-to-person transmission is unlikely because the parasite is not immediately infectious when excreted.

TREATMENT

The treatment of choice is trimethoprim-sulfamethoxazole. Travelers may also be advised to consult with an infectious disease specialist. Physicians may consult CDC about patients who are allergic to or intolerant of sulfa-containing medications. For more information, see the Division of Parasitic Diseases' website at http://www.cdc.gov/ncidod/dpd/parasites/cyclospora/factsht_cyclospora.htm and http://www.cdc.gov/ncidod/dpd/parasites/cyclospora/healthcare_cyclospora.htm.

Bibliography

Herwaldt BL. *Cyclospora cayetanensis:* a review, focusing on the outbreaks of cyclosporiasis in the 1990s. Clin Infect Dis 2000;31:1040–57.

Hoge CW, et al. Placebo-controlled trial of co-trimoxazole for *Cyclospora* infections among travellers and foreign residents in Nepal. Lancet 1995;345:691–3.

Ortega YR, Shlim DL, Ghimire M, et al. *Cyclospora* species — a new protozoan pathogen of humans. N Engl J Med 1993;328:1308–12.

–BARBARA HERWALDT

>>Dengue

DESCRIPTION

Dengue fever and dengue hemorrhagic fever (DHF) are viral diseases transmitted by *Aedes* mosquitoes, usually *Ae. aegypti.* The four dengue viruses (DEN-1 through DEN-4) are immunologically related, but do not provide cross-protective immunity against each other.

OCCURRENCE

Dengue, a rapidly expanding disease in most tropical and subtropical areas of the world, has become the most important arboviral disease of humans. More than 2.5 billion persons now live in areas at risk of infection, and attack rates for reported disease in epidemics are in the range of 1 per thousand to 1 per hundred of the population. Infection rates (that is, proportion of the population that is infected, including persons who do not get severe symptoms or are not reported) can be five- to ten-fold greater. The case-fatality ratio for DHF averages about 5% worldwide, but can be kept below 1% with proper clinical management. Epidemics caused by all four virus serotypes have become progressively more frequent and larger in the past 25 years. As of 2004, dengue fever is endemic in most tropical countries of the South Pacific, Asia, the Caribbean, the Americas, and Africa (see Maps 4–1 and 4–2). Additionally, most tropical urban centers in these regions have multiple dengue virus serotypes co-circulating (hyperendemicity), which increases dengue transmission and the risk of DHF. Future dengue incidence in specific locales cannot be predicted accurately, but a high level of dengue transmission is anticipated in all tropical areas of the world for the indefinite future. The incidence of the severe disease, DHF, has increased dramatically in Southeast Asia, the South Pacific, and the American tropics in the past 25 years, with major epidemics occurring in many countries every 3–5 years. The first major epidemic in the Americas occurred in Cuba in 1981, and a second major epidemic of DHF occurred in Venezuela in 1989–1990. Since then, outbreaks, sporadic cases, or both, of confirmed DHF have occurred in most tropical American countries. After an absence of 35 years, several autochthonous cases of dengue fever occurred in southern Texas in 1980, 1986, 1995, 1997, 1998 and 1999, associated with imported cases and epidemic dengue in adjacent states in Mexico. After an absence of 56 years, a limited outbreak of dengue fever occurred in Hawaii in 2001, associated with imported cases and epidemic dengue in the South Pacific.

RISK FOR TRAVELERS

The principal vector mosquito, *Ae. aegypti*, is most frequently found in or near human habitations and prefers to feed on humans during the daytime. It has two peak periods of biting activity: in the morning for several hours after daybreak and in the late afternoon for several hours before dark. The mosquito may feed at any time during the day, however, especially indoors, in shady areas, or when it is overcast. Mosquito breeding sites include artificial water containers such as discarded tires, uncovered barrels, buckets, flower vases or pots, cans, and cisterns.

Estimates derived from studies of military and relief workers allow for an estimate of risk near one illness per thousand travelers. This estimate may overstate the danger for tourists who will have less contact with the vector, who stay only a few days in air-conditioned hotels with well-kept grounds, and who participate in outdoor recreational activities where the vector mosquito may be absent (such as sunbathing or playing golf in the middle of the day). Travelers who stay at other types of accommodations

MAP 4-1. DISTRIBUTION OF DENGUE, WESTERN HEMISPHERE

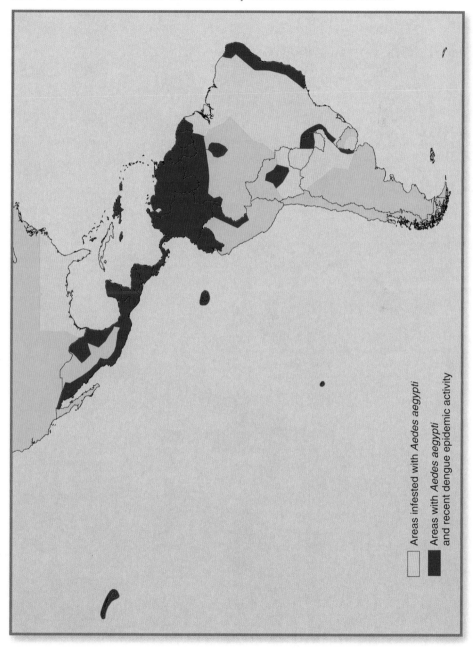

Areas infested with *Aedes aegypti*

Areas with *Aedes aegypti* and recent dengue epidemic activity

MAP 4-2. DISTRIBUTION OF DENGUE, EASTERN HEMISPHERE

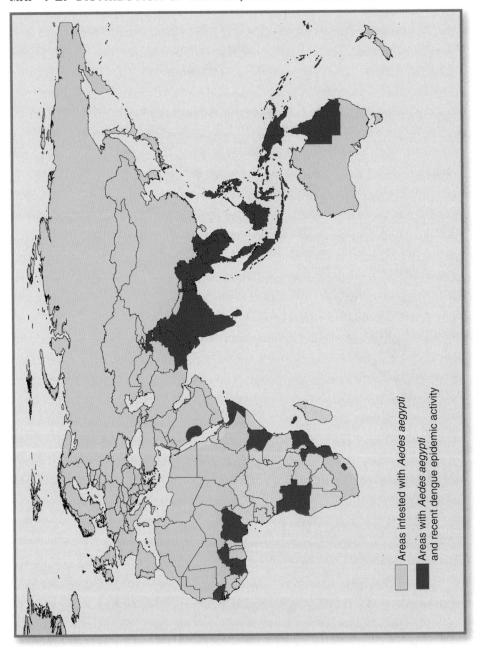

Areas infested with *Aedes aegypti*

Areas with *Aedes aegypti* and recent dengue epidemic activity

or with friends and relatives in locations with intense disease transmission may have a higher risk of illness. Cases of dengue are confirmed every year in travelers returning to the United States after visits to tropical and subtropical areas. Travelers to endemic and epidemic areas, therefore, should take precautions to avoid mosquito bites.

Current data suggest that virus strain, the immune status (i.e., having had a previous dengue infection), age, and genetic background of the human host are the most important risk factors for developing DHF. In Asia, where a high proportion of the population has experienced a dengue infection early in life, DHF is observed most commonly in infants and children <15 years of age who are experiencing a second dengue infection. In the Americas and the Pacific, where herd immunity is lower, DHF is more commonly observed in older children and adults. International travelers from nonendemic areas (such as the United States) are generally at low risk for DHF.

There is little information in published reports about the consequences of dengue infection for pregnant women. In spite of many epidemics, no increase in congenital malformations has been noted after dengue epidemics. A small number of recently reported cases suggests that if the mother is ill with dengue at the time of delivery, the child can be born with dengue infection or can acquire dengue through the delivery process itself, and then develop the manifestations of dengue fever or DHF.

CLINICAL PRESENTATION

Dengue fever is characterized by sudden onset after an incubation period of 3–14 days (most commonly 4–7 days), high fevers, severe frontal headache, and joint and muscle pain. Many patients have nausea, vomiting, and rash. The rash appears 3–5 days after onset of fever and can spread from the torso to the arms, legs, and face. The disease is usually self-limited, although convalescence can be prolonged. Many cases of nonspecific viral syndrome or even subclinical infection occur, but dengue can also present as a severe, sometimes fatal disease characterized by hemorrhagic manifestations and hypotension (DHF/dengue shock syndrome).

Physicians should consider dengue in the differential diagnosis of all patients who have fever and a history of travel to a tropical area within

2 weeks of onset of symptoms. Commercial tests are available for serologic diagnosis, but their results must be interpreted with care. Sensitivity and specificity of kits may vary among manufacturers, laboratories, and over time. IgM positivity indicates a recent dengue infection, but IgG positivity may only indicate infection at an indeterminate time in the past. In addition, either IgM or IgG positivity may result from cross-reactivity with anti-West Nile, yellow fever, Japanese encephalitis, and other flavivirus antibodies, so the possibility of exposure to other flaviviruses must be considered. If testing at CDC is requested, acute- and convalescent-phase serum samples should be obtained and sent through state or territorial health department laboratories to CDC's Dengue Branch, Division of Vector-Borne Infectious Diseases (DVBID), National Center for Infectious Diseases, 1324 Calle Cañada, San Juan, Puerto Rico 00920-3860. Serum samples should be accompanied by clinical and epidemiologic information, including the date of disease onset, the date of collection of the sample, and a detailed recent travel history. For additional information, the Dengue Branch can be contacted at telephone 1-787-706-2399; fax 1-787-706-2496; e-mail hseda@cdc.gov; or the DVBID website at http://www.cdc.gov/ncidod/ dvbid/dengue/index.htm.

PREVENTION

No vaccine is available. Travelers should be advised that they can reduce their risk of acquiring dengue by remaining in well-screened or air-conditioned areas when possible, wearing clothing that adequately covers the arms and legs, and applying insect repellent to both skin and clothing. The most effective repellents are those containing N,N-diethylmetatoluamide (DEET). (See *Protection against Mosquitoes and Other Arthropods.*)

TREATMENT

Acetaminophen products are recommended for managing fever. Acetylsalicyclic acid (aspirin) and nonsteroidal anti-inflammatory agents (such as ibuprofen) should be avoided because of their anticoagulant properties. Patients should be encouraged to rest and take abundant fluids. In severe cases, the prompt infusion of intravenous fluids is necessary to maintain adequate blood pressure. Because shock may develop suddenly, vital signs must be monitored frequently. Hypotension is a more frequent complication of DHF than severe hemorrhage.

Bibliography

CDC. Imported dengue —United States, 1999 and 2000. MMWR Morbid Mortal Wkly Rep 2002; 5:281–3.

Ellerin T, Hurtado R, Lockman S, Baden L. Fever in a returned traveler: an "off the cuff" diagnosis. Clin Infect Dis 2003; 36:1004–5, 10-74–75.

García-Rivera EJ, Rigau-Pérez JG. Dengue severity in the elderly in Puerto Rico. Rev Panam Salud Pública/ Pan Am J Public Health 2003; 13:362–8.

Gubler DJ. Cities spawn epidemic dengue viruses. Nature Med 2004; 10:129–30.

Harris E, Pérez L, Phares CR, Pérez MA, Idiaquez W, Rocha J, et al. Fluid intake and decreased risk of hospitalization. Emerg Infect Dis 2003; 9:1003–6.

Kroeger A, Nathan M, Hombach J. Disease Watch: Dengue — Nature Reviews. Microbiology 2004; 2:360–1.

Rigau-Pérez JG, Gubler DJ, Vorndam AV, Clark GG. Dengue: A literature review and case study of travelers from the United States, 1986-1994. J Travel Med 1997; 4:65–71.

–JOSÉ G. RIGAU-PÉREZ, DUANE J. GUBLER, AND GARY G. CLARK

>>Diphtheria, Tetanus, and Pertussis

DESCRIPTION

Diphtheria is an acute bacterial disease caused by toxigenic strains of *Corynebacterium diphtheriae* and occasionally *C. ulcerans.* It is transmitted through respiratory droplets and personal contact. Diphtheria affects the mucous membranes of the respiratory tract (respiratory diphtheria), the skin (cutaneous diphtheria), and occasionally other sites (eyes, nose, or vagina).

Tetanus, an acute disease caused by *Clostridium tetani,* is characterized by muscle rigidity and painful spasms, often starting in the muscles of the jaw and neck. Severe tetanus can lead to respiratory failure and death. The disease is caused by a neurotoxin produced by anaerobic tetanus bacilli growing in contaminated wounds. Lesions that are considered "tetanus prone" are wounds contaminated with dirt, feces or saliva, deep wounds, burns, crush injuries or those with necrotic tissue. However, tetanus has also been associated with apparently clean superficial wounds, surgical procedures, insect bites, dental infections, chronic sores and infections, and intravenous drug use. In 5%–10% of reported cases in the United States, no antecedent wound was identified.

Pertussis, caused by the bacterium *Bordetella pertussis,* is a highly communicable respiratory illness characterized by prolonged paroxysmal coughing. Persons in all age groups can be infected. Complications and deaths from pertussis are most common among unvaccinated infants.

OCCURRENCE

Diphtheria remains a serious disease throughout much of the world. In particular, large outbreaks of diphtheria occurred in the 1990s throughout Russia and the other former Soviet republics. Most life-threatening cases occurred in inadequately immunized persons. Travelers to disease-endemic areas are at increased risk for exposure to toxigenic strains of *C. diphtheriae*. Areas with known endemic diphtheria include *Africa –* Algeria, Egypt, and the countries in sub-Saharan region; *Americas –* Brazil, Colombia, Dominican Republic, Ecuador, Haiti and Paraguay; *Asia/South Pacific –* Afghanistan, Bangladesh, Bhutan, Cambodia, China, India, Indonesia, Laos, Mongolia, Burma (Myanmar), Nepal, Pakistan, Papua New Guinea, Philippines, Thailand, and Vietnam; *Middle East –* Iran, Iraq, Syria, Turkey, and Yemen; *Europe –* Albania and all countries of the former Soviet Union.

Tetanus is a global health problem because *C. tetani* spores are ubiquitous. The disease occurs almost exclusively in persons who are inadequately immunized. In developing countries, tetanus occurring in neonates born to unvaccinated mothers (neonatal tetanus) is the most common form of the disease.

B. pertussis circulation occurs worldwide, but disease rates are highest among young children in countries where vaccination coverage is low. In developed countries, severe disease is usually limited to unvaccinated infants. Immunity from childhood vaccination, as well as from natural disease, wanes with time so adolescents and adults can become infected or re-infected.

RISK FOR TRAVELERS

Diphtheria and pertussis are more frequent in parts of the world where vaccination levels are low. Tetanus can occur anywhere in the world in inadequately vaccinated persons.

CLINICAL PRESENTATION

Diphtheria

The incubation period is 2–5 days (range 1–10 days); symptom onset is typically gradual. Early symptoms of respiratory diphtheria include malaise, sore throat, loss of appetite, and a moderate fever (rarely >103° F). If the larynx is involved, persons may become hoarse and have a barking cough. Within 2–3 days, an adherent, gray membrane forms over the mucous membrane of the tonsils and/or pharynx. Attempts to remove the membrane cause bleeding. Extensive membrane formation may result in airway obstruction. In severe cases of respiratory diphtheria, there is cervical lymphadenopathy and a swollen neck ("bull-neck" appearance). Toxin absorbed from the respiratory tract can cause serious complications, including myocarditis and neuropathies. The case-fatality rate of respiratory diphtheria is 5%–10%. Cutaneous diphtheria is characterized by a scaling rash or chronic non-healing ulcers with a gray membrane. Cutaneous and nasal diphtheria are localized infections rarely associated with systemic toxicity.

Tetanus

There are three clinical syndromes associated with tetanus infection: 1) generalized, 2) localized, and 3) cephalic. Generalized tetanus is the most common form, accounting for more than 80% of cases. In generalized tetanus, the average incubation period between injury and symptom onset is 7–8 days (range 3 days–3 weeks). The most common initial sign is trismus (spasm of the muscles of mastication or "lockjaw"). Trismus may be followed by painful spasms in other muscle groups in the neck, trunk, and extremities and by generalized tonic tetanic seizure-like activity or frank convulsions in severe cases. Generalized tetanus can be accompanied by autonomic nervous system abnormalities, as well as a variety of complications related to severe spasm and prolonged hospitalization. Neonatal tetanus is generalized tetanus occurring in neonates, usually due to umbilical stump infections. The clinical course of generalized tetanus is variable and depends on the degree of prior immunity, the amount of toxin present, and the age and general health of the patient. Even with modern intensive care, generalized tetanus is associated with mortality rates of 10%–20%.

Localized tetanus is an unusual form of the disease consisting of spasm of muscles in a confined area close to the site of the injury. Although localized tetanus often occurs in persons with partial immunity and is usually mild, progression to generalized tetanus can occur. Cephalic tetanus is the rarest form of tetanus. It is associated with lesions of the head or face, and also has been described in association with ear infections (i.e., otitis media). The incubation period is short, usually 1–2 days. Unlike generalized and localized tetanus, cephalic tetanus results in flaccid cranial nerve palsies rather than spasm. Trismus may also be present. Like localized tetanus, cephalic tetanus can progress to the generalized form.

Pertussis
In classic disease, mild upper respiratory tract symptoms begin 7–10 days (range 6–21 days) after exposure, followed by development of a cough that becomes paroxysmal. Coughing paroxysms can be frequent or relatively infrequent and are often followed by vomiting. Fever is absent or minimal. Young infants may present with apnea before significant cough develops. In older infants and young children, an inspiratory whoop may be generated at the end of a coughing spell. Recently immunized children may have mild cough illness; older children and adults may have prolonged cough with or without paroxysms. The cough gradually wanes over several weeks to months. Serious complications are most common in young, unvaccinated infants and include apnea, seizures, pneumonia, weight loss, and rarely, death.

PREVENTION

Vaccine
Immunizations for Infants and Children <7 Years of Age
Simultaneous immunization against diphtheria, tetanus, and pertussis during infancy (see Tables 8–2 and 8–3) is recommended. Combination vaccines contain diphtheria and tetanus toxoids and either whole-cell

pertussis antigens (DTwP) or acellular pertussis antigens (DTaP). Neither DTwP nor DTaP pertussis vaccine is licensed for persons 7 or more years of age. DTwP vaccine is no longer available in the United States.

Three brands of DTaP currently are approved for use and are available in the United States. Whenever possible, the same brand of DTaP vaccine should be used for all doses of the vaccination series; however, any licensed DTaP vaccine may be used to continue or complete the vaccination series if the type of vaccine previously administered is not known or the type of vaccine used for earlier doses is not available.

Immunization for infants and children up to the seventh birthday consists of five doses of DTaP vaccine. The first three doses are usually given at ages 2, 4 and 6 months, the fourth dose at age 15–18 months, and the fifth dose at age 4–6 years. The fifth dose is not necessary if the fourth dose was given after the child's fourth birthday.

Three—and preferably four—doses of DTaP are necessary for protection against diphtheria, tetanus and pertussis. Travelers should be advised to complete as many doses as possible of the primary series before traveling. If an accelerated schedule is required to complete the series of DTaP vaccine, the schedule may be started as soon as the infant is 6 weeks of age, with the second and third doses given 4 weeks after each preceding dose (Table 8–3). The fourth dose should not be given before the child is age 12 months and should be separated from the third dose by at least 6 months. The fifth dose should not be given before the child is age 4 years. Interruption of the recommended schedule or delay in doses does not lead to a reduction in the level of immunity reached on completion of the primary series. There is no need to restart a series regardless of the time that has elapsed between doses. For infants and children age <7 years with a contraindication to the pertussis component of DTaP, diphtheria-tetanus (DT) should be used (Table 8–2).

Immunizations for Children 7 or More Years of Age, Adolescents, and Adults

Children ≥7 years of age, adolescents, and adults should receive the adult formulation of tetanus and diphtheria toxoids (Td) whenever either tetanus or diphtheria toxoid is indicated (Tables 8–2 and 8–3; no pertussis vaccine is licensed for use in adults). Anyone ≥7 years of age who has not received a primary series against tetanus and diphtheria should receive three doses of Td; the first two doses should be given 4–8 weeks apart and the third dose 6–12 months after the second. Two doses of Td received at intervals of at least 4 weeks can provide some protection, but a single dose is of little benefit. In the rare instance when administration of the third dose following a 6- to 12-month interval cannot be ensured, the third Td dose can be given 4–8 weeks after the second dose to complete the primary series. Anyone whose history of primary tetanus and diphtheria vaccination is uncertain should be considered unvaccinated and should receive the three-dose series. Anyone who has received only one or two prior doses of tetanus and diphtheria toxoids should receive additional doses to complete the three-dose series. The first booster dose of Td should be given when the child is 11 or 12 years of age if at least 5 years has elapsed since the last dose of DTaP or pediatric DT. Thereafter, routine booster doses of Td should be given every 10 years.

Adverse Reactions

Local reactions (erythema and induration with or without tenderness) are common after the administration of vaccines containing diphtheria, tetanus, and pertussis antigens. Mild systemic reactions such as fever, drowsiness, fretfulness, and low-grade fever can occur after vaccination with DTaP. These reactions are self-limited and can be managed with symptomatic treatment of acetaminophen or ibuprofen. Reports of moderate to severe systemic events (e.g., fever 40.5° C or higher [105° F or higher], febrile seizures, persistent crying lasting 3 hours or more, and hypotonic-hyporesponsive episodes) have been uncommon after administration of DTaP and they have occurred less frequently among children administered DTaP than those administered DTwP. Swelling involving the entire thigh or upper arm has occurred after the fourth and fifth doses of DTaP. These reactions are also self limited.

Anaphylactic and other serious adverse reactions are rare after receipt of preparations containing diphtheria, tetanus or pertussis components, or a combination of these. Arthus-type hypersensitivity reactions, characterized by severe local reactions, have been reported in adults who received frequent boosters of tetanus or diphtheria toxoids.

Precautions and Contraindications

An immediate anaphylactic reaction to a prior dose of vaccine or vaccine component is a contraindication to further vaccination with DTaP,

DT, or adult Td. Encephalopathy not due to another identifiable cause within 7 days of vaccination is a contraindication to further vaccination with a pertussis-containing vaccine.

Moderate or severe acute illness is a precaution to vaccination. Anyone with mild illnesses, such as otitis media or upper respiratory infection, should be vaccinated. Anyone for whom vaccination is deferred because of moderate or severe acute illness should be vaccinated when the condition improves.

Certain infrequent adverse events following pertussis vaccination are considered precautions (not contraindications) to additional doses of pertussis vaccine: a seizure, with or without fever, occurring within 3 days of immunization; temperature >40.5° C (>105° F) not resulting from another identifiable cause within 48 hours of immunization; collapse or a shock-like state (hypotonic-hyporesponsive episode) within 48 hours of immunization, or persistent, inconsolable crying lasting >3 hours and occurring within 48 hours of immunization. These events have not been proven to cause permanent sequelae. In certain circumstances (e.g., during a communitywide outbreak of pertussis), the benefit of additional vaccination with DTaP may outweigh the risk of another reaction.

Progressive neurologic conditions characterized by changing developmental findings are considered contraindications to receipt of pertussis vaccine. Such disorders include infantile spasms and other epilepsies beginning in infancy. Refer to the American Academy of Pediatrics Red Book for additional information. Infants and children with stable neurologic conditions such as cerebral palsy or controlled seizures should be vaccinated.

TREATMENT

Patients with respiratory diphtheria require hospitalization, immediate treatment with diphtheria antitoxin, appropriate antibiotics, and supportive care. Such patients should also receive a dose of a diphtheria toxoid-containing vaccine during the convalescent period.

Close contacts of diphtheria cases should be tested for C. *diphtheriae* infection, may require antibiotic prophylaxis, and may need vaccination with a diphtheria toxoid-containing vaccine if immunization status is not up to date.

Tetanus is a medical emergency requiring hospitalization, immediate treatment with tetanus immune globulin (human TIG, or equine anti-toxin if human immune globulin is not available) a tetanus toxoid booster, agents to control muscle spasm, and, if indicated, aggressive wound care and antibiotics. Depending on the severity of disease, mechanical ventilation and agents to control autonomic nervous system instability may be required.

Young infants with pertussis often require hospitalization to manage apnea, hypoxia and feeding difficulties. Antibiotic therapy with a macrolide antibiotic (or trimethoprim/sulfamethoxazole if macrolide is contraindicated) may ameliorate the cough illness if given during the catarrhal stage; once paroxysmal cough has developed, however, anti-biotics usually have no effect on the course of illness but are recommended to limit transmission to others. Antibiotic treatment is therefore recommended for persons with pertussis who have cough duration of ≤3 weeks. Prophylaxis (with antibiotics listed above) for close contacts and high-risk contacts of such cases is generally recommended within 3 weeks of exposure, regardless of the age and vaccination status of the contacts. Initiating prophylaxis 3 weeks or more after exposure is usually not of benefit, but can be considered for high-risk contacts (e.g., newborn infants) up to 6 weeks after exposure.

Bibliography

CDC. Diphtheria acquired by U.S. citizens in the Russian Federation and Ukraine —1994. MMWR Morb Mortal Wkly Rep 1995; 44:243–44.

CDC. Fatal respiratory diphtheria in a U.S. traveler to Haiti —2003. MMWR Morb Mortal Wkly Rep 2003;52:1285–86.

Farizo KM, Strebel PM, Chen RT, et al. Fatal respiratory disease due to *Corynebacterium diphtheriae*: case report and review of guidelines for management, investigation, and control. Clin Infect Dis 1993;16:59–68.

Galazka AM. The immunologic basis for immunization: Tetanus (WHO/EPI/GEN/13.13). Geneva, World Health Organization,

1993. Available at: http://whqlibdoc.who.int/hq/1993/WHO_EPI_GEN_93.13_mod3.pdf

Long SS, Pertussis. In: Behrman RE, Kliegman R, Jenson HB, editors. Nelson Textbook of Pediatrics: 16th ed. Philadelphia: W.B. Saunders; 2000. p. 779–84.

Lumio J, Olander RM, Grounstorem K, et al. Epidemiology of three cases of severe diphtheria in Finnish patients with low antitoxin antibody levels. Eur J Clin Microbiol Infect Dis 2001; 20:705–10.

–MARGARET CORTESE, MARTHA H. ROPER, AND TEJPRATAP TIWARI

>>Encephalitis, Japanese

DESCRIPTION

Japanese encephalitis (JE), a mosquito-borne flaviviral infection, is the leading cause of childhood encephalitis in Asia, where up to 50,000 cases may be reported annually. Most infections are asymptomatic, but when encephalitis develops, the case-fatality rate can be as high as 30%. Neuropsychiatric sequelae are reported in 50% of survivors. Although children are at greatest risk of infection in endemic areas, outdoor occupation, recreational exposure, and male gender are also risk factors for infection. Immunity to JE virus from previous vaccination or naturally acquired immunity reduces the risk of illness. Although most adults living in endemic areas have acquired natural immunity and older persons rarely develop illness, a high case-fatality rate has also been reported in the elderly.

JE virus is transmitted chiefly by mosquitoes in the *Culex vishnui* complex; the specific species depends on the geographic area. In China and other endemic areas in Asia, *C. tritaeniorhyncus* is the principal vector. This species feeds outdoors beginning at dusk and during evening hours until dawn. Larvae are found in flooded rice fields, marshes, and other small stable collections of water found around cultivated fields. In temperate zones, this vector is present in greatest density from June through September; it is inactive during winter months. It has a wide host range that includes domestic mammals, birds, and humans. Swine and certain species of wading birds are the amplifying hosts in an enzootic transmission cycle. Because JE virus primarily cycles among animals and mosquitoes and because national JE vaccination programs are present in many affected countries (e.g., Thailand, Taiwan, Japan, Korea), the absence of human infections alone should not be used to gauge a traveler's risk for infection.

OCCURRENCE

JE transmission principally occurs in rural agricultural locations where flooding irrigation is practiced. In many areas of Asia, these ecologic conditions may occur near or occasionally within urban centers. Transmission is seasonal and occurs in the summer and autumn in the temperate regions of China, Japan, Korea, and eastern Russia. Elsewhere, seasonal patterns of disease may be extended or vary with the rainy season and irrigation practices. Risk of JE varies by season and geographic area (Table 4–1 and Map 4–3).

RISK FOR TRAVELERS

The risk to short-term travelers and those who confine their travel to urban centers is very low. Expatriates and travelers living for prolonged periods in rural areas where JE is endemic or epidemic are at greater risk. Travelers with extensive unprotected outdoor, evening, and night-time exposure in rural areas, such as might be experienced while bicycling, camping, or engaging in certain occupational activities, may be at high risk even if their trip is brief.

PREVENTION

Vaccine
An inactivated JE vaccine produced from infected mouse brains has been licensed for use in the U.S. civilian population since 1992. This vaccine is manufactured by Biken (Osaka, Japan) and distributed in the United States by Aventis Pasteur. Other JE vaccines are made by other Asian companies but not licensed for use in the United States.

Vaccination should be considered by persons who plan to live in areas where JE is endemic or epidemic and by travelers whose activities include trips into rural farming areas. Short-term travelers, especially those whose visits are restricted to major urban areas, are at lower risk for infection and generally should not be advised to receive the vaccine. Evaluation of

Text continued on p. 138

TABLE 4-1. RISK OF JAPANESE ENCEPHALITIS, BY COUNTRY, REGION, AND SEASON

COUNTRY	AFFECTED AREAS	TRANSMISSION SEASON	COMMENTS
Australia	Islands of Torres Strait	Probably year-round transmission risk	Localized outbreak in Torres Strait in 1995 and sporadic cases in 1998 in Torres Strait and one case on mainland Australia at Cape York Peninsula
Bangladesh	Little data, but probably widespread	Possibly July to December, as in northern India	Outbreak reported from Tangail District, Dhaka Division in 1977; more recently, sporadic cases in Rajshahi Division
Bhutan	No data	No data	No comments
Brunei	Presumed to be sporadic-endemic, as in Malaysia	Presumed year-round transmission	No comments
Burma (Myanmar)	Presumed to be endemic-hyperendemic countrywide	Presumed to be May to October	Repeated outbreaks in Shan State
Cambodia	Presumed to be endemic-hyperendemic countrywide	Presumed to be May to October	Cases reported from refugee camps on Thai border

NOTE: Assessments are based on publications, surveillance reports, and personal correspondence. Extrapolations have been made from available data. Transmission patterns can change.

TABLE 4-1. RISK OF JAPANESE ENCEPHALITIS, BY COUNTRY, REGION, AND SEASON-CONT'D

COUNTRY	AFFECTED AREAS	TRANSMISSION SEASON	COMMENTS
China	Cases in all provinces except Xizang (Tibet), Xinjiang, Qinghai. Hyperendemic in southern China. Endemic-periodically epidemic in temperate areas. Hong Kong: Rare cases in new territories Taiwan: Endemic, sporadic cases islandwide[1]	Northern China: May to September Southern China: April to October (Guangxi, Yunnan, Guangdong, and Southern Fujian, Sichuan, Guizhou, Hunan, and Jiangxi provinces) Hong Kong: April to October Taiwan: April to October, with a June peak[1]	Vaccine not routinely recommended for travelers to urban areas only Taiwan: Cases reported in and around Taipei and the Kao-hsiung-Pingtung river basins
India	Reported cases from all states except Arunachal, Dadra, Daman, Diu, Gujarat, Himachal, Jammu, Kashmir, Lakshadweep, Meghalaya, Nagar Haveli, Orissa, Punjab, Rajasthan, and Sikkim	South India: May to October in Goa; October to January in Tamil Nadu; and August to December in Karnataka. Second peak, April to June in Mandya District Andrha Pradesh: September to December North India: July to December	Outbreaks in West Bengal, Bihar, Karnataka, Tamil Nadu, Andrha Pradesh, Assam, Uttar Pradesh, Manipur, and Goa. Urban cases reported (e.g., in Luchnow)
Indonesia	Kalimantan, Bali, Nusa, Tenggara, Sulawesi, Mollucas, Irian Jaya (Papua), and Lombok	Probably year-round risk; varies by island; peak risks associated with rainfall, rice cultivation, and presence of pigs Peak periods of risk: November to March; June and July in some years	Human cases recognized on Bali and Java, and possibly in Lombok

[1]Local JE incidence rates may not accurately reflect risks to nonimmune visitors because of high vaccination rates in local populations. Humans are incidental to the transmission cycle. High levels of viral transmission can occur in the absence of human disease.

TABLE 4-1. RISK OF JAPANESE ENCEPHALITIS, BY COUNTRY, REGION, AND SEASON-CONT'D

COUNTRY	AFFECTED AREAS	TRANSMISSION SEASON	COMMENTS
Japan[1]	Rare-sporadic cases on all islands except Hokkaido	June to September, except April to December on Ryuku Islands (Okinawa)	Vaccine not routinely recommended for travel to Tokyo and other major cities. Enzootic transmission without human cases observed on Hokkaido
Korea	North Korea: No data. South Korea: Sporadic-endemic with occasional outbreaks	July to October	Last major outbreaks in 1982 and 1983. Sporadic cases reported in 1994 and 1998.
Laos	Presumed to be endemic-hyperendemic countrywide	Presumed to be May to October	No comments
Malaysia	Sporadic-endemic in all states of Peninsula, Sarawak, and probably Sabah	Year-round transmission	Most cases from Penang, Perak, Salangor, Johore, and Sarawak
Nepal	Hyperendemic in southern lowlands (Terai)	July to December	Vaccine not recommended for travelers visiting only high-altitude areas
Pakistan	May be transmitted in central deltas	Presumed to be June to January	Cases reported near Karachi; endemic areas overlap those for West Nile virus. Lower Indus Valley might be an endemic area.
Papua New Guinea	Normanby Islands and Western Province	Probably year-round risk	Localized sporadic cases

TABLE 4-1. RISK OF JAPANESE ENCEPHALITIS, BY COUNTRY, REGION, AND SEASON-CONT'D

COUNTRY	AFFECTED AREAS	TRANSMISSION SEASON	COMMENTS
Philippines	Presumed to be endemic on all islands	Uncertain; speculations based on locations and agroecosystems. West Luzon, Mindoro, Negros, Palawan: April to November Elsewhere: year-round, with greatest risk April to January	Outbreaks described in Nueva Ecija, Luzon, and Manila
Russia	Far Eastern maritime areas south of Khabarousk	Peak period July to September	First human cases in 30 years recently reported
Singapore	Rare cases	Year-round transmission, with April peak	Vaccine not routinely recommended
Sri Lanka	Endemic in all but mountainous areas Periodically epidemic in northern and central provinces	October to January; secondary peak of enzootic transmission May to June	Recent outbreaks in central (Anuradhapura) and northwestern provinces
Thailand	Hyperendemic in north; sporadic-endemic in south	May to October	Annual outbreaks in Chiang Mai Valley; sporadic cases in Bangkok suburbs
Vietnam	Endemic-hyperendemic in all provinces	May to October	Highest rates in and near Hanoi
Pacific Islands	Two epidemics reported in Guam & Saipan since 1947	Uncertain; possibly September to January	Enzootic cycle might not be sustainable; epidemics might follow introductions of virus.

MAP 4-3. GEOGRAPHIC DISTRIBUTION OF JAPANESE ENCEPHALITIS

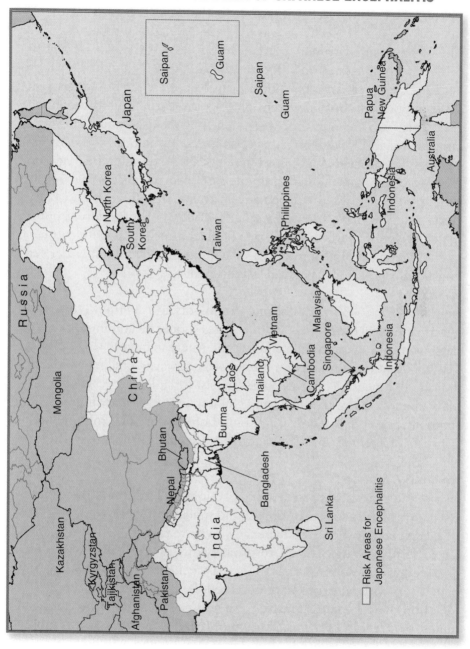

an individual traveler's risk should take into account itinerary and activities and the current level of JE activity in the travel area (see Table 4–1).

The recommended primary immunization series is three doses of 1.0 mL each, administered subcutaneously on days 0, 7, and 30. An abbreviated schedule of days 0, 7, and 14 can be used when the longer schedule is impractical. Both regimens produce similar immunity among recipients. Two doses given a week apart may be used in unusual circumstances and will confer short-term immunity in 80% of vaccinees. The last dose should be administered at least 10 days before beginning travel to ensure an adequate immune response and access to medical care in the event of any delayed adverse reactions (Table 4–2). Many Asian countries have adopted a schedule of two primary doses approximately 4 weeks apart, followed by a booster after 1 year, with subsequent boosters at 3-year intervals. The duration of immunity after serial booster doses has not been well established.

Immunization routes and schedules for infants and children 1–3 years of age are identical except that 0.5-mL doses should be administered. No data are available on vaccine efficacy and safety in infants <1 year of age. The full duration of protection is unknown; however, preliminary data indicate that neutralizing antibodies persist for at least 2 years after primary immunization. In infants and children whose primary immunization series included 0.5-mL doses, a 1.0-mL booster dose (0.5 mL for children <3 years of age) may be administered 2 years after the primary series.

Adverse Reactions

JE vaccine is associated with local reactions and mild systemic side effects (fever, headache, myalgias, and malaise) in approximately 20% of vaccinees. More serious hypersensitivity reactions, including generalized urticaria, angioedema, respiratory distress, and anaphylaxis have occurred within minutes to as long as 1 week after immunization. Such hypersensitivity reactions have occurred in up to 0.6% of vaccinees. Reactions have been responsive to therapy with epinephrine, antihistamines, or steroids, or a combination of these. Vaccine recipients should be observed for 30 minutes after immunization and warned about the possibility of delayed allergic reactions. The full course of immunization should be completed at least 10 days before departure, and vaccinees should be advised to remain in areas with access to medical care. Persons with a history of urticaria or angioedema appear to have a

TABLE 4-2. JAPANESE ENCEPHALITIS VACCINE

DOSES[1]	1-2 YEARS OF AGE	≥3 YEARS OF AGE	COMMENTS
Primary series 1, 2, and 3	0.5 mL	1.0 mL	Days 0, 7, and 30
Booster	0.5 mL	1.0 mL	1 dose at 24 months or later[2]

[1]Administered by the subcutaneous route

[2]For vaccinees who have completed a three-dose primary series, the full duration of protection is unknown; therefore, definitive recommendations cannot be given.

greater risk for developing more serious allergic reactions; this factor must be considered when weighing the risks and benefits of the vaccine. A history of allergy to JE or other mouse-derived vaccines is a contraindication to further immunization.

Although the use of mouse brains as the substrate for virus growth has always elicited concern about post-vaccination neurologic side effects, the evidence of an association between JE vaccine and demyelinating neurologic events such as acute disseminated encephalomyelitis or polyneuritis remains circumstantial and primarily based on case reports.

Precautions and Contraindications
Persons with known hypersensitivity to the vaccine should not be vaccinated. Persons with multiple allergies or with a history of urticaria or angioedema for any reason are at higher risk for allergic complications from the JE vaccine. Vaccination during pregnancy should be avoided unless the risk of acquiring JE outweighs the theoretical risk of vaccination.

Personal Protection Measures
Although JE vaccination is very effective against developing infection, travelers should still avoid mosquito bites to reduce the risk of other vector-borne infectious diseases. Travelers should be advised to stay in screened or air-conditioned rooms, to use bed nets when such quarters are unavailable, to use area aerosol insecticides and mosquito coils as necessary, and to use personal insect repellents containing DEET and protective clothing to avoid mosquito bites (see Chapter 2, *Protection against Mosquitoes and Other Arthropods*).

Bibliography

Burke DS, Leake CJ. Japanese encephalitis. In: Monath TP, editor. The arboviruses: epidemiology and ecology, Vol 3. Boca Raton, FL: CRC Press; 1998. p. 63–92.

CDC. General Recommendations on Immunization Recommendations of the Advisory Committee on Immunization Practices (ACIP). MMWR Recomm Rep. 1994; 43(RR-1):1–38.

Halstead SB, Jacobson J. Japanese encephalitis. Adv Virus Res. 2003;61:103–38

Konishi E, Shoda M, Kondo T. Prevalence of antibody to Japanese encephalitis virus nonstructural 1 protein among racehorses in Japan: indication of natural infection and need for continuous vaccination. Vaccine. 2004;22:1097–103.

Monath TP. Japanese encephalitis vaccines: current vaccines and future prospects. Curr Top Microbiol Immunol. 2002;267:105–38.

Plesner AM. Allergic reactions to Japanese encephalitis vaccine. Immunol Allergy Clin North Am. 2003;23:665–97.

Tsai TF. New Initiatives for the control of Japanese encephalitis by vaccination: minutes of a WHO/CVI meeting, Bangkok, Thailand, 13–15 October 1998. Vaccine. 2000;18 Suppl 2:1–25.

World Health Organization. Japanese Encephalitis vaccine [monograph on the Internet]. Geneva: WHO; 1998 [cited 2004 Nov 5]. Available from: http://childrensvaccine.org/files/JE_position_paper_WHO.pdf

—MICHAEL BUNNING AND ANTHONY MARFIN

>>Encephalitis, Tickborne

DESCRIPTION

Tickborne encephalitis (TBE), also known as spring-summer encephalitis, is a flavivirus infection of the central nervous system. The two main serotypes, European and Far Eastern, are transmitted by the hard ticks *Ixodes ricinus* and *I. persulcatus*, respectively. Humans acquire disease by the bite of an infected tick or rarely, by ingesting unpasturized dairy products primarily from infected goats, but also sheep or cows.

OCCURRENCE

TBE disease occurs in endemic foci correlated with the distribution of the tick vectors in the temperate regions of Europe and Asia between latitudes 39–65 degrees, extending from western France to Hokkaido in Japan. The countries most heavily impacted are Austria, Belarus, Czech Republic, Estonia, Germany, Hungary, Kazakhastan, Latvia, Lithuania, Poland, Romania, Russia, Slovakia, and the Ukraine. There are also foci in the southern portions of Finland, Norway, Sweden, and the island of Bornholm in Denmark, as well as the northern portions of Albania, Bosnia, Croatia, Italy, Greece, and Slovenia. Sporadic cases have also been reported in Turkey. In China the known endemic areas are Hunchun in Jilin province and western Yunan near the Burmese border.

The tick vectors are most active in warm, moist conditions; thus, there are two peaks of disease in Central Europe: April/May and September/October. In cooler climates there is a single peak in summer. Infected ticks are generally localized in transition zones between different types of vegetation (e.g., forest fringes with adjacent grassland and the transition zones between deciduous and coniferous forests). Individual ticks are suspended on the edges of leaves adjacent to trails and attach to passing mammals.

RISK FOR TRAVELERS

The risk for travelers to urban or nonforested areas who do not consume unpasteurized dairy products is thought to be negligible. Travelers who sustain unprotected exposure via bicycling, camping, hiking, or fishing; collecting flowers, berries, or mushrooms; or certain occupational activities, such as forestry in endemic areas, might be at high risk, even if the visit is brief.

The number of cases reported from individual countries (see www.tbe-info.com) is not always a reliable predictor of risk to the traveler, as it is dependent not only on the ecology within that geographic area, but also on the level of surveillance and the percentage of the population that have been vaccinated. For example, the number of cases in Austria declined from >600 per year to 60 in 2000, when 84% of the population had been vaccinated. Vaccination prevents disease in humans but does not eradicate the virus in the tick population. An unvaccinated tourist staying four months in a highly endemic province in Austria is estimated to have a risk of acquiring TBE of about 1 per 10,000 person-months of exposure. Based on the number of tourist overnight stays in Austria, this would equate to 60 travel-associated clinical TBE cases per summer. Members of a US military unit that trained in a highly endemic area in Bosnia had an infection rate of 0.9/1,000 person-months of exposure.

CLINICAL PRESENTATION

TBE usually has a biphasic course. The median incubation period is a week. The first phase consists of a few days of fever, fatigue, headache, and muscle pain. This may be followed by a week-long asymptomatic interval before signs of CNS involvement develop, including meningitis, encephalitis, and myelitis, which can result in severe neurologic sequelae. The European form seems to be milder with only 20%–30% experiencing the second phase and a mortality rate less than 1%. Case-fatality rates of 20%–40% have been reported during outbreaks of the Far Eastern subtype, which tends to be monophasic. A slow progressive form in 2%–5% of cases of the Far Eastern subtype is characterized by a long incubation period of years.

TBE should be suspected in travelers who return from an endemic area and present with uncharacteristic influenza-like illness that progresses to aseptic meningitis or encephalitis within 1–4 weeks of return. More than 50% of infected persons will not remember a tick bite. Diagnosis is made by demonstration of specific IgM, which is usually detectable by ELISA during the second (neurologic) phase of the illness. As TBE virus antibodies cross-react with other flaviviruses the laboratory that performs the test will want to know whether there is a prior history of dengue infection or flavivirus vaccination.

PREVENTION

Travelers may reduce their risk by avoiding exposure to tick-infested areas of forest and woodland during the spring and summer, when ticks are active. They may also protect themselves from tick bites by barrier methods, such as wearing clothing with long sleeves and taping trouser legs or tucking them into socks or shoes. Light-colored clothing makes it easier to detect ticks, and smoothly woven clothing makes it more difficult for ticks to attach. Clothing and camping gear can be impregnated with compounds containing permethrin, which have an acaricidal and repellent effect. These compounds can be used with repellents containing N,N-diethylmetatoluamide (DEET), which can be directly applied to exposed skin (see *Protection against Mosquitoes and Other Arthropods*). Travelers should also inspect their bodies and clothing for ticks daily during exposure and should avoid unpasteurized dairy products.

Two effective vaccines are available in Europe from Baxter (Vienna, Austria) and Chiron (Marburg, Germany). However, since protection lasting 3 years requires 3 doses (the first 2 separated by 4–12 weeks, and the last at least 9 months after the second), it will be the rare traveler who will be in the position to benefit by immunization. An accelerated schedule is used by some clinicians. Travelers anticipating high-risk exposures, such as working or camping in forested areas or farmland, adventure travelers, expatriates or those planning to live in disease-endemic countries for an extended period of time may need special consideration.

TREATMENT

The only treatment currently available is supportive. Post-exposure prophylaxis with specific immune globulin is no longer recommended.

Bibliography

Beran J, Asokliene L, Lucenko I. Tickborne encephalitis in the Czech Republic, Lithuania, and Latvia. Eurosurveillance Weekly [serial on the Internet]. 2004 Jun [cited 2004 Nov 5]. Available from: http://www.eurosurveillance.org/ew/2004/040624.asp.

Gritson TS, Laskevich VA, Gould EA. Tick-borne encephalitis. Antiviral Res 2003;57:129–46.

Haglund M, Gunther G. Tick-borne encephalitis—pathogenesis, clinical course and long-term follow-up. Vaccine 2003;21 Suppl 1:S11–18.

Holzmann H. Diagnosis of tick-borne encephalitis. Vaccine 2003;21 Suppl 1:S36–40.

Reinhild S, Samuelsson S, Nohynek H, et al. Tickborne encephalitis in Europe: basic information, country by country. Eurosurveillance Weekly [serial on the Internet]. 2004 Jun [cited 2004 Nov 5]. Available from: http://www.eurosurveillance.org/ew/2004/040715.asp.

Rendi-Wagner P. Risk and prevention of tick-borne encephalitis in travelers. J Travel Med. 2004;11:307–12.

Sanchez JL Jr, Craig SC, Kohlhase K, et al. Health assessment of U.S. military personnel deployed to Bosnia-Herzegovina for operation joint endeavor. Military Med. 2001;166:470–4.

Suss J. Epidemiology and ecology of TBE relevant to the production of effective vaccines. Vaccine 2003;21 Suppl 1:S19–35.

TBE-info.com [homepage on the Internet]. International Scientific Working Group on Tick-Borne Encephalitis; c2000 [cited 2004 Nov 5]. Available from: http://www.tbe-info.com.

–CHRISTIE REED

>>Filariasis, Lymphatic

DESCRIPTION

Lymphatic filariasis is caused primarily by adult worms (filariae) that live in the lymphatic vessels. The female worms release microfilariae that circulate in the peripheral blood and are ingested by mosquitoes; thus, infected mosquitoes transmit the infection from person to person. The two major species of filariae that cause lymphatic disease in humans are *Wuchereria bancrofti and Brugia malayi.*

OCCURRENCE

Lymphatic filariasis affects an estimated 120 million persons in tropical areas of the world, including sub-Saharan Africa, Egypt, southern Asia, the western Pacific islands, the northeastern coast of Brazil, Guyana, and the Caribbean island of Hispaniola.

RISK FOR TRAVELERS

Short-term travelers to endemic areas are at low risk for this infection. Travelers who visit endemic areas for extended periods of time and who are intensively exposed to infected mosquitoes can become infected. Most infections seen in the United States are in immigrants from endemic countries.

CLINICAL PRESENTATION

Most infections are asymptomatic, but the living adult worm causes progressive lymphatic vessel dilation and dysfunction. Lymphatic dysfunction may lead to lymphedema of the leg, scrotum, penis, arm, or breast, which can increase in severity as a result of recurrent secondary bacterial infections. Tropical pulmonary eosinophilia is a potentially serious progressive lung disease with nocturnal cough, wheezing, and fever, resulting from immune hyperresponsiveness to microfilariae in the pulmonary capillaries.

PREVENTION

No vaccine is available, nor has the effectiveness of chemoprophylaxis been well documented. Protective measures include avoidance of mosquito bites through the use of personal protection measures (see *Protection against Mosquitoes and Other Arthropods*).

TREATMENT

The drug of choice for treatment of travelers with *W. bancrofti or B. malayi* infections is diethylcarbamazine (DEC). DEC, which is available to U.S.-licensed physicians for this purpose, can be obtained from the CDC Parasitic Diseases Drug Service at 404-639-3670. (See Immunobiologics Distributed by the Centers for Disease Control and Prevention website, which is available at: http://www.cdc.gov/ncidod/srp/drugs/drug-service.html.) DEC kills circulating microfilariae and is partially effective against the adult worms and tropical pulmonary eosinophilia. Many patients with lymphedema are no longer infected with the filarial parasite and do not benefit from antifilarial drug treatment. For chronic manifestations of lymphatic filariasis, such as lymphedema and hydrocele, specific lymphedema treatment (including hygiene, skin care, physical therapy, and in some cases, antibiotics) and surgical repair, respectively, are recommended. To ensure correct diagnosis and treatment, travelers should be advised to consult an infectious disease or tropical medicine specialist.

Bibliography

Dreyer G, Addiss D, Dreyer P, Noroes J. Basic lymphoedema management: Treatment and prevention of problems associated with lymphatic filariasis. Hollis, NH: Hollis Publishing Co.; 2002.

Dreyer G, Addiss D, Roberts J, Noroes J. Progression of lymphatic vessel dilatation in the presence of living adult *Wuchereria bancrofti*. Trans R Soc Trop Med Hyg. 2002; 96:157–61.

Dreyer G, Medeiros Z, Netto MJ, Leal NC, de Castro LG, Piessens WF. Acute attacks in the extremities of persons living in an area endemic for bancroftian filariasis: differentiation of two syndromes. Trans R Soc Trop Med Hyg. 1999;93:413–7.

Michael E, Bundy DAP, Grenfell BT. Re-assessing the global prevalence and distribution of lymphatic filariasis. Parasitology. 1996;112:409–28.

Ottesen, EA. Efficacy of diethylcarbamazine in eradicating infection with lymphatic-dwelling filariae in humans. Rev Infect Dis. 1985;7:341–56.

Shenoy RK, Suma TK, Rajan K, Kumaraswami V. Prevention of acute adenolymphangitis in brugian filariasis: comparison of the efficacy of ivermectin and diethylcarbamazine, each combined with local treatment of the affected limb. Ann Trop Med Parasitol. 1998;92:587–94.

Weil GJ, Lammie PJ, Weiss N. The ICT filariasis test: a rapid format antigen test for diagnosis of bancroftian filariasis. Parasitol Today. 1997;13:401–4.

–DAVID ADDISS

>>Giardiasis

DESCRIPTION

Giardiasis is a diarrheal illness caused by the protozoan *Giardia intestinalis,* which lives in the intestines of persons and animals and is passed in their feces. Transmission occurs from ingestion of fecally contaminated food or drinking water, swallowing recreational water, from exposure to fecally contaminated environmental surfaces, and from person to person by the fecal-oral route.

OCCURRENCE

Giardiasis occurs worldwide.

RISK FOR TRAVELERS

Risk of infection increases with duration of travel and is highest for those who live in or visit rural areas, trek in backcountry areas, or frequently eat, drink, or swim in areas that have poor sanitation and inadequate drinking water treatment facilities.

CLINICAL PRESENTATION

Symptoms, which occur approximately 1–2 weeks after ingestion of the parasite, include diarrhea, abdominal cramps, bloating, fatigue, weight loss, flatulence, anorexia, or nausea, in various combinations. Symptoms usually last >5 days and can become chronic, resulting in malabsorption. Fever and vomiting are uncommon.

PREVENTION

No vaccine is available, and there is no known chemoprophylaxis. To prevent infection, travelers to disease-endemic areas should be advised to follow the precautions included in the section *Risks from Food and Water.*

TREATMENT

Several effective antimicrobial drugs (e.g., tinidazole, metronidazole, quinacrine, albendazole, nitazoxanide) are now available. Treatment recommendations are available in textbooks on internal medicine and infectious diseases; consultation with a travel or tropical medicine specialist can also be sought.

Bibliography

Hardie RM, Wall PG, Gott P, et al. Infectious diarrhea in tourists staying in a resort hotel. Emerg Infect Dis. 1999;5:168–71.

Stuart JM, Orr HJ, Warburton FG, et al. Risk factors for sporadic giardiasis: a case-control study in southwestern England. Emerg Infect Dis. 2003;9:229–33.

–MICHAEL BEACH

>>*Haemophilus influenzae* Type b Meningitis and Invasive Disease

DESCRIPTION

Haemophilus influenzae type b (Hib) causes meningitis and other severe infections (e.g., pneumonia, bacteremia, septic arthritis, and epiglottitis) primarily among infants and children <5 years of age. Because Hib vaccine is used widely in the United States, the highest rate of reported invasive Hib disease is now among infants too young to be fully vaccinated (<6 months of age); the incidence among infants and children 1–4 years of age is much lower than among infants <1 year of age. The disease is uncommon in anyone 5 years of age or older. Most cases occur in infants and children who are unvaccinated or incompletely vaccinated.

OCCURRENCE

In the early 1980s (before licensure of conjugate Hib vaccines), approximately 20,000 cases of invasive Hib disease occurred annually in the United States, primarily among infants and children <5 years of age. As a result of the widespread use of conjugate Hib vaccines, the disease is now uncommon in the United States, with <200 cases reported annually.

RISK FOR TRAVELERS

Invasive Hib disease occurs throughout the world. Few countries routinely use Hib vaccine, so invasive Hib disease remains common in infants and young children in many countries, and unvaccinated children who travel may be at risk.

CLINICAL PRESENTATION

The presentation of Hib disease in children depends on the localization of the infection, which usually occurs after the organism enters the bloodstream from the nasopharynx. Meningitis, pneumonia, sepsis, or arthritis caused by Hib resemble these conditions caused by other bacteria. Epiglottitis presents as sudden onset of fever, drooling, and difficulty in swallowing, and rapidly progresses to airway obstruction.

PREVENTION

Vaccine

Three conjugate Hib vaccines are licensed for use in infants and children in United States: HbOC (HibTiTER, Wyeth-Lederle), PRP-OMP (PedvaxHIB, Merck & Co., Inc.), and PRP-T (ActHIB, Aventis Pasteur; OmniHIB, GlaxoSmithKline). PRP-OMP vaccine is available combined with hepatitis B vaccine (Comvax). PRP-T (ActHIB) is also available combined with acellular pertussis vaccine (DTaP Tripedia); the combined product is called TriHIBit. TriHIBit is licensed for use only as the fourth dose of the Hib and DTaP series, and should not be given for the first, second, or third doses of the Hib series.

All infants should receive a primary series of conjugate Hib vaccine beginning at age 2 months (Table 8–2). The number of doses in the primary series depends on the type of vaccine used. A primary series of PRP-OMP vaccine is two doses; HbOC and PRP-T require a three-dose primary series (Table 4–3). A booster should be given at age 12–15 months, regardless of which vaccine is used for the primary series.

The optimal interval between doses is 2 months, with a minimum interval of 1 month. At least 2 months should separate the booster dose from the previous (second or third) dose. Hib vaccines may be given simultaneously with all other vaccines.

Limited data suggest that Hib conjugate vaccines given to infants <6 weeks of age may result in a reduced antibody response to additional doses of Hib vaccine. Therefore, Hib vaccines, including combination vaccines that contain Hib conjugate, should not be given to infants <6 weeks of age.

All three conjugate Hib vaccines licensed for use in infants are interchangeable. If it is necessary to change the type of vaccine, three doses of any combination constitute the primary series. Any licensed conjugate vaccine may be used for the booster dose regardless of what type was received in the primary series.

TABLE 4-3. RECOMMENDED *HAEMOPHILUS INFLUENZAE* TYPE b (Hib) ROUTINE VACCINATION SCHEDULE

VACCINE	2 MONTHS	4 MONTHS	6 MONTHS	12-15 MONTHS
HbOC/PRP-T	Dose 1	Dose 2	Dose 3	Booster
PRP-OMP	Dose 1	Dose 2	–	Booster

Unvaccinated infants and children ages 7 months and older might not require a full series of three or four doses (Table 8–2). The number of doses an infant or a child needs to complete the series depends on the infant's or child's age and, to a lesser degree, on the number of prior doses of Hib vaccine received. Previously unvaccinated children 15–59 months of age should receive a single dose of any conjugate Hib vaccine. In general, children >59 months of age do not need Hib vaccination. Refer to the American Academy of Pediatrics Red Book for additional information on late or lapsed Hib vaccination schedules.

Adverse Reactions
Adverse events following vaccination with Hib conjugates are uncommon. Swelling, redness, or pain, or a combination of these, have been reported in 5%–30% of recipients and usually resolve within 12–24 hours. Systemic reactions such as fever and irritability are infrequent.

Precautions and Contraindications
Vaccination with Hib conjugate vaccine is contraindicated in anyone known to have experienced anaphylaxis following a prior dose of that vaccine. Vaccination should be delayed in infants and children with moderate or severe acute illnesses. Minor illnesses (for example, mild upper respiratory infection) are not contraindications to vaccination. Contraindications and precautions for the use of TriHIBit and Comvax are the same as those for their individual component vaccines (i.e., DTaP, Hib, and hepatitis B).

TREATMENT

Specific parenteral antibiotic treatment is necessary for invasive Hib disease, and immediate airway stabilization is necessary for epiglottitis. In certain circumstances, antibiotic prophylaxis is indicated for household contacts. Refer to the American Academy of Pediatrics Red Book for additional information.

Bibliography

American Academy of Pediatrics. *Haemophilus influenzae* Infections. In: Pickering LK, editor. Red Book: 2003 Report of the Committee on Infectious Diseases. 26th ed. Elk Grove Village, IL: American Academy of Pediatrics; 2003:293–301.

Wenger JD, Ward JI. *Haemophilus influenzae* Vaccine. In: Plotkin SA, Orenstein WA, editors. Vaccines. 4th ed. Philadelphia: W.B. Saunders; 2004: 229–68.

−MARGARET M. CORTESE

>>Hepatitis, Viral, Type A

DESCRIPTION

Hepatitis A is a viral infection of the liver caused by hepatitis A virus (HAV). HAV infection may be asymptomatic or its clinical manifestations may range in severity from a mild illness lasting 1–2 weeks to a severely disabling disease lasting several months. Clinical manifestations of hepatitis A often include fever, malaise, anorexia, nausea, and abdominal discomfort, followed within a few days by jaundice.

OCCURRENCE

HAV is shed in the feces of persons with HAV infection. Transmission can occur through direct person-to-person contact; through exposure to contaminated water, ice, or shellfish harvested from sewage-contaminated water; or from fruits, vegetables, or other foods that are eaten uncooked and that were contaminated during harvesting or subsequent handling.

HAV infection is common (high or intermediate endemicity) throughout the developing world, where infections most frequently are acquired during early childhood and usually are asymptomatic or mild. In developed countries, HAV infection is less common (low endemicity), but communitywide outbreaks still occur in some areas of the United States. Map 4–4 indicates the seroprevalence of antibody to HAV (total anti-HAV) as measured in selected cross-sectional studies among each country's residents.

RISK FOR TRAVELERS

Hepatitis A is the most common vaccine-preventable infection acquired during travel. The risk for acquiring HAV infection for U.S. residents traveling abroad varies with living conditions, length of stay, and the incidence of HAV infection in the area visited. Travelers to North America (except Mexico), Japan, Australia, New Zealand, and developed countries in Europe are at no greater risk for infection than in the United States. For travelers to other countries, risk for infection increases with duration of travel and is highest for those who live in or visit rural areas, trek in back-country areas, or frequently eat or drink in settings of poor sanitation. Nevertheless, many cases of travel-related hepatitis A occur in travelers to developing countries with "standard" tourist itineraries, accommodations, and food consumption behaviors.

CLINICAL PRESENTATION

The incubation period for hepatitis A averages 28 days (range 15–50 days). Hepatitis A typically has an abrupt onset of symptoms that can include fever, malaise, anorexia, nausea, abdominal discomfort, dark urine, and jaundice. The likelihood of having symptoms with HAV infection is related to the infected person's age. In children <6 years old, most (70%) infections are asymptomatic; if illness does occur its duration is usually <2 months. No chronic or long-term infection is associated with hepatitis A, but 10% of infected persons will have prolonged or relapsing symptoms over a 6- to 9-month period. The overall case-fatality rate among cases reported to CDC is 0.3%; however, the rate is 1.8% among adults >50 years of age.

PREVENTION

Hepatitis A vaccine, immune globulin (IG), or both, are recommended for all susceptible persons traveling to or working in countries with an intermediate or high endemicity of HAV infection. Health-care providers should administer hepatitis A vaccination for persons traveling

MAP 4-4. GEOGRAPHIC DISTRIBUTION OF HEPATITIS A PREVALENCE, 2005

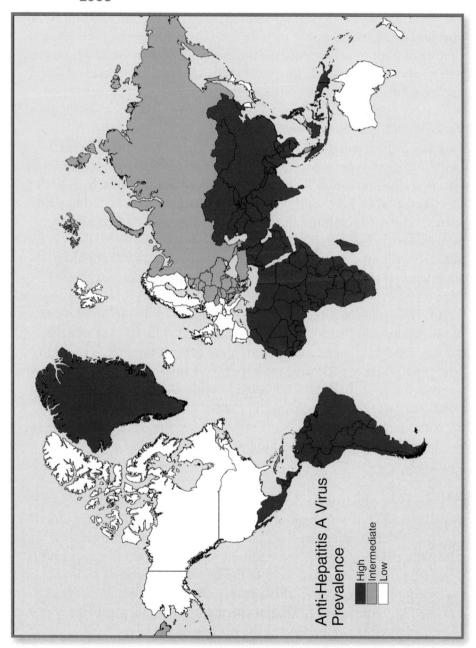

Anti-Hepatitis A Virus Prevalence

High
Intermediate
Low

for any purpose, frequency or duration to countries that have high or intermediate endemicity of HAV infection. In addition, health-care providers should be alert to opportunities to provide vaccination for all travelers whose plans might include travel at some time in the future to an area of high or intermediate endemicity, including those whose current medical evaluation is for travel to an area where hepatitis A vaccination is not currently recommended.

Vaccine and Immune Globulin

Two monovalent hepatitis A vaccines are currently licensed in the United States for persons >2 years of age: HAVRIX, manufactured by GlaxoSmithKline (Table 4–4), and VAQTA (manufactured by Merck & Co., Inc.) (Table 4–5). Both vaccines are made of inactivated hepatitis A virus adsorbed to aluminum hydroxide as an adjuvant. HAVRIX is prepared with 2-phenoxyethanol as a preservative, while VAQTA is formulated without a preservative. All hepatitis A vaccines should be administered intramuscularly in the deltoid muscle.

TWINRIX, manufactured by GlaxoSmithKline, is a combined hepatitis A and hepatitis B vaccine licensed for persons >18 years of age, containing 720 EL.U. of hepatitis A antigen (50% of the HAVRIX adult dose) and 20 μg of recombinant hepatitis B surface antigen protein (the same as the ENGERIX-B adult dose) (Table 4–6). Primary immunization consists of three doses, given on a 0-, 1-, and 6-month schedule, the same schedule as that commonly used for monovalent hepatitis B vaccine. TWINRIX contains aluminum phosphate and aluminum hydroxide as adjuvant and 2-phenoxyethanol as a preservative.

The first dose of hepatitis A vaccine should be administered as soon as travel to countries with high or intermediate endemicity is considered. One month after receiving the first dose of monovalent hepatitis A vaccine, 94%–100% of adults and children will have protective concentrations of antibody. The final dose in the hepatitis A vaccine series is necessary to promote long-term protection. The immunogenicity of TWINRIX is equivalent to that of the monovalent hepatitis vaccines when tested after completion of the licensed schedule.

Many persons will have a detectable antibody to hepatitis A virus (anti-HAV) response to the monovalent vaccine by 2 weeks after the first vac-

TABLE 4-4. LICENSED SCHEDULE FOR HAVRIX[1]

AGE GROUP (YRS)	DOSE (EL.U.)[2]	VOLUME	NO. OF DOSES	SCHEDULE (MONTHS)
2–18	720	0.5 mL	2	0, 6 to 12
≥19	1,440	1.0 mL	2	0, 6 to 12

[1]Hepatitis A vaccine, inactivated, GlaxoSmithKline
[2]EL.U. = enzyme-linked immunosorbent assay (ELISA) units

TABLE 4-5. LICENSED SCHEDULE FOR VAQTA[1]

AGE GROUP (YRS)	DOSE	VOLUME	NO. OF DOSES	SCHEDULE (MONTHS)
2–18	25 units	0.5 mL	2	0, 6 to 18
≥19	50 units	1.0 mL	2	0, 6 to 18

[1]Hepatitis A vaccine, inactivated, Merck & Co., Inc

TABLE 4-6. LICENSED SCHEDULE FOR TWINRIX[1]

AGE GROUP (YRS)	HEPATITIS A DOSE/ HEPATITIS B DOSE	VOLUME	NO. OF DOSES	SCHEDULE (MONTHS)
≥18	720 EL.U.[2]/ 20 μg	1.0 mL	3	0, 1, 6 months

[1]Combined hepatitis A and hepatitis B vaccine, GlaxoSmithKline
[2]EL.U. = enzyme-linked immunosorbent assay (ELISA) units

cine dose. The proportion of persons who develop a detectable antibody response at 2 weeks may be lower when smaller vaccine dosages are used, such as with the use of TWINRIX. Travelers who receive hepatitis A vaccine <2 weeks before traveling to an endemic area and who do not receive immune globulin either by choice or because of lack of availability likely will be at lower risk of infection than those who do not receive hepatitis A vaccine or IG. In the case of travel within 4 weeks of vaccine administration, a dose of immune globulin (0.02 mL/kg) may be given alone or in addition to hepatitis A vaccine, at a different site, for optimal protection. In the case of unavailability or refusal of immune globulin, administration of hepatitis A vaccine alone for this group is recommended, but they should be informed that they are not optimally protected from acquiring hepatitis A in the immediate future (i.e., the subsequent 2–4 weeks).

Although vaccination of an immune traveler is not contraindicated and does not increase the risk of adverse effects, screening for total anti-HAV before travel can be useful in some circumstances to determine susceptibility and eliminate unnecessary vaccination or IG prophylaxis of immune travelers. Such serologic screening for susceptibility might be indicated for adult travelers who are likely to have had prior HAV infection if the cost of screening (laboratory and office visit) is less than the cost of vaccination or IG prophylaxis and if testing will not delay vaccination and interfere with timely receipt of vaccine or IG before travel. Such travelers may include those >40 years of age and those born in areas of the world with intermediate or high endemicity. Post-vaccination testing for serologic response is not indicated.

Using the vaccines according to the licensed schedules is preferable. However, an interrupted series does not need to be restarted. Given their similar immunogenicity, a series that has been started with one brand of monovalent vaccine (i.e., HAVRIX or VAQTA) may be completed with the other brand. Hepatitis A vaccine may be administered at the same time as IG or other commonly used vaccines for travelers, at different injection sites.

In adults and children who have completed the vaccine series, anti-HAV has been shown to persist for at least 5–10 years after vaccination. Results of mathematical models indicate that after completion of the vaccination series, anti-HAV will likely persist for 20 years or more. For children and adults who complete the primary series, booster doses of vaccine are not recommended. Serologic testing to assess antibody levels after vaccination is not indicated.

Travelers who are <2 years of age, are allergic to a vaccine component, or otherwise elect not to receive vaccine should receive a single dose of IG (0.02 mL/kg), which provides effective protection against HAV infection for up to 3 months (Table 4–7). Those who do not receive vaccina-

TABLE 4-7. IMMUNE GLOBULIN FOR PROTECTION AGAINST VIRAL HEPATITIS A

LENGTH OF STAY	BODY WEIGHT		DOSE VOLUME (ML)[1]	COMMENTS
	Lb	Kg		
<3 months	<50	<23	0.5	Dose volume depends on body weight and length of stay.
	50–100	23–45	1.0	
	>100	>45	2.0	
3–5 months	<22	<10	0.5	
	22–49	10–22	1.0	
	50–100	23–45	2.5	
	>100	>45	5.0	

[1]For intramuscular injection

tion and plan to travel for >3 months should receive an IG dose of 0.06 mL/kg, which must be repeated if the duration of travel is >5 months.

Adverse Reactions

Among adults, the most frequently reported side effects occurring 3–5 days after a vaccine dose are tenderness or pain at the injection site (53%–56%) or headache (14%–16%). Among children, the most common side effects reported are pain or tenderness at the injection site (15%–19%), feeding problems (8% in one study), or headache (4% in one study). No serious adverse events in children or adults that could be definitively attributed to the vaccine or increases in serious adverse events among vaccinated persons compared with baseline rates have been identified.

Immune globulin for intramuscular administration prepared in the United States has few side effects (primarily soreness at the injection site) and has never been shown to transmit infectious agents (hepatitis B virus, hepatitis C virus [HCV], or HIV). Since December 1994, all IG products commercially available in the United States have had to undergo a viral inactivation procedure or be negative for HCV RNA before release.

Precautions and Contraindications

These vaccines should not be administered to travelers with a history of hypersensitivity to any vaccine component. HAVRIX or TWINRIX should not be administered to travelers with a history of hypersensitivity reactions to the preservative 2-phenoxyethanol. TWINRIX should not be administered to persons with a history of hypersensitivity to yeast. Because hepatitis A vaccine consists of inactivated virus and hepatitis B vaccine consists of a recombinant protein, no special precautions need to be taken for vaccination of immunocompromised travelers.

Pregnancy

The safety of hepatitis A vaccine for pregnant women has not been determined. However, because hepatitis A vaccine is produced from inactivated HAV, the theoretical risk to either the pregnant woman or the developing fetus is thought to be very low. The risk of vaccination should be weighed against the risk of hepatitis A in women travelers who might be at high risk for exposure to HAV. Pregnancy is not a contraindication to using IG.

Other Prevention Tips

Boiling or cooking food and beverage items for at least 1 minute to 185° F (85° C) inactivates HAV. Foods and beverages heated to this temperature and for this length of time cannot serve as vehicles for HAV infection unless they become contaminated after heating. Adequate chlorination of water as recommended in the United States will inactivate HAV. Travelers should be advised that, to minimize their risk of hepatitis A and other enteric diseases in developing countries, they should avoid potentially contaminated water or food. Travelers should also be advised to avoid drinking beverages (with or without ice) of unknown purity, eating uncooked shellfish, and eating uncooked fruits or vegetables that are not peeled or prepared by the traveler personally. (See Chapter 2, Risks from Food and Drink.)

TREATMENT

No specific treatment is available for persons with hepatitis A. Treatment is supportive.

Bibliography

Bell BP, Feinstone SM. Hepatitis A vaccine. In: Plotkin SA, Orenstein WA, editors. Vaccines. 4th edition. Philadelphia: W.B. Saunders, 2004.

CDC. Prevention of hepatitis A through active or passive immunization: recommendations of the Advisory Committee on Immunization Practices (ACIP). Morbid Mortal Wkly Rep MMWR.1999; RR 48:1–37.

Fiore AE. Hepatitis A transmitted by food. Clin Infect Dis. 2004;38:705–15.

Steffen R, Kane M, Shapiro C, et al. Epidemiology and prevention of hepatitis A in travelers. JAMA. 1994;272:885–9.

Van Damme P, Banatvala J, Fay O, et al. Hepatits A booster vaccination: is there a need? Lancet. 2003;362:1065–71.

Weinberg M, Hopkins J, Farrington L, et al. Hepatitis A in Hispanic children who live along the United States-Mexico border: the role of international travel and foodborne exposures. Pediatrics. 2004;114:e68–73.

Winokur PL, Stapleton JT. Immunoglobulin prophylaxis for hepatitis A. Clin Infect Dis. 1992;14:580–6.

—ANTHONY FIORE AND BETH BELL

>>Hepatitis, Viral, Type B

DESCRIPTION

Hepatitis B is caused by the hepatitis B virus (HBV). The clinical manifestations of HBV infection range in severity from no symptoms to fulminant hepatitis. Signs and symptoms of hepatitis B may include fever, malaise, anorexia, nausea, and abdominal discomfort, followed within a few days by jaundice.

OCCURRENCE

HBV is transmitted through activities that involve contact with blood or blood-derived fluids. Such activities can include unprotected sex with an

HBV-infected partner; shared needles used for injection of illegal drugs; work in health-care fields (medical, dental, laboratory, or other) that entails direct exposure to human blood; receiving blood transfusions that have not been screened for HBV; or having dental, medical, or cosmetic (e.g., tattooing or body piercing) procedures with needles or other equipment that are contaminated with HBV. In addition, open skin lesions, such as those due to impetigo, scabies, or scratched insect bites, can play a role in HBV transmission if direct exposure to wound exudates from HBV-infected persons occurs.

The prevalence of chronic HBV infection is low (<2%) in the general population in Northern and Western Europe, North America, Australia, New Zealand, Mexico, and Southern South America (Map 4–5). In the United States and many other developed countries, children and adolescents are routinely vaccinated against hepatitis B. The highest incidence of disease is in younger adults, and most HBV infections are acquired through unprotected sex with HBV-infected partners or through shared needles used for injection drug use. The prevalence of chronic HBV infection is intermediate (2%–7%) in South Central and Southwest Asia, Israel, Japan, Eastern and Southern Europe, Russia, most areas surrounding the Amazon River basin, Honduras, and Guatemala. The prevalence of chronic HBV infection is high (>8%) in all socioeconomic groups in certain areas: all of Africa; Southeast Asia, including China, Korea, Indonesia, and the Philippines; the Middle East, except Israel; South and Western Pacific islands; the interior Amazon River basin; and certain parts of the Caribbean (Haiti and the Dominican Republic).

RISK FOR TRAVELERS

The risk of HBV infection for international travelers is generally low, except for certain travelers in countries where the prevalence of chronic HBV infection is high or intermediate. Factors to consider in assessing risk include 1) the prevalence of chronic HBV infection in the local population, 2) the extent of direct contact with blood or secretions, or of sexual contact with potentially infected persons, and 3) the duration of travel. Modes of HBV transmission in areas with high or intermediate prevalence of chronic HBV infection that are important for travelers to consider are contaminated injection and other equipment used for health care-related procedures and blood transfusions from unscreened

MAP 4-5. GEOGRAPHIC DISTRIBUTION OF HEPATITIS B PREVALENCE, 2005

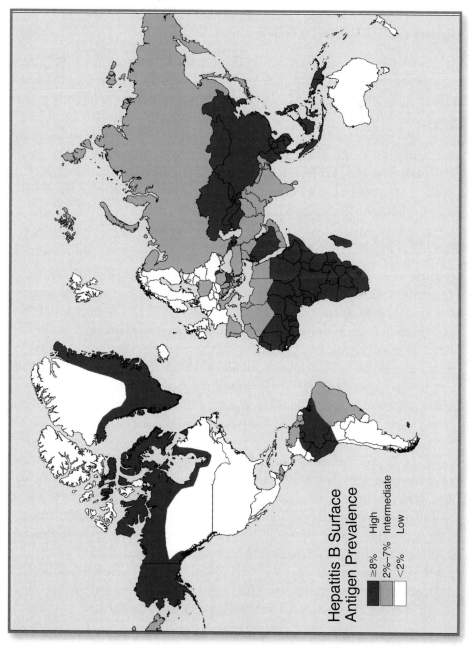

Hepatitis B Surface Antigen Prevalence

≥8% High
2%–7% Intermediate
<2% Low

donors. However, unprotected sex and sharing illegal drug injection equipment are also risks for HBV infection in these areas.

CLINICAL PRESENTATION

The incubation period of hepatitis B averages 120 days (range 45–160 days). Constitutional symptoms such as malaise and anorexia may precede jaundice by 1–2 weeks. Clinical symptoms and signs include nausea, vomiting, abdominal pain, and jaundice. Skin rashes, joint pains, and arthritis may occur. The case-fatality rate is approximately 1%. Acute HBV infection causes chronic (long-term) infection in 30%–90% of persons infected as infants or children and in 6%–10% of adolescents and adults. Chronic infection can lead to chronic liver disease, liver scarring (cirrhosis), and liver cancer.

PREVENTION

Vaccine

Hepatitis B vaccination should be administered to all unvaccinated persons traveling to areas with intermediate to high levels of endemic HBV transmission (i.e., with hepatitis B surface antigen [HBsAg] prevalence >2%) who will have close contact with the local populations. In particular, travelers who will have sex contact or will have daily physical contact with the local population; or who are likely to seek medical, dental, or other treatment in local facilities; or any combination of these activities during their stay should be advised to receive the vaccine.

Hepatitis B vaccination is currently recommended for all United States residents who work in health-care fields (medical, dental, laboratory, or other) that involve potential exposure to human blood. All unvaccinated United States children and adolescents (<19 years old) should receive hepatitis B vaccine. In addition, unvaccinated persons who have indications for hepatitis B vaccination independent of travel should be vaccinated, such as men who have sex with men, injection drug users, and heterosexuals who have recently had a sexually transmitted disease or have had more than one partner in the previous 6 months.

As part of the pre-travel education process, all travelers should be given information about the risks of hepatitis B and other bloodborne pathogens from contaminated medical equipment, injection drug use, or sexual activity, and informed of prevention measures (see below), including hepatitis B vaccination, that can be used to prevent transmission of HBV. Persons who might engage in practices that might put them at risk for HBV infection during travel should receive hepatitis B vaccination if previously unvaccinated. It is reasonable for physicians to consider their ability to accurately assess these potential risks, particularly among travelers to areas with intermediate or high levels of endemic HBV transmission, when considering if hepatitis B vaccine should be offered.

Two monovalent hepatitis B vaccines are currently licensed in the United States: Recombivax HB, manufactured by Merck and Co., Inc., and Engerix B, manufactured by GlaxoSmithKline. These vaccines are produced through recombinant DNA technology by baker's yeast into which the gene for HBsAg has been inserted. The usual schedule of primary vaccination consists of three intramuscular doses of vaccine. The recommended dose varies by product and the recipient's age (Table 4–8). The vaccine is usually administered as a three-dose series on a 0, 1, and 6 month schedule. The second dose should be given 1 month after the first dose; the third dose should be given at least 2 months after the second dose and at least 4 months after the first dose. Alternatively, the vaccine produced by GlaxoSmithKline is also approved for administration on a four-dose schedule at 0, 1, 2, and 12 months. There is also a two-dose schedule for a vaccine produced by Merck & Co., Inc., which has been licensed for children and adolescents 11–15 years of age. Using the two-dose schedule, the adult dose of Recombivax-HB is administered, with the second dose given 4-6 months after the first dose. An interrupted hepatitis B vaccine series does not need to be restarted. A three-dose series that has been started with one brand of vaccine may be completed with the other brand.

Twinrix, manufactured by GlaxoSmithKline, is a combined hepatitis A and hepatitis B vaccine licensed for persons 18 years of age or more. Primary immunization consists of three doses, given on a 0-, 1-, and 6-month schedule, the same schedule as that used for single-antigen hepatitis B vaccine (Table 4–6). Twinrix consists of inactivated hepatitis A virus and recombinant HBsAg protein, with aluminum phosphate and aluminum hydroxide as adjuvant and 2-phenoxyethanol as a preservative.

Individual clinicians may choose to use an accelerated schedule (for either the hepatitis B vaccine or Twinrix) (i.e., doses at days 0, 7,

TABLE 4-8. RECOMMENDED DOSES OF CURRENTLY LICENSED HEPATITIS B VACCINES[1]

| GROUP | DOSE | |
	RECOMBIVAX-HB[1,2]	ENGERIX-B[1]
All infants (regardless of mother's HBsAg status), children, adolescents, and adults, birth through 19 years	5 μg	10 μg
Adults ≥20 years of age	10 μg	20 μg
Dialysis patients and other immunocompromised persons	40 μg[3]	40 μg[4]

[1]Both vaccines are routinely administered in a three-dose series. Engerix-B also has been licensed for a four-dose series administered at 0, 1, 2, and 12 months.
[2]Recombivax-HB is now approved in a two-dose schedule for 11- to 15-year-olds (see "Preventive Measures").
[3]Special formulation (40 μg in 1.0 mL)
[4]Two 1.0-mL doses given at one site, in a four-dose schedule at 0, 1, 2, 6 months

and 21) for travelers who will depart before an approved vaccination schedule can be completed. The FDA has not approved accelerated schedules that involve vaccination at more than one time during a single month for hepatitis B vaccines currently licensed in the United States. Persons who receive a vaccination on an accelerated schedule that is not FDA approved should also receive a booster dose at one year after the start of the series to promote long-term immunity.

Ideally, vaccination should begin at least 6 months before travel so the full vaccine series can be completed before departure. Because some protection is provided by one or two doses, the vaccine series should be initiated, if indicated, even if it cannot be completed before departure. Optimal protection, however, is not conferred until after the final vaccine dose. There is no interference between hepatitis B vaccine and other simultaneously administered vaccine(s) or with IG. The optimum site of injection in adults is the deltoid muscle. Long-term studies of healthy adults and children indicate that immunologic memory remains intact for at least 15 years and confers protection against chronic HBV infection, even though hepatitis B surface antibody (anti-HBs) levels can become low or decline below detectable levels. For children and adults whose immune status is normal, booster doses of vaccine are not recommended. Serologic testing to assess antibody levels is not necessary for most vaccinees. (See *Vaccine Recommendations for Infants and Children,* for a discussion of the hepatitis B immunization schedule for infants who will be traveling.)

Adverse Reactions

Hepatitis B vaccines have been shown to be very safe for persons of all ages. Pain at the injection site (3%–29%) and elevated temperature >37.7° C (>99.9° F) (1%–6%) are the most frequently reported side effects among vaccine recipients. In placebo-controlled studies, these side effects were reported no more frequently among persons receiving hepatitis B vaccine than among those receiving placebo. Among children receiving both hepatitis B vaccine and diphtheria-tetanus-pertussis (DTP) vaccine, these mild side effects have been observed no more frequently than among children receiving DTP vaccine alone. For hepatitis A vaccine (a component of the combination hepatitis A/hepatitis B vaccine Twinrix), the most frequently reported adverse reactions occurring within 3–5 days were soreness or pain at the injection site (56% among adults and 8% among children) and headache (14% among adults and 4% among children). No serious adverse events among children or adults that could be definitively attributed to hepatitis A vaccine or increases in serious adverse events among vaccinated persons compared with baseline rates have been identified.

Precautions and Contraindications

These vaccines should not be administered to persons with a history of hypersensitivity to any vaccine component, including yeast. The vaccine contains a recombinant protein (HBsAg) that is noninfectious. Limited data indicate that there is no apparent risk of adverse events to the developing fetus when hepatitis B vaccine is administered to pregnant women. HBV infection affecting a pregnant woman can result in serious disease for the mother and chronic infection for the newborn. Neither pregnancy nor lactation should be considered a contraindication for vaccination.

Behavioral preventive measures are similar to those for HIV infection and AIDS. When seeking medical or dental care, travelers should be advised to be alert to the use of medical, surgical, and dental equipment that has not been adequately sterilized or disinfected, reuse of contaminated equipment, and unsafe injecting practices (e.g., reuse of disposable needles and syringes). HBV and other bloodborne pathogens can be transmitted if tools are not sterile or if the tattoo artist or piercer does not follow other proper infection-control procedures (e.g., washing hands, using latex gloves, and cleaning and disinfecting surfaces and instruments). Travelers should be advised to consider the health risks if they are considering getting a tattoo or body piercing in areas where adequate sterilization or disinfection procedures might not be available or practiced. (See *Seeking Health Care Abroad*.)

TREATMENT

No specific treatment is available for acute illness caused by hepatitis B. Antiviral drugs are approved for the treatment of chronic hepatitis B.

Bibliography

Bock HL, Loscher T, Scheiermann N, et al. Accelerated schedule for hepatitis B immunization. J Travel Med. 1995;2:213–7.

CDC. Hepatitis B virus: a comprehensive strategy for eliminating transmission in the United States through universal childhood vaccination. Recommendations of the Immunization Practices Advisory Committee (ACIP). Morbid Mortal Wkly Rep MMWR. 1991;40(RR-13):1–25.

CDC. Updated U.S. Public Health Service guidelines for the management of occupational exposures to HBV, HCV and HIV and recommendations for postexposure prophylaxis. Morbid Mortal Wkly Rep MMWR. 2001;50(RR-11):1–54.

CDC. Global progress toward universal childhood hepatitis B vaccination. MMWR. 2003;52:868–70.

Goldstein ST, Alter MJ, Williams IT, et al. Incidence and risk factors for acute hepatitis B in the United States, 1982-1998: implications for vaccination programs. J Infect Dis. 2002;185:713–9.

Lee WM. Hepatitis B virus infection. N Engl J Med. 1997;337:1733–45.

Mast E, Mahoney F, Kane M, et al. Hepatitis B vaccine. In: Plotkin SA, Orenstein WA, editors. Vaccines. 4th ed. Philadelphia: W.B. Saunders; 2004.

Simonsen L, Kane A, Lloyd J, et al. Unsafe injections in the developing world and transmission of bloodborne pathogens: a review. Bull World Health Organ. 1999;77:789–800.

Are booster immunisations needed for lifelong hepatitis B immunity? European Consensus Group on Hepatitis B Immunity. Lancet. 2000;355:561–5.

—ANTHONY FIORE AND BETH BELL

>>Hepatitis, Viral, Type C

DESCRIPTION

Hepatitis C is caused by the hepatitis C virus (HCV). Most persons who acquire acute HCV infection either have no symptoms or have a mild clinical illness. However, chronic HCV infection develops in 75%–85% of those acutely infected, with chronic liver disease developing in 60%–70% of chronically infected persons. Chronic hepatitis C is the leading cause for liver transplantation in the United States.

OCCURRENCE

HCV is transmitted primarily through activities that result in the exchange of blood; it is less commonly transmitted by sexual activity. The most frequent mode of transmission in the United States is through sharing of drug-injecting equipment among injecting drug users. For international travelers, the principal activities that can result in blood exposure include receiving blood transfusions that have not been screened for HCV; having medical or dental procedures or engaging in activities (e.g., acupuncture, tattooing, or injecting drug use) in which equipment has not been adequately sterilized or disinfected or in which contaminated equipment is reused; and working in health-care fields (e.g., medical, dental, or laboratory) that entail direct exposure to human blood.

Approximately 3% (170 million) of the world's population has been infected with HCV. For most countries, the prevalence of HCV infection is <3%. Prevalence is higher (up to 15%) in some countries in Africa and Asia, and highest (>15%) in Egypt.

RISK FOR TRAVELERS

Travelers' risk for contracting HCV infection is generally low. To assess risk, travelers should be advised to consider the extent of their direct contact with blood, particularly receipt of blood transfusions from unscreened donors, or exposure to contaminated equipment used in health care-related or cosmetic (e.g., tattooing) procedures.

CLINICAL PRESENTATION

Most persons (80%) with acute HCV infection have no symptoms. If symptoms occur, they may include loss of appetite, abdominal pain, fatigue, nausea, dark urine, and jaundice. Chronic infection occurs in 75%–85% of infected persons, leading to chronic liver disease in 60%–70%. The most common symptom of chronic hepatitis C is fatigue, although severe liver disease develops in 10%–20% of infected persons.

PREVENTION

No vaccine is available. When seeking medical or dental care, travelers should be advised to be alert to the use of medical, surgical, and dental equipment that has not been adequately sterilized or disinfected, reuse of contaminated equipment, and unsafe injecting practices (e.g., reuse of disposable needles and syringes). HCV and other bloodborne pathogens can be transmitted if tools are not sterile or if the tattoo artist or piercer does not follow other proper infection-control procedures (e.g., washing hands, using latex gloves, and cleaning and disinfecting surfaces and instruments). Travelers should be advised to consider the health risks if they are thinking about getting a tattoo or body piercing in areas where adequate sterilization or disinfection procedures might not be available or practiced. (See section on *Seeking Health Care Abroad.*)

TREATMENT

No specific treatment is available for acute hepatitis C. Antiviral drugs are available for the treatment of chronic hepatitis C in persons >18 years of age.

Bibliography

CDC. Recommendations for prevention and control of hepatitis C Virus (HCV) infection and HCV-related chronic disease. Morbid Mortal Wkly Rep MMWR. 1998; 47(RR-19):1–39.

Henderson DK. Managing occupational risks for hepatitis C transmission in the health care setting. Clin Microbiol Rev. 2003;16:546–68.

Simonsen L, Kane A, Lloyd J, et al. Unsafe injections in the developing world and transmission of bloodborne pathogens: a review. Bull World Health Organ. 1999;77:789–800.

Wasley A, Alter MJ. Epidemiology of hepatitis C: geographic differences and temporal trends. Semin Liver Dis. 2000; 20:1–16.

The Global Burden of Hepatitis C Working Group. Global burden of disease (GBD) for hepatitis C. J Clin Pharmacol. 2004;44:20–9.

–ANTHONY FIORE AND BETH BELL

>>Hepatitis, Viral, Type E

DESCRIPTION

Hepatitis E, which is caused by the hepatitis E virus (HEV), cannot be distinguished reliably from other forms of acute viral hepatitis except by specific serologic testing.

OCCURRENCE

HEV, which is transmitted by the fecal-oral route, occurs both in epidemic and sporadic forms. Transmission is associated primarily with ingestion of fecally contaminated drinking water. The potential for HEV transmission from contaminated food is still under investigation, and there is no evidence of transmission by percutaneous or sexual exposures.

Hepatitis E occurs primarily in adults. The highest rates of symptomatic disease (jaundice) have been reported in young to middle-aged adults. Lower disease rates in younger age groups may be the result of subclinical HEV infection. Chronic infection does not occur.

Epidemics and sporadic cases of hepatitis E have been reported from areas of Asia (Afghanistan, Bangladesh, Burma [Myanmar], China, India, Indonesia, Kazakhstan, Kyrgyzstan, Malaysia, Mongolia, Nepal, Pakistan, Tajikistan, Turkmenistan, and Uzbekistan), Mexico, the Middle East, Northern Africa, and sub-Saharan Africa. No outbreaks have been recognized in Europe, the United States, Australia, or South America. Hepatitis E usually occurs in persons who travel to or live in an endemic area. However, three cases have been identified in U.S. residents who had no history of recent international travel. Studies are in progress to determine if hepatitis E is an endemic disease in the United States.

RISK FOR TRAVELERS

The incidence of hepatitis E among travelers is unknown but likely low. As with hepatitis A, risk for infection is highest for those who frequently eat or drink in settings of poor sanitation.

CLINICAL PRESENTATION

The incubation period averages 40 days (range 15–60 days). Signs and symptoms, if they occur, include fatigue, loss of appetite, nausea, abdominal pain, and fever. Most patients with hepatitis E have a self-limiting course. Hepatitis E has a low (0.5%–4.0%) case-fatality rate in the general population. Fulminant hepatitis, however, is more commonly associated with hepatitis E than with other types of viral hepatitis, particularly among pregnant women in the second or third trimester. Fetal loss is common. Case-fatality rates as high as 15%–25% have been reported among pregnant women. Perinatal transmission of HEV has also been reported.

No FDA-approved diagnostic test is available, although some U.S. commercial laboratories offer serologic tests for HEV infection. Several of these tests have been shown to perform well in detecting anti-HEV in known positive sera, such as from travelers to an HEV-endemic country who develop acute hepatitis but have negative test results for other potential infectious and noninfectious causes of hepatitis. However, these tests provide highly discordant results when used on panels of U.S. blood donor sera, indicating that use of currently available serologic tests in persons without signs or symptoms of hepatitis and recent travel to an endemic country is unreliable, and results in this setting should be interpreted with caution.

PREVENTION

Vaccines to prevent hepatitis E are being developed, but none are yet available. Immune globulin prepared from plasma collected in HEV-endemic areas has not been effective in preventing clinical disease during HEV outbreaks. IG prepared from plasma collected from parts of the world where HEV is not an endemic disease is unlikely to be effective. The best prevention of infection is to avoid potentially contaminated water and food, using measures recommended to prevent hepatitis A and other enteric infections.

TREATMENT

No specific treatment is available for hepatitis E. Treatment is supportive.

Bibliography

CDC. Hepatitis E among U.S. travelers, 1989-1992. MMWR. 1993;42:1–4.

Krawczynski K, Aggarwal R, Kamili S. Hepatitis E. Infect Dis Clin North Am. 2000;14:669–87.

Labrique AB, Thomas DL, Stoszek SK, et al. Hepatitis E: an emerging infectious disease. Epidemiol Rev. 1999;21:162–79.

Mast EE, Alter MJ, Holland PV, et al. Evaluation of assays for antibody to hepatitis E virus by a serum panel. Hepatology. 1998;27:857–61.

Mast EE, Kuramoto IK, Favorov MO, et al. Prevalence of and risk factors for antibody to hepatitis E virus seroreactivity among blood donors in Northern California. J Infect Dis. 1997;176:34–40.

Schwartz E, Jenks NP, Van Damme P, et al. Hepatitis E virus infection in travelers. Clin Infect Dis. 1999;29:1312–4.

–ANTHONY FIORE AND BETH BELL

>>Histoplasmosis

DESCRIPTION

Histoplasmosis is a disease caused by the fungus *Histoplasma capsulatum*. The fungus usually grows in soil enriched with accumulations of bat or bird droppings. The disease is acquired via inhalation of spores (conidia) from soil contaminated with bat or bird droppings.

OCCURRENCE

In the United States, *H. capsulatum* var. *capsulatum* is found along the Ohio and Mississippi River valleys, mostly in the central and southeastern states. Its occurrence has been described on every continent except Antarctica. Autochthonous human cases have been reported throughout North, Central, and South America, the Caribbean, parts of the Middle East (Iran and Turkey), parts of Asia (Pakistan, India, China, Thailand, Indonesia, Vietnam, Malaysia, Philippines, Burma, and Japan); parts of Europe (northern Italy, Bulgaria, Spain, Hungary, Austria, France, Portugal, Romania, the countries of the former Soviet Union, Great Britain, Ireland, and Norway); parts of Africa; and Australia.

RISK FOR TRAVELERS

Persons who visit endemic areas and are exposed to accumulations of bat guano or bird droppings are at increased risk for infection. Not all sources of exposure are obvious when visiting endemic areas; however, activities such as spelunking, mining, construction, excavation, demolition, roofing, chimney cleaning, farming, gardening, and installing heating and air-conditioning systems are known to be associated with disease (high-risk activities). While in caves or mines, spending time close to the ground or kicking up dirt infested with bat guano containing *H. capsulatum* can increase the risk of infection. Histoplasmosis is not transmitted directly from person to person.

CLINICAL PRESENTATION

Ninety percent of infections are asymptomatic or result in a mild influenza-like illness. Some infections, however, cause acute pulmonary histoplasmosis, manifested by high fever, headache, nonproductive cough, chills, weakness, and pleuritic chest pain. Symptoms occur 3–17 days after exposure, and most persons recover spontaneously 2–3 weeks after symptom onset. Dissemination, especially to the gastrointestinal tract and central nervous system, can occur in persons with severe immunocompromising conditions (e.g., HIV infection). Reinfection and reactivation can occur.

PREVENTION

Persons at increased risk for severe disease should be advised to avoid high-risk areas, such as bat-inhabited caves. If exposure cannot be avoided, persons should be advised to decrease dust generation in infested areas by watering the areas before engaging in dust-generating activities and to wear masks and special protective equipment. Hosing off footwear and placing clothing in airtight plastic bags to be laundered after engaging in high-risk activities could also decrease the potential for exposure. Further details about protective equipment can be obtained from http://www.cdc.gov/niosh/97-146.html. No effective vaccine for histoplasmosis is currently available.

TREATMENT

For persons with acute, localized pulmonary histoplasmosis, specific antifungal treatment is not usually necessary because the disease is self-limited. Persons with persistent symptoms can be treated with itraconazole or Amphotericin B. All persons with severe disease, including diffuse pulmonary and disseminated histoplasmosis, should be treated with either itraconazole or Amphotericin B. Pregnant women for whom treatment is indicated should be given Amphotericin B. Consultation with an infectious diseases specialist is advised.

Bibliography

Cano MV, Hajjeh RA. The epidemiology of histoplasmosis: a review. Semin Respir Infect. 2001;16:109–18.

Panackal AA, Hajjeh RA, Cetron MS, et al. Fungal infections among returning travelers. Clin Infect Dis. 2002;35:1088–95.

Wheat LJ, Kaufmann CA. Histoplasmosis. Infect Dis Clin North Am. 2003;17:1–19.

Wheat J, Sarosi G, McKinsey D, et al. Practice guidelines for the management of patients with histoplasmosis. Infectious Diseases Society of America. Clin Infect Dis. 2000;30:688–95.

–JULIETTE MORGAN

>>Influenza

DESCRIPTION

Influenza is caused by infection with either influenza A or B viruses. Influenza A viruses are further classified into subtypes on the basis of two surface proteins: hemagglutinin (H) and neuraminidase (N). Both influenza A and B viruses undergo continual minor antigenic change (i.e., drift), but influenza B viruses evolve more slowly and are not divided into subtypes. Influenza A (H1N1), A (H1N2), A (H3N2), and influenza B viruses currently circulate globally.

OCCURRENCE

In the Northern Hemisphere, seasonal epidemics of influenza generally occur during the winter months on an annual or near annual basis and are responsible for approximately 36,000 deaths in the United States each year. Influenza virus infections cause disease in all age groups. Rates of infection are highest among infants, children, and adolescents, but rates of serious morbidity and mortality are highest among persons ≥65 years of age and persons of any age who have medical conditions that place them at high risk for complications from influenza (e.g., chronic cardiopulmonary disease). Children aged <2 years have rates of influenza-related hospitalization that are as high as those in the elderly. The emergence of a novel human influenza A virus could lead to a global pandemic, during which rates of morbidity and mortality from influenza-related complications could increase dramatically.

RISK FOR TRAVELERS

The risk for exposure to influenza during international travel depends on the time of year and destination. In the tropics, influenza can occur throughout the year, while in the temperate regions of the Southern Hemisphere most activity occurs from April through September. In temperate climates, travelers can also be exposed to influenza during the summer, especially when traveling as part of large tourist groups with travelers from areas of the world where influenza viruses are circulating. Influenza vaccine should be recommended before travel for persons at high risk for complications of influenza if 1) influenza vaccine was not received during the preceding fall or winter, 2) travel is planned to the tropics, 3) travel is planned with large groups of tourists at any time of year, or 4) travel is planned to the Southern Hemisphere from April through September. In North America, travel-related influenza vaccination should take place by spring when possible, because influenza vaccine may not be available during the summer. Travelers at high risk for influenza-related complications who plan summer travel should consult with their physicians to discuss the symptoms and risks of influenza before embarking.

CLINICAL PRESENTATION

Uncomplicated influenza illness is characterized by the abrupt onset of constitutional and respiratory signs and symptoms (e.g., fever, myalgia, headache, malaise, nonproductive cough, sore throat, and rhinitis). Among children, otitis media, nausea, and vomiting are also commonly reported with influenza illness. Respiratory illness caused by influenza is difficult to distinguish from illness caused by other respiratory pathogens on the basis of symptoms alone, and laboratory testing can aid in diagnosis. Influenza illness typically resolves relatively quickly for most persons, although cough and malaise can persist for >2 weeks. Influenza can exacerbate chronic conditions (e.g., pulmonary or cardiac disease), leading to secondary infections and severe complications. Influenza-related deaths can result from pneumonia as well as from exacerbations of cardiopulmonary conditions and other chronic diseases.

PREVENTION

Vaccines

Annual vaccination of persons at high risk for complications before the influenza season is the most effective measure for preventing influenza and associated complications. Two types of influenza vaccine are currently available for use in the United States: inactivated vaccine, administered by intramuscular injection, and live, attenuated influenza vaccine (LAIV), administered by nasal spray. LAIV is approved for use only in healthy persons 5–49 years of age. Annual influenza vaccination is recommended for the following groups who are at high risk for complications from influenza:

- Persons ≥50 years of age.
- Residents of nursing homes and other chronic-care facilities that house people of any age who have chronic medical conditions.

- Anyone ≥6 months of age who has a chronic disorder of the pulmonary or cardiovascular system, including asthma.
- Anyone ≥6 months of age who has required regular medical follow-up or hospitalization during the preceding year because of a chronic metabolic disease (including diabetes mellitus), renal dysfunction, hemoglobinopathy, or immunosuppression (including immuno-suppression caused by medications and HIV).
- Anyone 6 months to 18 years of age who is receiving long-term aspirin therapy and might be at risk for developing Reye syndrome after influenza.
- Women who will be pregnant during the influenza season.
- Children aged 6–23 months.
- Health-care workers and others (including household members) in close contact with persons at high risk for developing influenza-related complications.

Dosing, Timing, and Route of Vaccination

For persons at high risk for complications from influenza, annual vaccination is recommended because vaccine-derived immunity declines during the year and because the vaccine strains are continually updated to reflect ongoing antigenic changes among circulating influenza viruses. Dosage recommendations differ according to age group and type of vaccine used. For inactivated vaccine, two doses administered at least 1 month apart are required for previously unvaccinated infants and children <9 years of age. For previously unvaccinated children aged 5–8 years receiving LAIV, two doses are administered at least 6 weeks apart. For situations in which a child receives two different vaccine types, 4 weeks should separate doses if inactivated vaccine is used first, and 6 weeks should separate doses if LAIV is used first. In adults, studies have indicated little or no improvement in antibody response when a second dose of inactivated vaccine is administered during the same season; therefore, a booster is not recommended. For inactivated vaccine, infants and young children should be vaccinated in the anterolateral aspect of the thigh; all other recipients should be vaccinated in the deltoid muscle. LAIV is administered by nasal spray.

The target groups for influenza and pneumococcal vaccination overlap considerably. For travelers at high risk who have not previously been vaccinated with pneumococcal vaccine, health-care providers should strongly consider administering pneumococcal and influenza vaccines concurrently. Both vaccines can be administered at the same time at different sites without increasing side effects. Infants and children can receive influenza vaccine at the same time they receive other routine vaccinations.

Composition of the Vaccines
Both influenza vaccines contain three strains of inactivated influenza viruses. Viruses in inactivated vaccines are killed, while those in LAIV are live. These live viruses are attenuated and do not cause disease. The viruses used in both vaccines are representative of viruses likely to circulate in the upcoming season, and usually one or more vaccine strains are updated annually. Because the vaccine is grown in hen eggs, the vaccine may contain small amounts of egg protein. Influenza vaccine distributed in the United States may also contain thimerosal, a mercury-containing preservative. The package insert should be consulted regarding the use of other compounds to inactivate the viruses or limit bacterial contamination.

Adverse Reactions
Inactivated Vaccine
The most frequent side effect of vaccination with inactivated vaccine is soreness at the vaccination site that lasts up to 2 days. These local reactions generally are mild and rarely interfere with the ability to conduct usual daily activities. Fever, malaise, myalgia, and other systemic symptoms can occur following vaccination and most often affect people who have had no previous exposure to the influenza virus antigens in the vaccine (e.g., young children). These reactions begin 6 to 12 hours after vaccination and can persist for 1 to 2 days.

LAIV
The most frequent side effects of vaccination with LAIV include nasal congestion, headache, fever, vomiting, abdominal pain, and myalgia. These symptoms are associated more often with the first dose and are self-limited. There may be an increase in asthma or reactive airway disease in children aged <5 years, and LAIV is not approved for use among children in this age group.

Other Reactions
Allergic
Immediate reactions (e.g., hives, angioedema, allergic asthma, and systemic anaphylaxis) rarely occur after influenza vaccination. These reac-

tions probably result from hypersensitivity to some vaccine component; most reactions likely are caused by residual egg protein and occur among people who have severe egg allergy. People who have developed hives, have had swelling of the lips or tongue, or have experienced acute respiratory distress or collapse after eating eggs should consult a physician for appropriate evaluation to determine if vaccine should be administered. People who have documented immune globulin E (IgE)-mediated hypersensitivity to eggs, including those who have had occupational asthma or other allergic responses due to exposure to egg protein, may also be at increased risk for reactions from influenza vaccine, and similar consultation should be advised. Protocols have been published for safely administering influenza vaccine to people with egg allergies.

Guillain-Barré Syndrome (GBS)
Investigations to date indicate no substantial increase in GBS associated with influenza vaccines (other than the "swine flu" vaccine of 1976). A study of the 1992–93 and 1993–94 influenza seasons estimated a risk of GBS of slightly more than 1 case per million people vaccinated. The potential benefits of influenza vaccination in preventing serious illness, hospitalization, and death greatly outweigh the possible risks for developing vaccine-associated GBS.

Precautions and Contraindications
Pregnancy
Many experts consider influenza vaccination with inactivated vaccine safe during any stage of pregnancy. A study of influenza vaccination of more than 2,000 pregnant women demonstrated no adverse fetal effects associated with influenza vaccine. Influenza vaccine does not affect the safety of mothers who are breastfeeding or their infants. Breastfeeding does not adversely affect immune response and is not a contraindication for vaccination.

Persons Infected with HIV
Information is limited on the frequency and severity of influenza illness or the benefits of influenza vaccination among HIV-infected persons. On the basis of a risk-modeling study, the risk for influenza-related death among persons with AIDS appears higher than among those without AIDS. In addition, symptoms of influenza might be prolonged and the risk for complications from influenza increased for certain HIV-infected persons. HIV-infected persons who have minimal AIDS-related

symptoms and high CD4+ T-lymphocyte cell counts can develop protective influenza antibody titers from influenza vaccine, and vaccination has been shown to prevent influenza in this group. However, influenza vaccine might not induce protective antibody titers in people who have advanced HIV disease and low CD4+ T-lymphocyte cell counts; a second dose of vaccine does not improve the immune response in these persons. Deterioration of CD4+ T-lymphocyte cell counts and progression of HIV disease have not been demonstrated among HIV-infected people who receive the vaccine. The effect of antiretroviral therapy on potential increases in HIV ribonucleic acid (RNA) levels following either natural influenza infection or influenza vaccine is unknown. Because influenza can result in serious illness and complications and because influenza vaccination can result in the production of protective antibody titers, vaccination will benefit many HIV-infected persons, including HIV-infected pregnant women.

Antiviral Medications

Influenza-specific antiviral drugs for chemoprophylaxis of influenza are important adjuncts to vaccine. The four currently licensed U.S. antiviral agents are amantadine, rimantadine, zanamivir, and oseltamivir. Amantadine and rimantadine are active against influenza A viruses but not influenza B viruses. Both drugs are approved by the U.S. Food and Drug Administration for the prophylaxis of influenza A virus infections. Oseltamivir has activity against both influenza A and B viruses and has been approved for prophylaxis. Amantadine and rimantadine are approved for prophylaxis in persons aged ≥1 year, and oseltamivir is approved for prophylaxis in persons aged ≥13 years.

TREATMENT

Amantadine and rimantadine are approved by the U.S. Food and Drug Administration for the treatment of influenza A virus infections. Zanamivir and oseltamivir are currently approved for treatment of both influenza A and B virus infections. These four drugs differ in dosing, approved age groups for use, side effects, and cost. The package inserts should be consulted for more information.

Bibliography

Harper SA, Fukuda K, Uyeki T, et al. Prevention and control of
     influenza: recommendations of the Advisory Committee on Immu-

nization Practices (ACIP). Morbid Mortal Wkly Rep MMWR. 2004 May 28;53(RR-6):1–40.

Marsden AG. Influenza outbreak related to air travel. Med J Aust. 2003 Aug 4;179(3):172–3.

O'Brien D, Tobin S, Brown GV, et al. Fever in returned travelers: review of hospital admissions for a 3-year period. Clin Infect Dis. 2001 Sep 1;33(5):603–9.

Uyeki TM, Zane SB, Bodnar UR, et al. Large summertime influenza A outbreak among tourists in Alaska and the Yukon Territory. Clin Infect Dis. 2003 May 1;36(9):1095–102.

Uyeki TM. Influenza diagnosis and treatment in children: a review of studies on clinically useful tests and antiviral treatment for influenza. Pediatr Infect Dis J. 2003;22(2):164–77.

–SCOTT HARPER

>>Legionellosis

DESCRIPTION

Legionellosis encompasses two diseases, Legionnaires' disease and Pontiac fever, caused by bacteria in the genus *Legionella*. The bacterium grows in warm, freshwater environments. Under specific conditions, it can be inhaled into the lungs, the principal site of infection.

OCCURRENCE

Legionellae are ubiquitous worldwide in freshwater environments. However, concentrations of the organism do not reach sufficient levels to cause disease unless three environmental conditions are met. First, the aquatic environment must be somewhat stagnant. For example, plumbing systems in large buildings (e.g., hotels) sometimes have sections that are infrequently used. Second, the water must be warm enough (25°–42° C, 77°–108° F) to promote bacterial growth to sufficient numbers to cause disease. Third, the water must be aerosolized so that the bacteria can be inhaled into the lungs. These three conditions are met almost exclusively in developed or industrialized settings. Disease does not occur in association with natural settings such as waterfalls, lakes, or streams. Outbreaks of legionellosis have been described in numerous countries throughout the world.

RISK FOR TRAVELERS

Travelers who visit developed settings (e.g., hotels, even in developing countries) and are exposed to aerosolized, warm water are at risk for infection. Despite the presence of *Legionella* bacteria in many aquatic environments, the risk of developing legionellosis for most individuals is low. Elderly and immunocompromised travelers, such as those being treated for cancer, are at higher risk. Exposures can occur during activities such as recreation in or near a whirlpool spa (e.g., on a cruise ship), while showering in a hotel, or touring in cities with buildings that have cooling towers. The largest outbreak (449 cases) ever reported was traced to a cooling tower on the roof of a city hospital in Murcia, Spain, in 2001.

CLINICAL PRESENTATION

The first sign of Legionnaires' disease is pneumonia which usually requires hospitalization and can be fatal in 10%–15% of cases. Symptoms occur 2–10 days after exposure. In outbreak settings, fewer than 5% of persons exposed to the source of the outbreak actually develop Legionnaires' disease. Pontiac fever is different from Legionnaires' disease in that Pontiac fever presents as an influenza-like illness, with fever, headache, and myalgias, but no signs of pneumonia. Pontiac fever can affect healthy individuals as well as those with underlying illnesses, and symptoms occur within 72 hours of exposure. Full recovery is the rule. Up to 95% of people exposed in outbreak settings can develop symptoms of Pontiac fever. Infrequently, simultaneous outbreaks of Legionnaires' disease and Pontiac fever can be traced to the same source. Person-to-person transmission does not occur with either Legionnaires' disease or Pontiac fever.

PREVENTION

Travelers at increased risk for infection, such as the elderly or those with immunocompromising conditions (e.g., cancer, diabetes), may choose to avoid high-risk areas, such as whirlpool spas. If exposure cannot be avoided, travelers should be advised to seek medical attention promptly if they develop symptoms of Legionnaires' disease or

Pontiac fever. There is no vaccine for legionellosis and antibiotic prevention is not effective.

TREATMENT

For travelers with Legionnaires' disease, specific antibiotic treatment is necessary and should be administered promptly while diagnostic tests are being processed. Appropriate antibiotics include quinolones and macrolides. Treatment may be necessary for up to 3 weeks. In severe cases, patients may have prolonged stays in intensive-care units. Consultation with an infectious diseases specialist is advised. Pontiac fever is a self-limited illness that requires supportive care only; antibiotics have no benefit.

Bibliography

Benin AL, Benson RF, Arnold KE, et al. An outbreak of travel-associated Legionnaires' disease and Pontiac fever: the need for enhanced surveillance of travel-associated legionellosis in the United States. J Infect Dis. 2002;185:237–43.

Benin AL, Benson RF, Besser RE. Trends in Legionnaires' disease, 1980-1998: declining mortality and new patterns of diagnosis. Clin Infect Dis. 2002;35:1039–46.

Fields BS, Benson RF, Besser RE. *Legionella* and Legionnaires' disease: 25 years of investigation. Clin Microbiol Rev. 2002;15:506–26.

Jernigan DB, Hoffman J, Cetron MS, et al. Outbreak of Legionnaires' disease among cruise ship passengers exposed to a contaminated whirlpool spa. Lancet. 1996;347:494–9.

Joseph CA. Legionnaires' disease in Europe 2000–2002. Epidemiol Infect. 2004;132:417–24.

Joseph C, Morgan D, Birtles R, et al. An international investigation of an outbreak of Legionnaires' disease among UK and French tourists. Eur J Epidemiol. 1996;12:215–9.

–MATTHEW MOORE

>>Leishmaniasis

DESCRIPTION

Leishmaniasis, a parasitic disease caused by obligate intracellular protozoa, is transmitted by the bite of some species of phlebotomine sand flies. The disease most commonly manifests as either a cutaneous (skin) form or a visceral (internal organ) form.

OCCURRENCE

Leishmaniasis is found in approximately 90 countries around the world, including countries in the tropics, subtropics, and southern Europe. More than 90% of the world's cases of cutaneous leishmaniasis are in Afghanistan, Algeria, Brazil, Iran, Iraq, Peru, Saudi Arabia, and Syria. More than 90% of the world's cases of visceral leishmaniasis occur in Bangladesh, Brazil, India, Nepal, and Sudan. Leishmaniasis is not found in Australia, the South Pacific, or Southeast Asia. The geographic distribution of cases of leishmaniasis evaluated in the developed world reflects travel and immigration patterns. For example, approximately 75% of the cases of leishmaniasis that are evaluated in the United States (non-military associated) and are reported to CDC are cases of cutaneous leishmaniasis that were acquired in Latin America, where it occurs from northern Mexico (rarely in rural south-central Texas) to northern Argentina.

RISK FOR TRAVELERS

Travelers of all ages are at risk for leishmaniasis if they live in or travel to leishmaniasis-endemic areas. Leishmaniasis usually is more common in rural than urban areas, but it is found in the outskirts of some cities. In the Old World, transmission of a particular species of the parasite *(Leishmania tropica)* that usually causes cutaneous leishmaniasis is common in some urban areas (e.g., Kabul, Afghanistan and Baghdad, Iraq). Risk is highest between dusk and dawn. Adventure travelers, Peace Corps volunteers, missionaries, ornithologists, and other persons who do research outdoors at night, and soldiers are examples of those who might have an increased risk for leishmaniasis, especially the cutaneous form. Even persons with short stays in leishmaniasis-endemic areas can become infected.

CLINICAL PRESENTATION

Cutaneous leishmaniasis is characterized by one or more skin sores (either painful or painless, with or without a scab) that develop weeks to months after a person is bitten by infected sand flies. If untreated, the sores can last from weeks to years and often eventually develop raised edges and a central crater. The manifestations of visceral leishmaniasis, such as fever, weight loss, enlargement of the spleen and liver, and anemia, typically develop months, but sometimes years, after a person becomes infected. If untreated, symptomatic visceral leishmaniasis typically is fatal.

PREVENTION

No vaccines or drugs for preventing infections are currently available. Preventive measures for the individual traveler are aimed at reducing contact with sand flies. Travelers should be advised to avoid outdoor activities when sand flies are most active (dusk to dawn). Although sand flies are primarily nighttime biters, infection can be acquired during the daytime if resting sand flies are disturbed. Sand fly activity in an area can easily be underestimated because sand flies are noiseless fliers and rare bites might not be noticed.

Travelers should be advised to use protective clothing and insect repellent for supplementary protection. Clothing should cover as much of the body as possible and be tolerable in the climate. Repellent with N,N-diethylmetatoluamide (DEET) should be applied to exposed skin and under the edges of clothing, such as sleeves and pant legs. DEET should be applied according to the manufacturer's instructions; repeated applications may be necessary under conditions of excessive perspiration and washing. (See *Protection against Mosquitoes and Other Arthropods.*) Impregnation of clothing with permethrin can provide additional protection, but it does not eliminate the need for repellent on exposed skin and should be repeated after every five washings.

Contact with sand flies can be reduced by using bed nets and screens on doors and windows. Fine-mesh netting (at least 18 holes to the linear inch; some sources advise even finer) is required for an effective barrier against sand flies, which are about one-third the size of mosquitoes. However, such closely woven bed nets might be difficult to tolerate in hot climates. Impregnating bed nets and window screens with permethrin can provide some protection, as can spraying dwellings with insecticide.

TREATMENT

Travelers should be advised to consult with an infectious disease or tropical medicine specialist for diagnosis and treatment. The relative merits of various treatments, including parenteral, oral, local, or topical treatments, can be discussed with the specialist. Physicians may consult with CDC to obtain information about the diagnosis and treatment of leishmaniasis. The parenteral drug sodium stibogluconate is available from the CDC Drug Service (404-639-3670) under an Investigational New Drug protocol. Additional information can be found on the Division of Parasitic Diseases' website: http://www.cdc.gov/ncidod/dpd/parasites/leishmania/factsht_leishmania.htm.

Bibliography

Berman JD. Human leishmaniasis: clinical, diagnostic, and chemotherapeutic developments in the last 10 years. Clin Infect Dis 1997;24:684–703.

Desjeux P. Leishmaniasis: public health aspects and control. Clin Dermatol 1996;14:417–23.

Herwaldt BL. Leishmaniasis. Lancet 1999;354:1191–9.

Herwaldt BL, Stokes SL, Juranek DD. American cutaneous leishmaniasis in U.S. travelers. Ann Intern Med 1993;118:779–84.

–BARBARA HERWALDT

>>Leptospirosis

DESCRIPTION

Leptospirosis is a bacterial zoonosis that is endemic worldwide, with a higher incidence in tropical climates. A variety of wild and domestic animals may excrete the organism in their urine or in the fluids of parturition. Humans may be infected through direct exposure to urine or fluids of parturition of infected animals, or through exposure to contaminated water or soil. A variety of occupational and recreational activities have been associated with leptospirosis, including farming, veterinary and abattoir work, and canoeing, kayaking, and swimming in contaminated water.

OCCURRENCE

Leptospira proliferate in fresh water, damp soil, vegetation, and mud. The occurrence of flooding after heavy rainfall facilitates the spread of the organism because, as water saturates the environment, *Leptospira* present in the soil pass directly into surface waters. *Leptospira* can enter the body through cut or abraded skin, mucous membranes, and conjunctivae. Ingestion of contaminated water can also lead to infection.

RISK FOR TRAVELERS

Travelers participating in recreational water activities, such as whitewater rafting, adventure racing, or kayaking, in areas where leptospirosis is endemic or epidemic could be at increased risk for the disease, particularly during periods of flooding. Travelers who might be at increased risk for leptospirosis and who have a febrile illness should be advised to consider leptospirosis as a possible cause and to seek appropriate medical care.

CLINICAL PRESENTATION

The acute, generalized illness associated with infection can mimic other tropical diseases (e.g., dengue fever, malaria, and typhus), and common symptoms include fever, chills, myalgia, nausea, diarrhea, cough, and conjunctival suffusion. Manifestations of severe disease can include jaundice, renal failure, hemorrhage, pneumonitis, and hemodynamic collapse. The laboratory diagnosis of leptospirosis requires culture of the organism or demonstration of serologic conversion by the microagglutination test (MAT). However, culture is relatively insensitive and requires specialized media, and the MAT is difficult to perform. Therefore, availability of these techniques has been restricted to reference laboratories. Recently, several rapid, simple serologic tests have been developed that are reliable and commercially available.

PREVENTION

No vaccine is available to prevent leptospirosis in the United States. Travelers who might be at an increased risk for the disease should be advised to consider preventive measures such as wearing protective clothing and minimizing contact with potentially contaminated water.

Such travelers also might benefit from chemoprophylaxis. Until further data become available, CDC recommends that travelers who might be at increased risk for leptospirosis be advised to consider chemoprophylaxis with doxycycline (200 mg orally, once a week), begun 1 to 2 days before exposure and continuing through the period of exposure. Travelers who may be at increased risk for leptospirosis and who are also in need of malaria chemoprophylaxis may consider using doxycycline for both indications. (See Table 4–9 for recommended doses).

TREATMENT

Treatment with antimicrobial agents (e.g., penicillin, amoxicillin, or doxycycline) should be initiated early in the course of the disease. An infectious diseases or tropical medicine specialist should be consulted.

Bibliography

Bajani MD, Ashford DA, Bragg SL, et al. Evaluation of four commercially available rapid serologic tests for diagnosis of leptospirosis. J Clin Microbiol. 2003;41:803–9.

Haake DA, Dundoo M, Cader R, et al. Leptospirosis, water sports, and chemoprophylaxis. Clin Infect Dis. 2002;34:e40–3.

Levett PN. Leptospirosis. Clin Microbiol Rev. 2001;14:296–326.

Morgan J, Bornstein SL, Karpati AM, et al. Outbreak of leptospirosis among triathlon participants and community residents in Springfield, Illinois, 1998. Clin Infect Dis. 2002; 34:1593–9.

Sejvar J, Bancroft E, Winthrop K, et al. Leptospirosis in "Eco-Challenge" athletes, Malaysian Borneo. Emerg Infect Dis. 2003;6:702–7.

—DAVID ASHFORD AND THOMAS CLARK

>>Lyme Disease

DESCRIPTION

Lyme disease results from infection with spirochetes belonging to the *Borrelia burgdorferi* sensu lato complex. In Europe and Asia, most cases of Lyme disease are caused by *B. burgdorferi* sensu stricto, *B. afzelii*, or

B. garinii; however, in the United States, all cases are caused by *B. burgdorferi* sensu stricto. The spirochetes are transmitted to humans through the bite of infected ticks of the *Ixodes ricinus* complex.

OCCURRENCE

Lyme disease occurs in temperate forested regions of Europe and Asia and in the northeastern, north central, and Pacific coastal regions of North America. It is not transmitted in the tropics.

RISK FOR TRAVELERS

Travelers to endemic areas who have exposure to tick habitats may be at risk for Lyme disease.

CLINICAL PRESENTATION

Manifestations of Lyme disease include a characteristic expanding rash called erythema chronicum migrans at the site of tick attachment, fever, arthritis, and neurologic manifestations, including facial palsy.

PREVENTION

Vaccine
A safe and efficacious vaccine was, until recently, available for protection from Lyme disease in endemic areas of the United States. However, the vaccine was withdrawn from the market by the manufacturer in February 2002 because of low sales and is no longer commercially available.

Other
Travelers to endemic areas should be advised to avoid tick habitats if possible. If exposure to tick habitats cannot be avoided, the application of repellents to skin and Permethrin to clothing (See *Protection Against Mosquitoes and Other Arthropods*) can reduce the risk of infection, as can daily tick checks and prompt removal of any attached ticks. Remove ticks by grasping them firmly with tweezers as close to the skin as possible and lifting gently.

TREATMENT

Travelers who have erythema chronicum migrans or other manifestations of Lyme disease should be advised to seek early medical attention.

In general, it should not be necessary to seek care from a specialist in travel or tropical medicine. Lyme disease can usually be cured by a course of antibiotic treatment.

Bibliography

Gern L, Humair PF. Ecology of *Borrelia burgdorferi* sensu lato in Europe. In: Gray JS, Kahl O, Lane RS, Stanek G, editors. Lyme borreliosis: biology, epidemiology and control. 1st ed. New York: CABI Publishing; 2002. p. 149–74.

Korenberg EI, Gorelova NB, Kovalevskii YV. Ecology of *Borrelia burgdorferi* sensu lato in Russia. In: Gray JS, Kahl O, Lane RS, Stanek G, editors. Lyme borreliosis: biology, epidemiology and control. 1st ed. New York: CABI Publishing; 2002. p. 175–200.

Miyamoto K, Masuzawa T. Ecology of *Borrelia burgdorferi* sensu lato in Japan and East Asia. In: Gray JS, Kahl O, Lane RS, Stanek G, editors. Lyme borreliosis: biology, epidemiology and control. 1st ed. New York: CABI Publishing; 2002. p. 201–22.

Stanek G, Strle F. Lyme borreliosis. Lancet. 2003;362:1639–47.

Steere AC. Lyme disease. N Eng J Med. 2001;345:115–25.

Weber K. Aspects of Lyme borreliosis in Europe. Eur J Clin Microbiol Infect Dis. 2001;20:6–13.

Wormser GP, Nadelman RB, Dattwyler RJ, et al. Practice guidelines for the treatment of Lyme disease. The Infectious Diseases Society of America. Clin Infec Dis. 2000;31 Suppl 1:S1–14.

–EDWARD B. HAYES AND PAUL MEAD

>>Malaria

DESCRIPTION

Malaria in humans is caused by one of four protozoan species of the genus *Plasmodium*: *P. falciparum*, *P. vivax*, *P. ovale*, or *P. malariae*. All species are transmitted by the bite of an infected female *Anopheles* mosquito. Occasionally, transmission occurs by blood transfusion, organ transplantation, needle-sharing, or congenitally from mother to fetus.

Although malaria can be a fatal disease, illness and death from malaria are largely preventable.

OCCURRENCE

Malaria is a major international public health problem, causing 300–500 million infections worldwide and approximately 1 million deaths annually. Information about malaria risk in specific countries (Yellow Fever Vaccine Requirements and Information on Malaria Risk and Prophylaxis, by Country) is derived from various sources, including WHO. The information presented herein was accurate at the time of publication; however, factors that can change rapidly and from year to year, such as local weather conditions, mosquito vector density, and prevalence of infection, can markedly affect local malaria transmission patterns. Updated information may be found on the CDC Travelers' Health website: http://www.cdc.gov/travel.

Malaria transmission occurs in large areas of Central and South America, the island of Hispaniola (the Dominican Republic and Haiti), Africa, Asia (including the Indian Subcontinent, Southeast Asia, and the Middle East), Eastern Europe, and the South Pacific.

The estimated risk for a traveler's acquiring malaria differs substantially from area to area. This variability is a function of the intensity of transmission within the various regions and of the itinerary and time and type of travel. From 1985 through 2002, 11,896 cases of malaria among U.S. civilians were reported to CDC. Of these, 6,961 (59%) were acquired in sub-Saharan Africa; 2,237 (19%) in Asia; 1,672 (14%) in the Caribbean and Central and South America; and 822 (7%) in other parts of the world. During this period, 76 fatal malaria infections occurred among U.S. civilians; 71 (93%) were caused by *P. falciparum*, of which 52 (73%) were acquired in sub-Saharan Africa.

Thus, most imported *P. falciparum* malaria among U.S. travelers was acquired in Africa, even though only 467,940 U.S. residents traveled to countries in that region in 2002. In contrast, that year 21 million U.S. residents traveled from the United States to other countries where malaria is endemic (including 19 million travelers to Mexico). This disparity in the risk for acquiring malaria reflects the fact that the predominant species of malaria transmitted in sub-Saharan Africa is *P. falciparum*, that malaria transmission is generally higher in Africa than in other parts of the world, and that malaria is often transmitted in urban areas as well as rural areas in sub-Saharan Africa. In contrast, malaria transmission is generally lower in Asia and South America, a larger proportion of the malaria is *P. vivax*, and most urban areas do not have malaria transmission.

RISK TO TRAVELERS

Estimating the risk for infection for various types of travelers is difficult. Risk can differ substantially even for persons who travel or reside temporarily in the same general areas within a country. For example, travelers staying in air-conditioned hotels may be at lower risk than backpackers or adventure travelers. Similarly, long-term residents living in screened and air-conditioned housing are less likely to be exposed than are persons living without such amenities, such as Peace Corps volunteers. Travelers should also be reminded that even if one has had malaria before, one can get it again and so preventive measures are still necessary.

Persons who have been in a malaria risk area, either during daytime or nighttime hours, are not allowed to donate blood in the United States for a period of time after returning from the malarious area. Persons who are residents of nonmalarious countries are not allowed to donate blood for 1 year after they have returned from a malarious area. Persons who are residents of malarious countries are not allowed to donate blood for 3 years after leaving a malarious area. Persons who have had malaria are not allowed to donate blood for 3 years after treatment for malaria.

CLINICAL PRESENTATION

Malaria is characterized by fever and influenza-like symptoms, including chills, headache, myalgias, and malaise; these symptoms can occur at intervals. Malaria may be associated with anemia and jaundice, and *P. falciparum* infections can cause seizures, mental confusion, kidney failure, coma, and death. Malaria symptoms can develop as early as 7 days after initial exposure in a malaria-endemic area and as late as several months after departure from a malarious area, after chemoprophylaxis has been terminated.

MAP 4-6. MALARIA-ENDEMIC COUNTRIES IN THE WESTERN HEMISPHERE

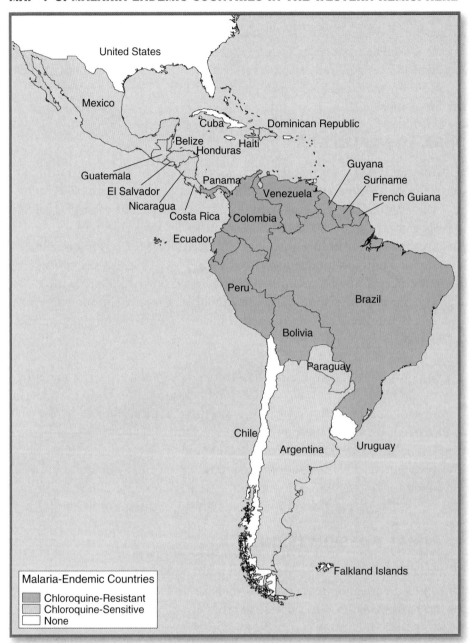

Malaria-Endemic Countries
- Chloroquine-Resistant
- Chloroquine-Sensitive
- None

MAP 4-7. MALARIA-ENDEMIC COUNTRIES IN THE EASTERN HEMISPHERE

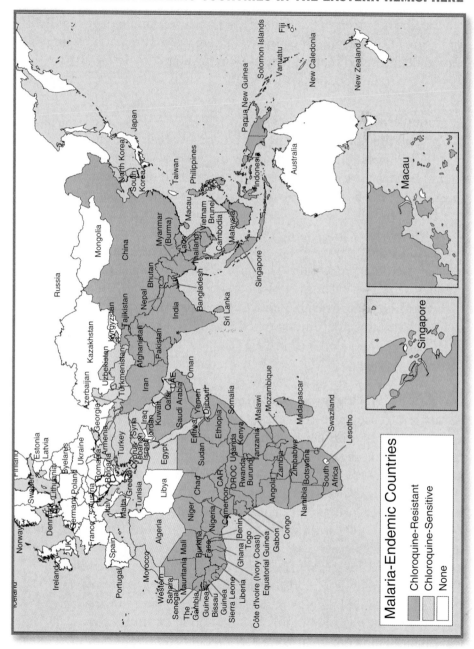

PREVENTION

No vaccine is currently available. Taking an appropriate drug regimen and using anti-mosquito measures will help prevent malaria. Travelers should be informed that no method can protect completely against the risk for contracting malaria.

Personal Protection Measures

Because of the nocturnal feeding habits of *Anopheles* mosquitoes, malaria transmission occurs primarily between dusk and dawn. Travelers should be advised to take protective measures to reduce contact with mosquitoes, especially during these hours. Such measures include remaining in well-screened areas, using mosquito bed nets (preferably insecticide-treated nets), and wearing clothes that cover most of the body. Additionally, travelers should be advised to purchase insect repellent for use on exposed skin. The most effective repellent against a wide range of vectors is DEET (N,N-diethylmetatoluamide), an ingredient in many commercially available insect repellents. The actual concentration of DEET varies widely among repellents. DEET formulations as high as 50% are recommended for both adults and children >2 months of age (See *Protection against Mosquitoes and Other Arthropods*).

Travelers not staying in well-screened or air-conditioned rooms should be advised to use a pyrethroid-containing flying-insect spray in living and sleeping areas during evening and nighttime hours. They should take additional precautions, including sleeping under bed nets (preferably insecticide-treated bed nets). In the United States, permethrin (Permanone) is available as a liquid or spray. Overseas, either permethrin or another insecticide, deltamethrin, is available and may be sprayed on bed nets and clothing for additional protection against mosquitoes. Bed nets are more effective if they are treated with permethrin or deltamethrin insecticide; bed nets may be purchased that have already been treated with insecticide. Information about ordering insecticide-treated bed nets is available at http://www.travmed.com, telephone 1-800-872 8633, fax: 413-584-6656; or http://www.travelhealthhelp.com, telephone 1-866-621-6260.

Chemoprophylaxis

Chemoprophylaxis is the strategy that uses medications before, during, and after the exposure period to prevent the disease caused by malaria parasites. The aim of prophylaxis is to prevent or suppress symptoms caused by blood-stage parasites. In addition, presumptive anti-relapse therapy (also known as terminal prophylaxis) uses medications towards the end of the exposure period (or immediately thereafter) to prevent relapses or delayed-onset clinical presentations of malaria caused by hypnozoites (dormant liver stages) of *P. vivax* or *P. ovale*.

In choosing an appropriate chemoprophylactic regimen before travel, the traveler and the health-care provider should consider several factors. The travel itinerary should be reviewed in detail and compared with the information on areas of risk in a given country (Yellow Fever Vaccine Requirements and Information on Malaria Risk and Prophylaxis, by Country) to determine whether the traveler will actually be at risk for acquiring malaria. Whether the traveler will be at risk for acquiring drug-resistant *P. falciparum* malaria should also be determined. Resistance to antimalarial drugs has developed in many regions of the world. Health-care providers should consult the latest information on resistance patterns before prescribing prophylaxis for their patients. (See section "Malaria Hotline" below for details about accessing this information from CDC.)

The resistance of *P. falciparum* to chloroquine has been confirmed in all areas with *P. falciparum* malaria except the Dominican Republic, Haiti, Central America west of the Panama Canal, Egypt, and some countries in the Middle East. In addition, resistance to sulfadoxine-pyrimethamine (e.g., Fansidar) is widespread in the Amazon River Basin area of South America, much of Southeast Asia, other parts of Asia, and, increasingly, in large parts of Africa. Resistance to mefloquine has been confirmed on the borders of Thailand with Burma (Myanmar) and Cambodia, in the western provinces of Cambodia, and in the eastern states of Burma (Myanmar).

Tolerability
Malaria chemoprophylaxis with mefloquine or chloroquine should begin 1–2 weeks before travel to malarious areas; prophylaxis with doxycycline, atovaquone/proguanil, or primaquine can begin 1–2 days before travel. Beginning the drug before travel allows the antimalarial agent to be in the blood before the traveler is exposed to malaria parasites. Chemoprophylaxis can be started earlier if there are particular concerns about tolerating one of the medications. Starting the medication 3–4

CHECKLIST FOR TRAVELERS TO MALARIOUS AREAS

The following is a checklist of key issues to be considered in advising travelers.

Risk for Malaria (Yellow Fever Vaccine Requirements and Information on Malaria Risk and Prophylaxis, by Country)

Travelers should be informed about the risk of malaria infection and the presence of drug-resistant *Plasmodium falciparum* malaria in their areas of destination.

Personal Protective Measures (Protection against Mosquitoes and Other Arthropods Vectors)

Travelers should be told how to protect themselves against mosquito bites.

Chemoprophylaxis
Travelers should be–

- Advised to start chemoprophylaxis before travel and to use prophylaxis continuously while in malaria-endemic areas and for 4 weeks (chloroquine, doxycycline, or mefloquine) or 7 days (atovaquone/proguanil) after leaving such areas.

- Questioned about drug allergies and other contraindications for use of drugs to prevent malaria.

- Advised which drug to use for chemoprophylaxis and whether atovaquone/ proguanil should be carried for presumptive self-treatment.

- Informed that any antimalarial drug can cause side effects and, if these side effects are serious, that medical help should be sought promptly and use of the drug discontinued.

- Advised that, while using chemoprophylaxis greatly decreases their risk of acquiring malaria, preventive measures cannot guarantee complete protection.

In Case of Illness, travelers should be–

- Informed that symptoms of malaria can be mild to severe and that they should suspect malaria if they experience fever, chills, or other influenza-like symptoms such as persistent headaches, muscle aches and weakness, vomiting, or diarrhea.

- Informed that malaria can be fatal if treatment is delayed. Medical help should be sought promptly if malaria is suspected, and a blood sample should be taken and examined for malaria parasites on one or more occasions.

- Reminded that self-treatment should be taken only if prompt medical care is not available and that medical advice should still be sought as soon as possible after self-treatment.

Special Categories
Pregnant women and young children require special attention because of the potential effects of malaria illness and their inability to take certain drugs (e.g., doxycycline).

weeks in advance allows potential adverse events to occur before travel. If unacceptable side effects develop, there would be time to change the medication before the traveler's departure.

The drugs used for antimalarial chemoprophylaxis are generally well tolerated. However, side effects can occur. Minor side effects usually do not require stopping the drug. Travelers who have serious side effects should see a health-care provider. See the section below on "Adverse Reactions and Contraindications" for more detail on safety and tolerability of the drugs used for malaria prevention. The health-care provider should establish whether the traveler has previously experienced an allergic or other reaction to one of the antimalarial drugs of choice. In addition, the health-care provider should determine whether medical care will be readily accessible during travel should the traveler develop intolerance to the drug being used and need to change to a different agent.

General Recommendations for Prophylaxis
Chemoprophylaxis should continue during travel in the malarious areas and after leaving the malarious areas (4 weeks after travel for chloroquine, mefloquine, and doxycycline, and 7 days after travel for atovaquone/proguanil and primaquine). In comparison with drugs with short half-lives, which are taken daily, drugs with longer half-lives, which are taken weekly, offer the advantage of a wider margin of error if the traveler is late with a dose. For example, if a traveler is 1–2 days late with a weekly drug, prophylactic blood levels can remain adequate; if the traveler is 1–2 days late with a daily drug, protective blood levels are less likely to be maintained.

Travel to Areas without Chloroquine-Resistant *P. falciparum*
For travel to areas of risk where chloroquine-resistant *P. falciparum* has NOT been reported, once-a-week use of chloroquine alone is recommended for prophylaxis. Persons who experience uncomfortable side

effects after taking chloroquine may tolerate the drug better by taking it with meals. As an alternative, the related compound hydroxychloroquine sulfate may be better tolerated. Travelers unable to take chloroquine or hydroxychloroquine should take atovaquone/proguanil, doxycycline, or mefloquine; these antimalarial drugs are also effective against chloroquine-sensitive parasites.

Chloroquine prophylaxis should begin 1–2 weeks before travel to malarious areas. It should be continued by taking the drug once a week, on the same day of the week, during travel in malarious areas and for 4 weeks after a traveler leaves these areas (Table 4–9).

Travel to Areas with Chloroquine-Resistant *P. falciparum*

For travel to areas of risk where chloroquine-resistant *P. falciparum* exists, three efficacious options are available, listed in alphabetical order below. In addition, there are new recommendations for the use of primaquine for prophylaxis in special situations.

Atovaquone/proguanil (Malarone). Atovaquone/proguanil is a fixed combination of the two drugs, atovaquone and proguanil. Atovaquone/proguanil prophylaxis should begin 1–2 days before travel to malarious areas and should be taken daily, at the same time each day, while in the malarious areas and daily for 7 days after leaving the area. (See Table 4–9 for recommended dosages.)

Doxycycline (many brand names and generic). Doxycycline prophylaxis should begin 1–2 days before travel to malarious areas. It should be continued once a day, at the same time each day, during travel in malarious areas and daily for 4 weeks after the traveler leaves such areas. Insufficient data exist on the antimalarial prophylactic efficacy of related compounds such as minocycline (commonly prescribed for the treatment of acne). Persons on a long-term regimen of minocycline who are in need of malaria prophylaxis should stop taking minocycline 1–2 days before travel and start doxycycline instead. The minocycline can be restarted after the full course of doxycycline is completed. (See Table 4–9 for recommended dosages.)

Either doxycycline or atovaquone/proguanil (see above) can be used by travelers to areas with mefloquine-resistant strains of *P. falciparum* (the borders of Thailand with Burma (Myanmar) and Cambodia, western Cambodia, and eastern Burma (Myanmar) (see Map 4–8).

Mefloquine (Lariam and generic). Mefloquine prophylaxis should begin 1–2 weeks before travel to malarious areas. It should be continued once a week, on the same day of the week, during travel in malarious areas and for 4 weeks after a traveler leaves such areas. (See Table 4–9 for recommended dosages.)

NOTE: In special circumstances and after consultation with malaria experts available through the CDC Malaria Hotline (770-488-7788), **primaquine** may be used for prophylaxis for travel to areas with or without chloroquine-resistant *P. falciparum*. This use should generally be reserved for travelers unable to take any of the other chemoprophylaxis regimens recommended for the region of travel. The traveler must have a documented level of G6PD in the normal range prior to being prescribed primaquine. Primaquine prophylaxis should begin 1–2 days before travel to malarious areas, be taken daily at the same time each day while in the malarious areas, and daily for 7 days after leaving such areas. (See Table 4–9 for recommended dosages.)

IN THOSE WHO ARE G6PD DEFICIENT, PRIMAQUINE CAN CAUSE HEMOLYSIS, WHICH CAN BE FATAL. BE SURE TO DOCUMENT A NORMAL G6PD LEVEL BEFORE PRESCRIBING PRIMAQUINE.

CDC no longer recommends chloroquine/proguanil as a preventive option for persons traveling to areas with chloroquine-resistant *P. falciparum*.

Prevention of Relapses of *P. vivax* and *P. ovale*: Presumptive anti-relapse therapy (terminal prophylaxis) with primaquine

P. vivax and *P. ovale* parasites can persist in the liver and cause relapses for as long as 4 years or more after departure from the malarious areas. Travelers to malarious areas should be alerted to this risk and, if they have malaria symptoms after leaving a malarious area, they should be advised to report their travel history and the possibility of malaria to a physician as soon as possible.

Presumptive anti-relapse therapy with primaquine decreases the risk of relapses by acting against the liver stages of *P. vivax* or *P. ovale*.

TABLE 4-9. DRUGS USED IN THE PROPHYLAXIS OF MALARIA

DRUG	USAGE	ADULT DOSE	PEDIATRIC DOSE	COMMENTS
Atovaquone/ proguanil (Malarone)	Prophylaxis in areas with chloroquine-resistant or mefloquine-resistant *P. falciparum*.	Adult tablets contain 250 mg atovaquone and 100 mg proguanil hydrochloride. 1 adult tablet orally, daily	Pediatric tablets contain 62.5 mg atovaquone and 25 mg proguanil hydrochloride. 11–20 kg: 1 tablet 21–30 kg: 2 tablets 31–40 kg: 3 tablets 41 kg or more: 1 adult tablet daily	Begin 1–2 days before travel to malarious areas. Take daily at the same time each day while in the malarious area and for 7 days after leaving such areas. Contraindicated in persons with severe renal impairment (creatinine clearance <30 mL/min). Atovaquone/proguanil should be taken with food or a milky drink. Not recommended for prophylaxis for children <11 kg, pregnant women, and women breastfeeding infants weighing <11 kg.
Chloroquine phosphate (Aralen and generic)	Prophylaxis only in areas with chloroquine-sensitive *P. falciparum*.	300 mg base (500 mg salt) orally, once/week	5 mg/kg base (8.3 mg/kg salt) orally, once/week, up to maximum dose of 300 mg base.	Begin 1–2 weeks before travel to malarious areas. Take weekly on the same day of the week while in the malarious area and for 4 weeks after leaving such areas. May exacerbate psoriasis.
Doxycycline (Many brand names and generic)	Prophylaxis in areas with chloroquine-resistant or mefloquine-resistant *P. falciparum*.	100 mg orally, daily	≥8 years of age: 2 mg/kg up to adult dose of 100 mg/day.	Begin 1–2 days before travel to malarious areas. Take daily at the same time each day while in the malarious area and for 4 weeks after leaving such areas. Contraindicated in children <8 years of age and pregnant women.
Hydroxychloroquine sulfate (Plaquenil)	An alternative to chloroquine for prophylaxis only in areas with chloroquine-sensitive *P. falciparum*.	310 mg base (400 mg salt) orally, once/week	5 mg/kg base (6.5 mg/kg salt) orally, once/week, up to maximum adult dose of 310 mg base.	Begin 1–2 weeks before travel to malarious areas. Take weekly on the same day of the week while in the malarious area and for 4 weeks after leaving such areas.

TABLE 4-9. DRUGS USED IN THE PROPHYLAXIS OF MALARIA-CONT'D

DRUG	USAGE	ADULT DOSE	PEDIATRIC DOSE	COMMENTS
Mefloquine (Lariam and generic)	Prophylaxis in areas with chloroquine-resistant P. falciparum.	228 mg base (250 mg salt) orally, once/week	≤9 kg: 4.6 mg/kg base (5 mg/kg salt) orally, once/week 10–19 kg: 1/4 tablet once/week 20–30 kg: 1/2 tablet once/week 31–45 kg: 3/4 tablet once/week ≥46 kg: 1 tablet once/week	Begin 1–2 weeks before travel to malarious areas. Take weekly on the same day of the week while in the malarious area and for 4 weeks after leaving such areas. Contraindicated in persons allergic to mefloquine or related compounds (e.g., quinine and quinidine) and in persons with active depression, a recent history of depression, generalized anxiety disorder, psychosis, schizophrenia, other major psychiatric disorders, or seizures. Use with caution in persons with psychiatric disturbances, or a previous history of depression. Not recommended for persons with cardiac conduction abnormalities.
Primaquine	An option for prophylaxis in special circumstances. Call Malaria Hotline (770-488-7788) for additional information.	30 mg base (52.6 mg salt) orally, daily	0.5 mg/kg base (0.8 mg/kg salt) up to adult dose orally, daily	Begin 1–2 days before travel to malarious areas. Take daily at the same time each day while in the malarious area and for 7 days after leaving such areas. Contraindicated in persons with G6PD[1] deficiency. Also contraindicated during pregnancy and lactation unless the infant being breastfed has a documented normal G6PD level. Use in consultation with malaria experts.
Primaquine	Used for presumptive anti-relapse therapy (terminal prophylaxis) to decrease the risk of relapses of P. vivax and P. ovale.	30 mg base (52.6 mg salt) orally, once/day for 14 days after departure from the malarious area.	0.5 mg/kg base (0.8 mg/kg salt) up to adult dose orally, once/day for 14 days after departure from the malarious area.	Indicated for persons who have had prolonged exposure to P. vivax and P. ovale or both. Contraindicated in persons with G6PD[1] deficiency. Also contraindicated during pregnancy and lactation unless the infant being breastfed has a documented normal G6PD level.

[1]Glucose-6-phosphate dehydrogenase. All persons who take primaquine should have a documented normal G6PD level prior to starting the medication.

MAP 4-8. GEOGRAPHIC DISTRIBUTION OF MEFLOQUINE-RESISTANT MALARIA

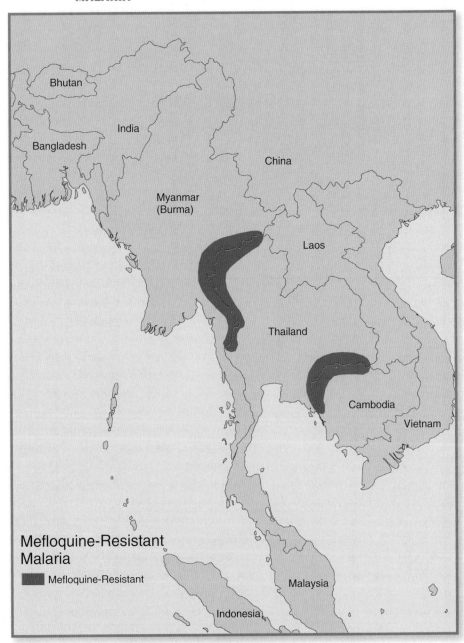

Mefloquine-Resistant Malaria

▨ Mefloquine-Resistant

Primaquine presumptive anti-relapse therapy is administered for 14 days after the traveler has left a malarious area. When chloroquine, doxycycline, or mefloquine is used for prophylaxis, primaquine is usually taken during the last 2 weeks of post-exposure prophylaxis, but may be taken immediately after those medications are completed. When atovaquone/ proguanil is used for prophylaxis, primaquine may be taken either during the final 7 days of atovaquone/ proguanil and then for an additional 7 days, or for 14 days after atovaquone/proguanil is completed. Note that the recommended dose of primaquine for terminal prophylaxis has been increased from 15 mg to 30 mg (base) for adults and from 0.3 mg/kg to 0.5 mg/kg (base) for children. (See Table 4–9 for additional details.)

Because most malarious areas of the world (except Haiti and the Dominican Republic) have at least one species of relapsing malaria, travelers to these areas have some risk for acquiring either *P. vivax* or *P. ovale*, although the actual risk for an individual traveler is difficult to define. Presumptive anti-relapse therapy with primaquine for prevention of relapses is generally indicated only for persons who have had prolonged exposure in malaria-endemic areas (e.g., missionaries and Peace Corps volunteers). Most persons can tolerate this regimen of primaquine (30 mg/day for adults if it is taken with food); the main exception is for persons who are deficient in G6PD. (See "Adverse Reactions and Contraindications" and Table 4–9 for recommended dosages.)

Chemoprophylaxis for Infants, Children, and Adolescents

Infants of any age or weight or children and adolescents of any age can contract malaria. Therefore, children traveling to malaria-risk areas should take an antimalarial drug. In the United States, antimalarial drugs are available only in tablet form and may taste quite bitter. Pediatric dosages should be carefully calculated according to body weight but should never exceed adult dosage. Pharmacists can pulverize tablets and prepare gelatin capsules for each measured dose. Parents should prepare the child's dose of medication by breaking open the gelatin capsule and mixing the drug with something sweet, such as applesauce, chocolate syrup, or jelly. Giving the dose on a full stomach may minimize stomach upset and vomiting.

OVERDOSE OF ANTIMALARIAL DRUGS CAN BE FATAL. MEDICATION SHOULD BE STORED IN CHILDPROOF CONTAINERS OUT OF THE REACH OF INFANTS AND CHILDREN.

Infants, Children, and Adolescents Traveling to Areas without Chloroquine-Resistant **P. falciparum.** Chloroquine is the drug of choice for children traveling to areas without chloroquine-resistant *P. falciparum.*

Infants, Children, and Adolescents Traveling to Areas with Chloroquine-Resistant **P. falciparum.** Mefloquine is an option for use in infants and children of all ages and weights who are traveling to areas with chloroquine-resistant *P. falciparum.* Doxycycline may be used for children ≥8 years of age. Atovaquone/proguanil may be used for prophylaxis for infants and children weighing ≥11 kg (≥24 lbs). At this time, insufficient data are available on the safety and efficacy of atovaquone/proguanil for prevention of malaria in children weighing <11 kg (<24 lbs). Atovaquone/proguanil is available in pediatric tablet form; dosage is based on weight. Pediatric dosing regimens are contained in Table 4–10; additional information on atovaquone/proguanil dosing is found in Table 4–9.

Chemoprophylaxis during Pregnancy

Malaria infection in pregnant women can be more severe than in non-pregnant women. Malaria can increase the risk for adverse pregnancy outcomes, including prematurity, abortion, and stillbirth. For these reasons and because no chemoprophylactic regimen is completely effective, women who are pregnant or likely to become pregnant should be advised to avoid travel to areas with malaria transmission if possible. (Also see Malaria during Pregnancy). If travel to a malarious area cannot be deferred, use of an effective chemoprophylaxis regimen is essential.

Travel during Pregnancy to Areas without Chloroquine-Resistant **P. falciparum.** Pregnant women traveling to areas where chloroquine-resistant *P. falciparum* has not been reported may take chloroquine prophylaxis. Chloroquine has not been found to have any harmful effects on the fetus when used in the recommended doses for malaria prophylaxis; therefore, pregnancy is not a contraindication

TABLE 4-10. PEDIATRIC PROPHYLACTIC DOSES OF ATOVAQUONE/PROGUANIL

BODY WEIGHT[1] (LB)	BODY WEIGHT[1] (KG)	ATOVAQUONE/PROGUANIL TOTAL DAILY DOSE (MG)	DOSAGE REGIMEN
24–45	11–20	62.5/25	1 pediatric tablet daily
46–67	21–30	125/50	2 pediatric tablets daily
68–88	31–40	187.5/75	3 pediatric tablets daily
≥89	≥41	250/100	1 adult tablet daily

[1]Insufficient data are available on the safety and efficacy of atovaquone/proguanil for prevention of malaria in children weighing <11 kg (24 lbs).

for malaria prophylaxis with chloroquine phosphate or hydroxychloroquine sulfate.

Travel during Pregnancy to Areas with Chloroquine-Resistant P. falciparum. Mefloquine is currently the only medication recommended for malaria chemoprophylaxis during pregnancy. A review of mefloquine use in pregnancy from clinical trials and reports of inadvertent use of mefloquine during pregnancy suggest that its use at prophylactic doses during the second and third trimesters of pregnancy is not associated with adverse fetal or pregnancy outcomes. More limited data suggest it is also safe to use during the first trimester.

Because of insufficient data regarding the use during pregnancy, atovaquone/proguanil is not currently recommended for the prevention of malaria in pregnant women. Doxycycline is contraindicated for malaria prophylaxis during pregnancy because of the risk of adverse effects of tetracycline, a related drug, on the fetus, which include discoloration and dysplasia of the teeth and inhibition of bone growth. Primaquine should not be used during pregnancy because the drug may be passed transplacentally to a glucose-6-phosphate dehydrogenase (G6PD)-deficient fetus and cause hemolytic anemia in utero. Health-care professionals who require additional assistance with the management of pregnant travelers who are unable to take mefloquine chemoprophylaxis should call the CDC Malaria Hotline (770-488-7788).

Antimalarial Drugs during Breastfeeding

Data are available for some antimalarial agents on the amount of drug excreted in breast milk of lactating women. Very small amounts of chloroquine and mefloquine are excreted in the breast milk of lactating women. The amount of drug transferred is not thought to be harmful to a nursing infant. Because the quantity of antimalarial drugs transferred in breast milk is insufficient to provide adequate protection against malaria, infants who require chemoprophylaxis must receive the recommended dosages of antimalarial drugs listed in Table 4–9.

Although there are very limited data about the use of doxycycline in lactating women, most experts consider the theoretical possibility of adverse events to be remote.

No information is available on the amount of primaquine that enters human breast milk; the mother and infant should be tested for G6PD deficiency before primaquine is given to a woman who is breastfeeding.

It is not known whether atovaquone is excreted in human milk. Proguanil is excreted in human milk in small quantities. Based on experience with other antimalarial drugs, the quantity of drug transferred in breast milk is likely insufficient to provide adequate protection against malaria for the infant. Because data are not yet available on the safety of atovaquone/proguanil prophylaxis in infants weighing <11 kg (24 lbs), CDC does not currently recommend it for the prevention of malaria in women breastfeeding infants weighing <11 kg. (Atovaquone/proguanil may be used for the treatment of malaria by women breastfeeding infants weighing >5 kg. However, it can be used for treatment of women who are breastfeeding infants of any weight when the potential benefit outweighs the potential risk to the infant, e.g., treating a breastfeeding woman who has acquired P. falciparum malaria in an area of multidrug-resistant strains and who cannot tolerate other treatment options.)

Adverse Reactions and Contraindications

Following is a summary of the frequent or serious side effects of recommended antimalarial drugs. In addition, physicians should review the prescribing information in standard pharmaceutical reference texts and in the manufacturers' package inserts.

Atovaquone/Proguanil
The most common adverse effects reported in persons using atovaquone/proguanil for prophylaxis or treatments are abdominal pain, nausea, vomiting, and headache. Atovaquone/proguanil should not be used for prophylaxis in children weighing <11 kg, pregnant women, women breastfeeding infants weighing <11 kg, or patients with severe renal impairment (creatinine clearance <30 mL/min).

Chloroquine and Hydroxychloroquine Sulfate
Reported side effects include gastrointestinal disturbance, headache, dizziness, blurred vision, insomnia, and pruritus, but generally these effects do not require that the drug be discontinued. High doses of chloroquine, such as those used to treat rheumatoid arthritis, have been associated with retinopathy; this serious side effect appears to be extremely unlikely when chloroquine is used for routine weekly malaria prophylaxis. Chloroquine and related compounds have been reported to exacerbate psoriasis.

Doxycycline
Doxycycline can cause photosensitivity, usually manifested as an exaggerated sunburn reaction. The risk of such a reaction can be minimized by avoiding prolonged, direct exposure to the sun and by using sunscreens that absorb long-wave UVA radiation. In addition, doxycycline use is associated with an increased frequency of *Candida* vaginitis. Gastrointestinal side effects (nausea or vomiting) may be minimized by taking the drug with a meal. To reduce the risk of esophagitis, travelers should be advised not to take doxycycline before going to bed. Doxycycline is contraindicated in persons with an allergy to tetracyclines, during pregnancy, and in infants and children <8 years of age. Vaccination with the oral typhoid vaccine Ty21a should be delayed for >24 hours after taking a dose of doxycycline.

Mefloquine
Mefloquine (Lariam) has been associated with rare serious adverse reactions (e.g., psychoses or seizures) at prophylactic doses; these reactions are more frequent with the higher doses used for treatment. Other side effects that have occurred in chemoprophylaxis studies include gastrointestinal disturbance, headache, insomnia, abnormal dreams, visual dis-

turbances, depression, anxiety disorder, and dizziness. Other more severe neuropsychiatric disorders occasionally reported during post-marketing surveillance include sensory and motor neuropathies (including paresthesia, tremor, and ataxia), agitation or restlessness, mood changes, panic attacks, forgetfulness, confusion, hallucinations, aggression, paranoia, and encephalopathy. On occasions, psychiatric symptoms have been reported to continue long after mefloquine has been stopped.

During prophylactic use, if psychiatric symptoms such as acute anxiety, depression, restlessness, or confusion occur, these may be considered prodromal to a more serious event. In these cases, the drug must be discontinued and an alternative drug substituted.

Mefloquine is contraindicated for use by travelers with a known hypersensitivity to mefloquine or related compounds (e.g., quinine and quinidine) and in persons with active depression, a recent history of depression, generalized anxiety disorder, psychosis, schizophrenia, other major psychiatric disorders, or seizures. It should be used with caution in persons with psychiatric disturbances or a previous history of depression. A review of available data suggests that mefloquine may be used in persons concurrently on beta blockers, if they have no underlying arrhythmia. However, mefloquine is not recommended for persons with cardiac conduction abnormalities. Any traveler receiving a prescription for mefloquine must also receive a copy of the FDA Medication Guide which can be found at the following website: http://www.fda.gov/cder/foi/label/2003/19591s19lbl_Lariam.pdf.

Primaquine
The most common adverse event in G6PD-normal persons is gastrointestinal upset if primaquine is taken on an empty stomach—this problem is minimized or eliminated if primaquine is taken with food. Primaquine can cause hemolysis that can be fatal, in G6PD-deficient persons. **Before primaquine is used, G6PD deficiency MUST be ruled out by appropriate laboratory testing.**

Medications Acquired Overseas
The medications recommended for chemoprophylaxis and treatment of malaria may also be available at overseas destinations. However, combinations of these medications and additional drugs that are not recommended may be commonly prescribed and used in other countries.

Travelers should be strongly discouraged from obtaining chemoprophylactic medications while abroad. These products may not be protective and may be dangerous. These medications may have been produced by substandard manufacturing practices, may be counterfeit, or may contain contaminants. Additional information on this topic can be found in a Food and Drug Administration document "Purchasing Medications Outside the United States" (http://www.fda.gov/ora/import/purchasing_medications.htm).

Medications that are not used in the United States, such as halofantrine (Halfan), are widely available overseas. CDC does not recommend halofantrine for treatment because of cardiac adverse events, including deaths, which have been documented following treatment doses. These adverse events have occurred in persons with and without preexisting cardiac problems and both in the presence and absence of other antimalarial drugs (e.g., mefloquine). Health-care providers should caution travelers not to use medications that are not recommended unless they have been diagnosed with life-threatening malaria and no other options are available.

Changing Medications during Chemoprophylaxis as a Result of Side Effects

The medications recommended for prophylaxis against malaria have different modes of action that affect the parasites at different stages of the life cycle. Thus, if the medication needs to be changed because of side effects before a full course has been completed, there are some special considerations. If a traveler starts prophylaxis with a medication such as mefloquine or doxycycline and then changes to atovaquone/proguanil during or after travel, the standard duration of prophylaxis for atovaquone/proguanil would be insufficient. The atovaquone/proguanil should be continued for 4 weeks after the drug change or 1 week after returning, whichever is longer. Health-care professionals who require additional assistance with the management of travelers who need to change medications during prophylaxis should call the CDC Malaria Hotline (770-488-7788).

TREATMENT

Specific treatment with antimalarial drugs is available. Travelers should be advised that malaria can be treated effectively early in the course of the disease but that delay of appropriate therapy can have serious or even fatal consequences. Travelers who have symptoms of malaria should be advised to seek prompt medical evaluation, including thick and thin blood smears, *as soon as possible*. If possible, it is advisable to consult with a provider who has specialized travel/tropical medicine expertise or with an infectious disease physician. CDC recommendations for malaria treatment can be found at http://www.cdc.gov/malaria/diagnosis_treatment/treatment.htm.

Self-Treatment

CDC recommends the use of malaria prophylaxis for travel to malarious areas. However, travelers who elect not to take prophylaxis, who do not choose an optimal drug regimen (e.g., chloroquine in an area with chloroquine-resistant *P. falciparum*) or who require a less than optimal drug regimen are at greater risk for acquiring malaria and needing prompt treatment. Travelers who are taking effective prophylaxis but who will be in very remote areas may decide, in consultation with their health-care provider, to take along a dose of antimalarial medication for self-treatment (Table 4–11). Travelers should be advised to take their presumptive self-treatment promptly if they have fever, chills, or other influenza-like illness and if professional medical care is not available within 24 hours. **Travelers should be advised that this self-treatment of a possible malarial infection is only a temporary measure and that prompt medical evaluation is imperative.**

Recommendations for Presumptive Self-Treatment

Atovaquone/proguanil may be used for presumptive self-treatment for travelers NOT taking atovaquone/proguanil for prophylaxis. The CDC Malaria Branch (Malaria Hotline 770-488-7788) can provide consultation to health-care providers on other potential options for self-treatment if atovaquone/proguanil cannot be used.

MALARIA HOTLINE

Detailed recommendations for the prevention of malaria are available from CDC 24 hours a day from the voice information service (1-877-FYI-TRIP; 1-877-394-8747), the fax information service (1-888-232-3299), or the Internet at http://www.cdc.gov/travel.

Health-care professionals who require assistance with the diagnosis or treatment of malaria should call the CDC Malaria Hotline (770-488-

TABLE 4-11. PRESUMPTIVE SELF-TREATMENT OF MALARIA

DRUG	ADULT DOSE	PEDIATRIC DOSE	COMMENTS
Atovaquone/ proguanil (Malarone). Self-treatment drug to be used if professional medical care is not available within 24 hours. Medical care should be sought immediately after treatment	4 tablets (each dose contains 1,000 mg atovaquone and 400 mg proguanil) orally as a single daily dose for 3 consecutive days	Daily dose to be taken for 3 consecutive days: 5–8 kg: 2 pediatric tablets 9–10 kg: 3 pediatric tablets 11–20 kg: 1 adult tablet 21–30 kg: 2 adult tablets 31–40 kg: 3 adult tablets ≥41 kg: 4 adult tablets	Contraindicated in persons with severe renal impairment (creatinine clearance <30 mL/min). Not recommended for self-treatment in persons on atovaquone/proguanil prophylaxis. Not currently recommended for children <5 kg,[1] pregnant women, and women breastfeeding infants weighing <5 kg

[1]Note: 5 kg is the cut-off weight for treatment with atovaquone/proguanil; 11 kg remains the recommended cut-off weight for prophylaxis.

7788) from 8:00 a.m. to 4:30 p.m. Eastern time. After hours or on weekends and holidays, health-care providers requiring assistance should call the CDC Emergency Operation Center at 770-488-7100 and ask the operator to page the person on call for the Malaria Branch. Information on diagnosis and treatment is available on the internet at www.cdc.gov/malaria.

Bibliography

Connor BA. Expert recommendations for antimalarial prophylaxis. J Travel Med. 2001;8 Suppl 3:S57–64.

Magill AJ. The prevention of malaria. Prim Care. 2002;29:815–42.

Newman RD, Parise ME, Barber AM, et al. Malaria-related deaths among U.S. travelers, 1963-2001. Ann Intern Med. 2004;141:547–55.

Parise ME, Lewis LS. Severe malaria: North American perspective. In: Feldman C, Sarosi GA, editors. Tropical and parasitic infections in the ICU. Springer Science+Business Media, Inc, 2005.

Powell VI, Grima K. Exchange transfusion for malaria and *Babesia* infection. Transfus Med Rev. 2002;16:239–50.

Re VL 3rd, Gluckman SJ. Prevention of malaria in travelers. Am Fam Physician. 2003;68:509–14.

Schlagenhauf-Lawlor P. Travelers' malaria. Hamilton, Ontario: BC Decker; 2001.

Schwartz E, Parise M, Kozarsky P, et al. Delayed onset of malaria—implications for chemoprophylaxis in travelers. N Engl J Med. 2003;349:1510–6.

Shah S, Filler S, Causer LM, et al. Malaria surveillance—United States, 2002. MMWR Surveill Summ. 2004;53:21–34.

–MONICA PARISE, ANN BARBER, AND SONJA MALI

>>Measles (Rubeola)

DESCRIPTION

Measles is an acute, highly communicable viral disease that begins with a prodromal fever, conjunctivitis, coryza, cough, and Koplik spots on the buccal mucosa. A characteristic red, blotchy rash appears around the third day of illness, beginning on the face and becoming generalized. Measles is frequently complicated by middle ear infection or diarrhea. The disease can be severe, with bronchopneumonia or brain inflammation (encephalitis) leading to death in approximately 2 of every 1,000 cases in developed countries. In the developing world, case-fatality rates often exceed 150 deaths per 1000 cases.

OCCURRENCE

Prior to widespread immunization, measles was common in childhood, with >90% of infants and children infected by 12 years of age. Since vaccine licensure in 1963, measles elimination efforts in the United States have resulted in record low numbers of reported measles cases. Since 1997, measles has not been endemic in the United States; the measles virus does not circulate in the United States except in limited chains of transmission following importation from other countries. Roughly half of imported measles cases occur in U.S. residents returning from visits to foreign countries. The risk of exposure to measles in the United States is low because of the high population immunity achieved through vaccination.

RISK FOR TRAVELERS

The risk of exposure to measles outside the United States can be high. Measles remains a common disease in many countries of the world, including some developed countries in Europe and Asia. International patterns of transmission of measles vary widely; CDC does not attempt to track levels of risk of exposure to measles in other countries. CDC recommends that all travelers leaving the United States should be immune to measles.

Unvaccinated infants and children in the United States are highly susceptible to measles. Children traveling internationally may be at higher risk than adults of exposure to measles. Special attention should be given to vaccinating infants and children according to the accelerated schedule listed in Vaccine Recommendations for Infants and Children. Because several recent outbreaks have been associated with international adoptions, families adopting children from other countries should ensure that all family members are immune to measles before the adoption.

PREVENTION

Prevention of Spread of Measles Virus

Persons who have a generalized rash and fever and persons who have fever and respiratory symptoms following exposure to a person with measles may be infectious with measles. Persons who are potentially infectious with measles should minimize the risk of spread of the disease by limiting contact with other people who may be susceptible to measles. Contact should be limited until a medical diagnosis has been established excluding measles, or the symptoms resolve completely, or 4 days have passed since the onset of the rash. Persons who are potentially infectious with measles should especially avoid public transportation (including commercial airlines) and crowded indoor areas. Patients who suspect they may have measles should call ahead before visiting a clinic or hospital so that arrangements may be made for the health-care provider to attend to the patient without exposing others in the facility to measles.

Vaccination

Measles vaccine contains live, attenuated measles virus. It is available as a single-antigen preparation or combined with live, attenuated mumps or rubella vaccines, or both. Combined measles, mumps, and rubella (MMR) vaccine is recommended whenever one or more of the individual components are indicated.

Although vaccination against measles, mumps, or rubella is not a requirement for entry into any country (including the United States), persons traveling or living abroad should ensure that they are immune to all three diseases. In general, travelers can be considered immune to measles if they have documentation of physician-diagnosed measles, laboratory evidence of measles immunity, or proof of receipt of two doses of live measles vaccine with the first dose received on or after their first birthday and the second dose at least 28 days later. Most persons born before 1957 have had measles disease and generally need not be considered susceptible. However, measles or MMR vaccine may be given to these persons if there is reason to believe they might be susceptible.

The recommended routine age for measles vaccination of infants in the United States is 12–15 months. A single dose of MMR vaccine induces antibody formation to all three viruses in at least 95% of susceptible persons vaccinated at ≥12 months of age. A second dose is expected to induce immunity in most vaccinees who do not respond to the first dose. The second dose should be separated from the first by at least 28 days and is routinely administered at 4–6 years of age. Because infants and children traveling internationally are at an increased risk of exposure to measles, earlier vaccination with the first and second doses is recommended. See the *Vaccine Recommendations for Infants and Children* section for a discussion of measles immunization schedule modifications for infants and children who will be traveling.

MMR may be administered simultaneously (but in a different site) with any other live or inactivated vaccine. Inactivated vaccines and typhoid vaccines may be administered at any time before or after live measles-containing vaccine. However, if MMR vaccine and live yellow fever vaccine are not administered simultaneously, they should be separated by an interval of at least 28 days.

Adverse Reactions to Vaccination

Fever and rash, the most common adverse reactions following MMR vaccine, are usually attributable to the measles component. Approximately 5% of vaccinees have fever >39.4° C (>103° F) or a generalized rash. Fever and rash usually occur 7–12 days after vaccination and last 1–2 days. Transient lymphadenopathy sometimes occurs after MMR and is attributable to the rubella component. Parotitis has been reported rarely after MMR receipt and is attributable to the mumps component of the vaccine. Joint symptoms (arthralgia or arthritis or both) are reported in ≤25% of rubella-susceptible postpubertal women who receive MMR or other rubella-containing vaccine. Joint symptoms are usually mild and transient. Allergic reactions have been reported after MMR vaccine, ranging from mild (urticaria or wheal and flare at the injection site, generalized rash, and pruritis) to severe anaphylactic reactions. Severe allergic reactions are estimated to occur less than once per million doses. Clinically apparent low platelet counts have been reported at a rate of <1 case per 30,000 doses. Central nervous system conditions, including aseptic meningitis, encephalitis, and encephalopathy, have been reported after MMR receipt, but are very uncommon (<1 case per million doses). Reactions following the second dose of MMR (except allergic reactions) are less frequent than reactions following the first dose and occur only primarily among the small proportion of persons who did not respond to the first dose.

Vaccine Precautions and Contraindications
Allergy

Persons with severe allergy (i.e., hives, swelling of the mouth or throat, difficulty breathing, hypotension, and shock) to gelatin or neomycin or who have had a severe allergic reaction to a prior dose of MMR should not be vaccinated with MMR except with extreme caution.

In the past, persons with a history of anaphylactic reactions after eating eggs were considered to be at increased risk of serious reactions after receipt of measles- and mumps-containing vaccines, which are produced in chick embryo fibroblasts. However, recent data suggest that anaphylactic reactions to measles- and mumps-containing vaccines are not associated with hypersensitivity to egg antigens, but to other components of the vaccines (such as gelatin). The risk for serious allergic reactions following receipt of these vaccines by egg-allergic persons is extremely low, and skin testing with vaccine is not predictive of allergic reaction to vaccination. MMR may be administered to egg-allergic persons without prior routine skin testing or the use of special protocols.

Pregnancy and Breastfeeding
Pregnant women should not receive MMR vaccine. Pregnancy should be avoided for 1 month after receipt of monovalent measles vaccine and MMR or other rubella-containing vaccines. Close contact with pregnant women is not a contraindication to MMR vaccination. Breastfeeding is not a contraindication to MMR vaccination of either a woman or an infant.

Immunosuppression
Replication of vaccine viruses can be prolonged in persons who are immunosuppressed or immunodeficient for any reason (e.g., who have congenital immunodeficiency, HIV infection, leukemia, lymphoma, or generalized malignancy, or who are receiving therapy with alkylating agents, antimetabolites, radiation, or large doses of corticosteroids). Evidence based on case reports has linked infection with measles vaccine virus to subsequent death in six severely immunosuppressed persons. For this reason, persons who are severely immunosuppressed for any reason should not be given MMR vaccine. Healthy, susceptible close contacts of severely immunosuppressed persons may be vaccinated.

In general, persons receiving large daily doses of corticosteroids (>2 mg per kg per day or >20 mg per day of prednisone) for ≥14 days should not receive MMR vaccine because of concern about vaccine safety. MMR and its component vaccines should be avoided for at least 1 month after cessation of high-dose therapy. Persons receiving low-dose or short-course (<14 days) therapy; alternate-day treatment; maintenance physiologic doses; or topical, aerosol, intra-articular, bursal, or tendon injections may be vaccinated. Although persons receiving high doses of systemic corticosteroids daily or on alternate days during an interval of <14 days generally can receive MMR or its component vaccines immediately after cessation of treatment, some experts prefer waiting until 2 weeks after completion of therapy. Persons receiving cancer chemotherapy or radiation who have not received these treatments for at least 3 months may receive MMR or its component vaccines.

Measles disease can be severe in persons with HIV infection. Available data indicate that vaccination with MMR has not been associated with severe or unusual adverse events in HIV-infected persons without evidence of severe immunosuppression, although antibody responses have been variable. MMR vaccine is recommended for all asymptomatic HIV-infected persons and should be considered for symptomatic persons who are not severely immunosuppressed. Asymptomatic persons do not need to be evaluated and tested for HIV infection before MMR or other measles-containing vaccines are administered. A theoretical risk of an increase (probably transient) in HIV viral load after MMR vaccination exists because such an effect has been observed with other vaccines. The clinical significance of such an increase is not known.

MMR and other measles-containing vaccines are not recommended for HIV-infected persons with evidence of severe immunosuppression (e.g., a very low CD4+ T-lymphocyte count), primarily because of the report of a case of measles pneumonitis in a measles vaccine recipient who had an advanced case of AIDS. Refer to the Advisory Committee on Immunization Practices (ACIP) recommendations on MMR for additional details on vaccination of persons with symptomatic HIV infection.

Acute Illness
Vaccination of travelers with moderate or severe acute illness should be postponed until their condition has improved. Minor illnesses, such as upper respiratory infections with or without low-grade fever, do not preclude vaccination.

Drug Interaction
MMR vaccination has no effect on antibiotics or antimalarial drugs, and the drugs do not reduce the immunogenicity of MMR. Persons taking these products should be vaccinated as usual.

Interaction with Immune Globulin or Other Antibody-Containing Blood Products
MMR or its component vaccines should be administered at least 14 days before the administration of antibody-containing blood products, such as immune globulin, because passively acquired antibodies may interfere with the response to the vaccine. Otherwise, MMR vaccination should be delayed until 3 to 11 months after administration of blood products, depending on the type of blood product received. (See Table 1–2 for details.)

Tuberculosis

Tuberculin skin testing is not a prerequisite for vaccination with MMR or other measles-containing vaccine. TB skin testing has no effect on the response to MMR vaccination. However, measles vaccine (and possibly mumps, rubella, and varicella vaccines) can suppress the response to skin testing in a person infected with *Mycobacterium tuberculosis*. To minimize the risk of a false-negative interpretation, TB skin testing should be done prior to MMR vaccination or at the same time MMR is administered, because the mild immunosuppressive effect of the vaccine will not occur for several days after vaccination. Otherwise, TB skin testing should be delayed for 4–6 weeks after MMR vaccination.

TREATMENT

There is no specific antiviral therapy for measles, and the basic treatment consists of providing necessary supportive therapy such as hydration and antipyretics and treating complications such as pneumonia. Multiple studies have shown that vitamin A supplementation improves outcome of measles in communities where vitamin A deficiency is known to occur. Although vitamin A deficiency is not a major problem in the United States, low serum concentrations have been found in children with severe measles. Therefore, the American Academy of Pediatrics recommends vitamin A supplementation be considered for children ≥6 months of age (limited data are available about the safety of vitamin A for infants <6 months of age) who have any of the following risk factors: immunodeficiency, clinical evidence of vitamin A deficiency, impaired intestinal absorption, moderate to severe malnutrition or recent immigration from areas where high measles mortality rates have been observed. All children 6 months to 2 years of age who are hospitalized with measles should also receive vitamin A. The recommended dosage, administered orally as a capsule, is a single dose of 100,000 IU for children 6–11 months of age or 200,000 IU for children ≥1 year of age. The dose should be repeated the next week and again 4 weeks later for children with evidence of vitamin A deficiency.

Bibliography

American Academy of Pediatrics. Measles. In: Pickering LK, editor. Red book: 2003 report of the Committee on Infectious Diseases. 26th ed. Elk Grove Village, IL: American Academy of Pediatrics; 2003. p. 419–29.

CDC. Epidemiology of Measles—United States, 2001–2003. Morbid
Mortal Wkly Rep MMWR. 2004;53:713–6.

Watson JC, Hadler SC, Dykewicz CA, et al. Measles, mumps and
rubella—vaccine use and strategies for elimination of measles, rubella,
and congenital rubella syndrome and control of mumps: recommendations of the Advisory Committee on Immunization Practices
(ACIP). Morbid Mortal Wkly Rep MMWR. 1998;47(RR-8):1–57.

–MARK PAPANIA

>>Meningococcal Disease

DESCRIPTION

Meningococcal disease is an acute bacterial disease characterized by
sudden onset with fever; intense headache; nausea and often vomiting;
stiff neck; and, frequently, a petechial rash with pink macules. Formerly,
the case-fatality ratio exceeded 50%, but early diagnosis, modern therapy, and supportive measures have lowered the case-fatality ratio to
about 10%. Among survivors, 11%–19% have long-term sequelae,
including hearing loss, neurologic disability, or loss of a limb. Up to 10%
of populations in countries with endemic disease carry the bacteria
(*Neisseria meningitidis*) asymptomatically in their nose and throat.

Meningococci are classified into serogroups based on the composition
of the capsular polysaccharide. Five major meningococcal serogroups
associated with disease are A, B, C, Y and W-135. In the past 30 years,
meningococci serogroups B and C have been responsible for most disease in the Americas and Europe. Serogroup A meningococci and, to a
lesser extent, serogroup C, account for most meningococcal disease
cases in Africa and some areas in Asia. During the past years, serogroup
Y has emerged as a cause of disease in Northern America, and
serogroup W-135 has been associated with meningococcal disease epidemics in Saudi Arabia and Burkina Faso.

OCCURRENCE

In the sub-Saharan African "meningitis belt," which extends from Mali
to Ethiopia, peaks of serogroup A meningococcal disease occur regu-

larly during the dry season (December through June). In addition, major epidemics occur every 8–12 years (see Map 4–9). In 2000, a serogroup W-135 epidemic occurred in Saudi Arabia in association with the Hajj pilgrimage. Cases also occurred in returning pilgrims and their families, including several cases in the United States. In 2002, a major meningococcal disease epidemic occurred in Burkina Faso caused by serogroup W-135. In 2003 and 2004, serogroup W-135 has been detected in several African countries, but it has not caused major epidemics. Meningococcal disease continues to cause epidemics outside the meningitis belt, including recent epidemics in the Great Lakes of Africa.

RISK FOR TRAVELERS

Travelers to sub-Saharan Africa may be at risk for meningococcal disease. Travelers to the meningitis belt during the dry season should be advised to receive meningococcal vaccine. Prompted by a serogroup A meningococcal disease outbreak associated with the 1987 Hajj, Saudi Arabia requires that Hajj and Umrah visitors have a certificate of vaccination against meningococcal disease before entering; however, the vaccine formulation varies by country.

CLINICAL PRESENTATION

Sudden onset of fever, intense headache, stiffness of the neck, nausea, and often vomiting are common symptoms of meningitis in anyone over the age of 2 years. These symptoms can develop over several hours, or they may take 1–2 days. Other symptoms may include photophobia and an altered mental status. In infants, a slower onset of symptoms may occur with nonspecific symptoms, and neck stiffness may be absent.

Early diagnosis and treatment are very important. If symptoms occur, the patient should see a doctor immediately. The diagnosis is usually made by growing bacteria collected from cerebrospinal fluid (CSF) or by detection of the meningococcal antigen through latex agglutination in fresh CSF. *Neisseria meningitidis* can also be identified in blood cultures. The signs and symptoms of meningococcal meningitis are similar to those of other causes of bacterial meningitis, such as *Haemophilus influenzae* and *Streptococcus pneumoniae*. Identification of the type of bacteria responsible is important for selection of correct antibiotics. Answers to frequently asked questions about meningitis can be found at

MAP 4-9. AREAS WITH FREQUENT EPIDEMICS OF MENINGOCOCCAL MENINGITIS

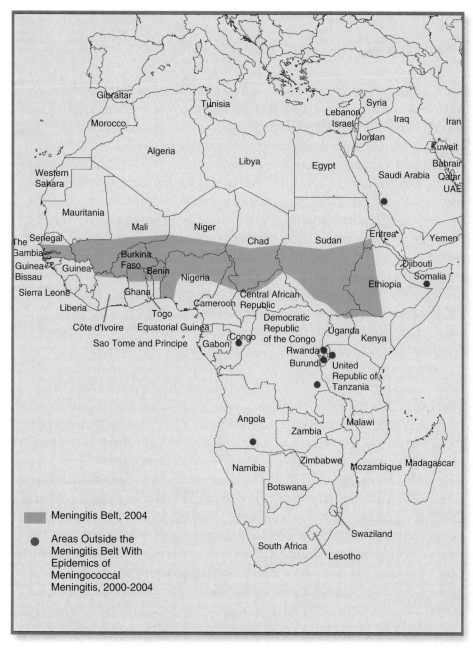

Meningitis Belt, 2004

Areas Outside the Meningitis Belt With Epidemics of Meningococcal Meningitis, 2000-2004

the following website: http://www.cdc.gov/ncidod/dbmd/diseaseinfo/
meningococcal_g.htm#What%20are%20the%20signs%20and%
20symptoms%20of%20meningitis.

PREVENTION

Vaccination against meningococcal disease is not a requirement for entry
into any country except Saudi Arabia, for travelers to Mecca during the
annual Hajj and Umrah pilgrimage. Vaccination is advised for travelers
to countries recognized as having epidemic meningococcal disease
caused by a vaccine-preventable serogroup (i.e., A, C, Y, and/or W-135)
during December through June. Advisories for travelers to other countries will be issued when epidemics of meningococcal disease caused by
vaccine-preventable serogroups are recognized. (See the CDC Travelers'
Health website at http://www.cdc.gov/travel/outbreaks.htm.) Vaccines
may benefit travelers to and persons residing in countries in which
meningococcal disease is hyperendemic or epidemic, particularly if contact with the local population will be prolonged. Vaccines are also recommended for high risk-travelers who have certain medical conditions,
particularly persons who have deficiencies in the terminal common
complement pathway (C3, C5-9) and those who have anatomic or
functional asplenia.

Serogroup A is the most common cause of epidemics outside the
United States, but serogroups C and B can also cause epidemic disease.
As of October 1, 2004, only one formulation of the meningococcal polysaccharide vaccine is available in the United States: quadrivalent
A/C/Y/W-135 vaccine (Table 4–12). The vaccine, which is available in
single- and 10-dose vials, is distributed in the United States by Aventis
Pasteur. Approximately 7–10 days are required following vaccination for
development of protective levels of antimeningococcal antibodies. No
vaccine is currently available to offer protection against serogroup B.
Meningococcal vaccines are chemically defined antigens consisting of
purified bacterial capsular polysaccharides, each inducing serogroup-
specific immunity. In general, use of meningococcal polysaccharide vaccine should be restricted to persons at least 2 years of age; however,
children as young as 3 months of age may be vaccinated to elicit short-
term protection against serogroup A meningococcal disease. The group
Y and W-135 polysaccharides have been shown to be safe and immuno-

genic in adults; however, the response of infants to these polysaccharides is unknown.

New meningococcal conjugate vaccines have recently been developed. These vaccines are expected to be highly efficacious in young children, confer long-term protection, and provide herd immunity by reducing carriage and disease transmission. Serogroup C polysaccharide conjugate vaccines are already licensed for use in infants and children in Europe and Canada. Studies in the United Kingdom (UK) have reported that these vaccines are safe and immunogenic in infants and children and can decrease transmission, thus protecting unvaccinated individuals by inducing herd immunity. In 2000, after introduction of the vaccine in the UK, the vaccine was shown to be highly efficacious and resulted in a dramatic decline in the number of serogroup C meningococcal disease cases. The vaccine also reduced carriage of serogroup C meningococci among young adults by 67%.

A new quadrivalent A/C/Y/W-135 meningococcal conjugate vaccine has been licensed in the United States for use among persons 11–55 years of age. Pre-licensure data on the new quadrivalent conjugate vaccine have shown that the vaccine appears to be safe and immunogenic and is expected to offer a duration of protection longer than polysaccharide vaccines. CDC's Advisory Committee on Immunization Practices (ACIP) is developing recommendations for use of this vaccine, including its use among travelers 11–55 years of age. The quadrivalent A/C/Y/W-135 polysaccharide vaccine will likely remain acceptable for ages 11-55, as well as for persons ages 2–11 and >55 years of age.

Antibiotic chemoprophylaxis among close contacts of a meningitis case may be recommended for control of secondary disease in the United States. Antimicrobial regimens for prophylaxis include rifampin, ciprofloxacin and ceftriaxone, although rifampin is not recommended for pregnant women. Antimicrobial chemoprophylaxis should be considered for passengers who have had direct contact with respiratory secretions from the index patient, and passengers seated directly next to the index patient on prolonged flights (>8 hours) (http://www.cdc.gov/travel/menin-guidelines.htm). A study in 2001 among U.S. Hajj pilgrims found that pathogenic meningococcal nasopharyngeal carriage was

TABLE 4-12. MENINGOCOCCAL VACCINE

TYPE OF VACCINE	DOSE	COMMENTS
Quadrivalent A,C,Y,W-135, for subcutaneous injection	0.5 mL	Duration of immunity is unknown, but appears to be at least 3 years in those ≥4 years of age. Revaccination after 2–3 years should be considered for children first vaccinated at <4 years of age who continue to be at high risk.

uncommon in this vaccinated population; CDC does not currently recommend antimicrobial chemoprophylaxis for returning pilgrims.

Adverse Reactions
Adverse reactions to meningococcal vaccine are infrequent and mild, consisting principally of localized erythema that lasts 1–2 days. Transient fever may develop in up to 2% of infants after vaccination. Data reported from prelicensure clinical trials from the A/C/Y/W-135 meningococcal conjugate vaccine show generally few mild adverse events, such as pain and redness at the injection site for 1–2 days.

Precautions and Contraindications
Studies of the meningococcal polysaccharide vaccine during pregnancy have not documented adverse events among either women or neonates (≤1 month of age). Based on data from studies involving the use of meningococcal vaccines and other polysaccharide vaccines administered during pregnancy, altering meningococcal vaccination recommendations during pregnancy is unnecessary.

TREATMENT

Meningococcal disease is potentially fatal and should always be viewed as a medical emergency. Admission to a hospital or health center is necessary. Standard and droplet precautions should be considered to reduce the risk of transmission of disease during hospitalization (http://www.cdc.gov/ncidod/hip/ISOLAT/isopart2.htm). Bacterial meningitis can be treated with a number of effective antibiotics. However, treatment must be started early in the course of the disease, as soon as possible after the lumbar puncture has been done (if started before, it may be difficult to grow the bacteria from the spinal fluid and thus confirm the diagnosis). Appropriate antibiotic treatment (including penicillin G, ampicillin, and third generation cephalosporins) of most common types of bacterial meningitis should reduce the risk of dying from meningitis to below 15%, although the risk is higher among the elderly.

Under epidemic conditions in Africa, the World Health Organization (WHO) recommends the use of intravenous chloramphenicol, ceftriaxone, or amipicillin. In situations with very limited resources, a single intramuscular dose of an oily suspension of chloramphenicol can be used to treat epidemic meningococcal meningitis. Further details of that treatment can be found at the following website: http://www.who.int/mediacentre/factsheets/fs141/en/.

Bibliography

American Academy of Pediatrics. Meningococcal infections. In: Pickering LK, editor. Red book: 2003 report of the Committee on Infectious Disease. 26th ed. Elk Grove Village, IL: American Academy of Pediatrics; 2003. p. 430–6.

CDC. Prevention and control of meningococcal disease: recommendations of the Advisory Committee on Immunization Practices (ACIP). MMWR Recomm Rep. 2000;49(RR-7):1–10.

CDC. Risk for meningococcal disease associated with the Hajj 2001. MMWR. 2001;50:97–8.

Dull P, Abdelwahab J, Sacchi CT, et al. Serogroup W-135 *Neisseria meningitidis* carriage among US travelers to the 2001 Hajj. J Infect Dis. In press 2004.

Greenwood B. Meningococcal meningitis in Africa. Trans R Soc Trop Med Hyg. 1999;93:341–53.

Lingappa JR, Rosenstein N, Zell ER, et al. Surveillance for meningococcal disease and strategies for use of conjugate meningococcal vaccines in the United States. Vaccine. 2001;19:4566–75.

Ramsay ME, Andrews N, Kaczmarski EB, et al. Efficacy of meningococcal serogroup C conjugate vaccine in teenagers and toddlers in England. Lancet. 2001; 357:195–6.

Rosenstein NE, Perkins BA, Stephens DS, et al. Meningococcal disease. N Engl J Med. 2001;344:1378–88.

Rosenstein NE, Perkins BA, Stephens DS, et al. The changing epidemiology of meningococcal disease in the United States, 1992–1996. J Infect Dis. 1999;180:1894–901.

–KRISTIN UHDE, NANCY ROSENSTEIN AND MONTSE SORIANO-GABARRÓ

>>Mumps

DESCRIPTION

Mumps is a viral illness characterized by parotitis preceded by a prodrome that may include fever, headache, malaise, myalgia, and anorexia.

OCCURRENCE

Following licensure of the vaccine in 1967, mumps cases in the United States have steadily decreased from an estimated 100,000 to 200,000 annually to fewer than 300 cases reported in 2003.

RISK FOR TRAVELERS

The risk for exposure outside the United States remains high. The WHO reports that 102 (53%) of their member states include mumps in their routine vaccination program; however, inclusion of mumps in the routine vaccination program of a country should not be interpreted as lowered risk for the traveler. Although incidence data are not generally available, mumps remains common in many parts of the world, including Western Europe.

CLINICAL PRESENTATION

Up to 50% of mumps infections may produce only nonspecific upper respiratory symptoms, 30%–40% result in parotitis, and 15%–20% are asymptomatic. Mild aseptic meningitis may affect 4%–6% persons infected, while more rare central nervous system complications can result in permanent sequelae, including deafness. Orchitis may occur in up to 50% of postpubertal males.

PREVENTION

Mumps vaccine contains live, attenuated mumps virus. In the United States, it is licensed as a single antigen preparation (Mumpsvax), combined with live attenuated measles vaccine (M-M-Vax), or combined with both live attenuated measles and rubella vaccine (M-M-R II or MMR). Currently, it is available only as single-antigen mumps vaccine (Mumpsvax) or combined with both measles and rubella vaccine (MMR).

Although not required for entry into any country, persons traveling or living abroad should ensure that they are immune to mumps. Travelers should receive MMR vaccine, which would offer immunity not only against mumps but measles and rubella as well. Persons may be considered immune to mumps if they have a) documentation of one or more doses of mumps-containing vaccine on or after their first birthday; b) physician-diagnosed mumps; c) laboratory evidence of mumps immunity; or d) were born before 1957. Mumps vaccine or MMR may be administered to any person if there is reason to believe they may be susceptible. Immunity to mumps is of particular importance for adolescent and adult males because of the risk of orchitis.

In the United States, a dose of MMR is recommended at 12-15 months of age and a second dose at age 4-6 years. A single dose of mumps vaccine, either as single antigen or in combination, has a protective efficacy of 90%-96% and the second dose should provide protection to most people who do not respond to the first dose.

Mumps vaccine has not been demonstrated to be effective in preventing infection after exposure; however, it can be administered post-exposure to provide protection against subsequent exposures. Immune globulin is not effective in preventing mumps infection following an exposure and is not recommended.

The most common adverse reactions to mumps vaccine are parotitis and low-grade fever. Typically, mumps vaccine in the US is administered as MMR vaccine. Refer to the travelers' health information on Measles (Rubeola) for information on reactions following MMR vaccine and additional precautions and contraindications.

TREATMENT

No specific treatment is available for persons with mumps. Treatment is supportive.

Bibliography

American Academy of Pediatrics. Mumps. In: Pickering LK, editor. Red book: 2003 report of the Committee on Infectious Diseases. 26th ed. Elk Grove Village, IL: American Academy of Pediatrics; 2003. p. 439–43.

CDC. Measles, mumps, and rubella— vaccine use and strategies for elimination of measles, rubella and congenital rubella syndrome and control of mumps: recommendations of the Advisory Committee on Immunization Practices (ACIP). MMWR. 1998;47(RR-8):1–57.

CDC [homepage on the Internet]. Atlanta: National Immunization Program; [updated 2003 Sept 6; cited 2004 Oct 7]. Available from http://www.cdc.gov/nip/diseases/mumps/default.htm.

Heymann DL, editor. Control of communicable diseases manual. 18th ed. Washington DC: American Public Health Association; 2004.

World Health Organization. Mumps virus vaccine. Wkly Epidemiol Rec. 2001;76:346–55.

—FRANCISCO AVERHOFF

>>Norovirus Infection

DESCRIPTION

Noroviruses (also referred to as "Norwalk-like viruses," Norwalk viruses, human caliciviruses, and small round-structured viruses) are a common cause of acute gastroenteritis worldwide. Norovirus infection presents as vomiting and diarrhea and usually occurs in large outbreaks propagated by fecal-oral transmission via contaminated food or water or by direct person-to-person contact. Evidence also suggests that norovirus can be transmitted via aerosolized vomit and contact with contaminated objects.

OCCURRENCE

In the United States, norovirus infections are estimated to cause 23 million illnesses a year. Seroprevalence studies in the Amazon, southern Africa, Mexico, Chile, and Canada have shown that norovirus infections are common throughout the world. Infection can occur year-round.

RISK TO TRAVELERS

Travelers of all ages are potentially at risk for norovirus infection, and previous infection does not reliably result in subsequent immunity.

Risk of infection is present anywhere where food is prepared unhygienically or drinking water is inadequately treated. Of particular risk are "ready-to-eat" cold foods, such as sandwiches and salads. Raw shellfish, especially oysters, are also a frequent source of infection. (Please see the *Risks from Food and Drink* section for additional information.)

Norovirus infection also has been associated with large outbreaks of gastroenteritis in various settings where persons living in close quarters, such as hotels, cruise ships, and camps, can easily infect each other over several days. Inapparent viral contamination of inanimate objects during outbreaks can also act as a source of infection.

CLINICAL PRESENTATION

Infected persons usually have acute-onset, violent vomiting and non-bloody diarrhea after an incubation period of 24–48 hours. Other symptoms include abdominal cramps, nausea, and occasionally a low-grade fever. Illness is generally self-limited, and full recovery can be expected in 1–4 days. In some cases, dehydration, especially in those who are very young or elderly, may require medical attention. (For infants, please refer to Table 8–1 for Assessment of Dehydration Levels for Infants.)

PREVENTION

No vaccines are available. Noroviruses are very common and highly contagious, but the risk of infection can be minimized by frequent and proper handwashing and avoidance of possibly contaminated food and water.

In addition to handwashing, measures to prevent transmission of noroviruses between persons traveling together include careful clean-up of fecal material or vomit and disinfection of contaminated surfaces with domestic bleach (at least a 1:50 solution of bleach and water). Soiled articles of clothing should be washed promptly and thoroughly and machine-dried at high heat. Confinement of ill persons to help prevent the spread of noroviruses has occasionally been implemented on cruise ships.

TREATMENT

No antiviral medication is available for treating norovirus infection. Supportive care, such as rest and oral rehydration, is the mainstay of management. (See Table 4–19, Composition of World Health Organization Oral Rehydration Solution (ORS) for Diarrheal Illness.)

Bibliography

Bresee JS, Widdowson M-A, Monroe SS, Glass RI. Foodborne viral gastroenteritis: challenges and opportunities. Clin Infect Dis 2002;35:748–53.

CDC. Norovirus activity, United States, 2002. MMWR Morbid Mortal Wkly Rep 2003;52:41–5.

CDC. Norwalk-like viruses: public health consequences and outbreak management. MMWR Morbid Mortal Wkly Rep 2001;50:(RR-9).

CDC. Outbreaks of gastroenteritis associated with noroviruses on cruise ships—United States, 2002. MMWR Morbid Mortal Wkly Rep 2002;l51:1112–5.

Mead PS, Slutsker L, Dietz V, et al. Food-related illness and death in the United States. Emerg Infect Dis 1999;5:607–25

–EILEEN LAU AND MARC-ALAIN WIDDOWSON

>>Onchocerciasis (River Blindness)

DESCRIPTION

Human onchocerciasis is caused by the prelarval (microfilaria) and adult stages of the filarial nematode *Onchocerca volvulus*. The disease is transmitted by the bite of certain species of female *Simulium* flies (black flies) that bite by day and are found near rapidly flowing rivers and streams.

OCCURRENCE

Onchocerciasis is endemic in more than 25 nations located in a broad band across the central part of Africa. Small endemic foci are also present in the Arabian Peninsula (Yemen) and in the Americas (Brazil, Colombia, Ecuador, Guatemala, southern Mexico, and Venezuela).

RISK FOR TRAVELERS

Persons traveling for short periods in onchocerciasis-endemic regions appear to be at very low risk for acquiring this condition. However, travelers who visit or live in endemic regions for >3 months and live or work near black fly habitats are at greater risk for infection. Infections tend to occur in expatriate groups such as missionaries, field scientists, and Peace Corps volunteers.

CLINICAL PRESENTATION

Infection with O. *volvulus* can result in a highly pruritic, papular dermatitis; subcutaneous nodules; lymphadenitis; and ocular lesions, which can progress to visual loss and blindness. Symptoms in travelers are almost always dermatologic and may occur months to years after departure from endemic areas. Immigrants from endemic areas may present with skin and/or ocular disease. Diagnosis is made by finding the microfilariae in superficial skin shavings, adult worms in histologic sections of excised nodules, or characteristic eye lesions. Serologic tests are nonspecific outside the research setting.

PREVENTION

No vaccine and no effective chemoprophylaxis are available. Protective measures include avoidance of black fly habitats and the use of personal protection measures against biting insects (the vectors of onchocerciasis bite by day) such as those outlined in the section on Protection against Mosquitoes and Other Arthropods).

TREATMENT

Ivermectin (150-200 μg/kg orally once or twice per year) is the drug of choice for onchocerciasis. Repeated annual or semiannual doses may be required because the drug kills the microfilariae but not the adult worms, which can live for many years. If subcutaneous nodules are present, they should be excised. Travelers who have a diagnosis of onchocerciasis should be advised to consult with a specialist in infectious diseases or tropical medicine.

Bibliography

Abiose A. Onchocercal eye disease and the impact of Mectizan treatment. Ann Trop Med Parasitol. 1998;92 Suppl 1: S11–22.

Albiez EJ, Buttner DW, Duke BO. Diagnosis and extirpation of nodules in human onchocerciasis. Trop Med Parasitol. 1988;39 Suppl 4:331–46.

Brieger WR, Awedoba AK, Eneanya CI, et al. The effects of ivermectin on onchocercal skin disease and severe itching: results of a multicentre trial. Tropical Med Int Health. 1998;3:951–61.

Burnham, G. Onchocerciasis. Lancet. 1998;351:1341–6.

Drugs for parasitic infections. The Medical Letter on Drugs and Therapeutics. 2004 Apr:1–12.

Murdoch ME, Asuzu MC, Hagan M, et al. Onchocerciasis: the clinical and epidemiological burden of skin disease in Africa. Ann Trop Med Parasitol. 2002;96:283–96.

World Health Organization. Onchocerciasis and its control: report of a WHO expert committee on onchocerciasis control. World Health Organ Tech Rep Ser. 1995;852:1–104.

–FRANK O. RICHARDS, JR.

>>Plague

DESCRIPTION

Plague is a zoonosis involving rodents and their fleas. The causative agent of plague is the bacterium *Yersinia pestis*. Humans are incidental hosts and are usually infected by the bite of rodent fleas. Plague can also be acquired by direct contact with infectious animals or other materials or inhalation of infective respiratory droplets.

Plague continues to be enzootic in wild rodent populations over large rural areas of the Americas, Africa, and Asia, with occasional outbreaks among commensal rats or other hosts in villages and small towns. Wild rodent plague poses a real, though limited, risk to persons. When infection spreads to rats in urban or populated areas, persons are at markedly increased risk of exposure. In recent decades, however, urban outbreaks have been rare and limited in size.

OCCURRENCE

Wild rodent plague exists in the western third of the United States and the immediately adjoining areas of Canada, widely scattered areas of South America; north-central, northwestern, eastern, and southern Africa; Madagascar; Iran; along the frontier between Yemen and Saudi Arabia; eastern Jordan, central and southeast Asia (Burma, China, India, Indonesia, Kazakhstan, and other former Soviet Republics of central Asia, Mongolia, and Vietnam); and in parts of extreme southern Russia. In recent years, human plague has been identified in Africa from Algeria, Angola, Botswana, Democratic Republic of the Congo, Kenya, Libya, Madagascar, Malawi, Mozambique, Namibia, Tanzania, Uganda, Zambia, and Zimbabwe; in Asia from Burma, China, India, Indonesia, Jordan, Kazakhstan, Laos, Mongolia, and Vietnam; and in the Americas from Bolivia, Brazil, Ecuador, and Peru to the United States.

RISK FOR TRAVELERS

Risk for travelers in any of these areas is small.

CLINICAL DESCRIPTION

Initial signs and symptoms of plague can be nonspecific, with fever, chills, headache, malaise, myalgia, nausea, and prostration. Bubonic plague, the most common form, usually presents with painful, swollen lymph nodes (buboes) that develop in the afferent lymphatic chain draining the site of the flea bite. Patients with pneumonic plague often have many of the above signs and symptoms, as well as cough, breathing difficulties and, in later stages of the illness, bloody sputum.

PREVENTION

Vaccine

Plague vaccine is no longer commercially available. Vaccination against plague is not required by any country as a condition for entry. In the past, vaccine was recommended only for persons who were at a particularly high risk of exposure because they worked with plague routinely in the laboratory or because of field exposures to rodents and their fleas in epizootic areas. In most of the countries of Africa, Asia, and the Americas where plague is reported, the risk of infection exists primarily in rural mountainous or upland areas. Persons who travel to plague-infected areas should follow the preventive measures described in the following section.

Other

Travelers considered at high risk for plague because of unavoidable exposures in active epizootic or epidemic areas should be advised to consider antibiotic chemoprophylaxis with tetracycline or doxycycline during periods of exposure. Trimethoprim-sulfamethoxazole is an acceptable substitute for use in infants and children <8 years of age. Personal protective measures should also be recommended, including the use of insect repellents containing DEET on skin and clothing. (See *Protection against Mosquitoes and Other Arthropods.*) Clothing also can be treated with insecticidal sprays containing permethrin. Travelers should be advised to avoid sick or dead animals or rodent nests and burrows. Whenever possible, travelers should also avoid visiting areas where recent plague epidemics or epizootics have occurred. Travelers are unlikely to be at high risk for plague while staying in modern accommodations.

TREATMENT

Human plague can be fatal unless cases are promptly treated with appropriate antibiotics. The preferred treatment is streptomycin, although gentamicin, tetracycline, and doxycycline are considered to be effective alternatives. Chloramphenicol has been used to treat human plague and is recommended for conditions that require high tissue penetration of the antibiotic agent, including plague meningitis, pleuritis, endophthalmitis, or myocarditis. Human plague cases also have been treated successfully with trimethoprim-sulfamethoxazole, but this agent is not considered to be a primary choice for therapy. An infectious diseases specialist should be consulted.

Bibliography

CDC. Prevention of plague. Recommendations of the Advisory Committee on Immunization Practices (ACIP). MMWR Morbid Mortal Wkly Rep 1996;45:RR–14.

Dennis DT. Plague. In: Guerrant RL, Krogstad DJ, Maguire JH, et al., eds. Tropical Infectious Diseases: Principles, Pathogens, and Practice, 1999. pp. 506–16.

Dennis DT. Plague, Method of. In: Rakel RE, ed., Conn's Current Therapy. W.B. Saunders, Co., Philadelphia, PA., 2001. pp. 115–7.

Dennis DT, Gage KL. Plague. In: Infectious Diseases, 2nd ed. Armstrong D, Cohen J. Mosby, Ltd. London. 2003. Vol. 2, Section 6:1641–8.

Dennis DT, Meier FA. Plague. In: Horsburgh CR, Nelson AM, eds. Pathology of Emerging Infections. Washington, DC: ASM Press, 1997. pp. 21–47.

Gage KL. Plague. In: Collier L, Balows A, Sussman M, general eds.; Hausler WJ, Sussman M, vol. eds. Topley and Wilson's Microbiology and Microbial Infections, 9th Edition. Volume 3, Bacterial Infections. London: Edward Arnold, Ltd. 1998. pp. 885–904.

World Health Organization. Human Plague in 2002 and 2003. Wkly Epidemiol Rec. 2004;79:301–8.

World Health Organization. Plague Manual. Dennis DT, Gage KL, Gratz N, Poland JD, and Tikhomirov E. (Principal authors). World Health Organization. Geneva, Switzerland. 1999. 172 pp. (Note: This manual is available online at the WHO website.)

—KENNETH GAGE

>>*Streptococcus pneumoniae* (Pneumococcal) Disease

DESCRIPTION

Streptococcus pneumoniae, also known as pneumococcus, is a bacterium that is often found in the noses and throats of healthy persons and is spread person-to-person through close contact. Pneumococcus is a common cause of mild illnesses, such as sinus and ear infections, but also causes life-threatening infections such as pneumonia, meningitis, and infections of the bloodstream. Many strains are resistant to antibiotics.

OCCURRENCE

Risk for pneumococcal disease is highest in young children, the elderly, and persons of any age who have chronic medical conditions such as heart disease, lung disease, or diabetes, or conditions that suppress the immune system, such as HIV. Smokers and those in close contact with small children are also at higher risk. Pneumococcal disease is more common in winter months and when respiratory viruses such as influenza are circulating. Outbreaks of pneumococcal disease are not common but can occur in child care centers, nursing homes, or other institutions. In the United States, most deaths from pneumococcal disease occur in older adults, although in developing countries many children die of pneumococcal pneumonia.

RISK TO TRAVELERS

Pneumococcal disease occurs worldwide. Crowded settings or situations with close, prolonged contact with young children may increase the risk of contracting pneumococcal disease while traveling.

CLINICAL PRESENTATION

Fever and malaise are typical symptoms for all forms of pneumococcal disease and may be the only symptoms in young children with blood infections. Patients with pneumonia usually have cough, often with purulent or blood-tinged sputum, and may have shaking chills, shortness of breath, or pleuritic chest pain. Fever and sputum production may be absent in elderly persons with pneumococcal pneumonia. Patients with pneumococcal meningitis have headache, photophobia, stiff or painful neck, vomiting, lethargy, or decreased consciousness. Persons with pneumococcal ear infections typically have pain in the infected ear and can have purulent drainage (pus) following perforation of the ear drum. Sinus infections cause pain over the sinuses or in the teeth.

PREVENTION

Vaccines

Two vaccines are available to prevent pneumococcal disease; the pneumococcal conjugate vaccine (PCV) (Prevnar, Wyeth Vaccines) and the pneumococcal polysaccharide vaccine (PPV) (Pneumovax, Merck). Both vaccines provide protection by inducing antibodies to specific types of pneumococcal capsule; 90 different types of pneumococcal capsule have been identified. The conjugate vaccine protects against the 7 serotypes most common in young children in the United States; the polysaccharide vaccine includes 23 types. Both vaccines are effective at preventing invasive disease; the severe form of pneumococcal disease in which the organism is found in blood, spinal fluid, or other typically sterile bodily fluids. The conjugate vaccine, licensed for use in young children, also prevents some pneumonia and ear infections.

Pneumococcal conjugate vaccine

The pneumococcal conjugate vaccine is part of the routine infant immunization schedule. Health-care visits to receive travel-related vaccines provide a good opportunity to make sure that all routine vaccines are up to date. The pneumococcal conjugate vaccine is recommended for all children <2 years of age and children 2–4 years of age who have:

- Sickle cell hemoglobinopathies,
- functional or anatomical asplenia,
- received or will receive a cochlear implant,
- HIV infection,
- chronic disease, including chronic cardiac and pulmonary disease (excluding asthma), diabetes mellitus, or cerebrospinal fluid leak; and
- immunocompromising conditions, including a) hematologic or other disseminated malignancies; b) chronic renal failure or nephrotic syndrome; c) ongoing immunosuppressive therapy; and d) solid organ transplant.

Pneumococcal conjugate vaccine also should be considered for healthy children 2–4 years of age, especially those 24–35 months old, those attending group child care, and those of African-American, Alaskan Native or Native American descent.

Pneumococcal polysaccharide vaccine

The pneumococcal polysaccharide vaccine is part of the routine adult immunization schedule, but many adults who should have received the vaccine have not. In 2003, only 62% of adults ≥65 years of age had received the vaccine.

Pneumococcal polysaccharide vaccine (Pneumovax) is recommended for all adults ≥65 years of age and for persons 2–64 years of age with certain chronic illnesses or immunocompromising conditions, including:

- chronic cardiovascular disease (e.g., congestive heart failure or cardiomyopathies)
- chronic pulmonary disease (e.g., chronic obstructive pulmonary disease or emphysema, but not asthma)
- diabetes mellitus
- alcoholism
- chronic liver disease (cirrhosis)
- cerebrospinal fluid leaks
- functional or anatomic asplenia
- cochlear implant (or those planning to receive a cochlear implant)
- HIV infection
- multiple myeloma
- immunocompromising conditions, including a) hematologic or other generalized malignancies; b) chronic renal failure or nephrotic syndrome; c) ongoing immunosuppressive therapy; and d) bone marrow or solid organ transplant.

The polysaccharide vaccine should also be given to those 2–64 years of age who are living in settings in which the risk for invasive pneumococcal disease or its complications is increased, such as certain Native American communities (e.g., Alaskan Natives and certain American Indian populations) and residents of nursing homes and other long-term care facilities.

TABLE 4-13. RECOMMENDED REGIMENS FOR USE OF PNEUMOCOCCAL CONJUGATE VACCINE IN CHILDREN <5 YEARS OF AGE

AGE AT EXAMINATION (MONTHS)		VACCINATION HISTORY	RECOMMENDED REGIMEN[1]
2–6		0 doses	3 doses 2 months apart, 4th dose at age 12–15 months
		1 dose	2 doses 2 months apart, 4th dose at age 12–15 months
		2 doses	1 dose 2 months after the most recent dose, 4th dose at age 12–15 months
7–11		0 doses	2 doses 2 months apart, 3rd dose at 12–15 months
		1 or 2 doses before age 7 months	1 dose at 7–11 months, with another dose at 12–15 months (≥2 months later)
12–23		0 doses	2 doses ≥2 months apart
		1 dose before age 12 months	2 doses ≥2 months apart
		1 dose at ≥12 months	1 dose ≥2 months after the most recent dose
		2 or 3 doses before age 12 months	1 dose ≥2 months after the most recent dose
24–59	Healthy children	Any incomplete schedule	Consider 1 dose ≥2 months after the most recent dose[2]
	High risk	Any incomplete schedule of <3 doses	1 dose ≥2 months after the most recent dose and another dose ≥2 months later
		Any incomplete schedule of 3 doses	1 dose ≥2 months after the most recent dose

[1]For children vaccinated at <1 year of age, the minimum interval between doses is 4 weeks. Doses given at ≥12 months should be at least 8 weeks apart.
[2]Providers should consider administering a single dose to unvaccinated, healthy children 24–59 months old, with priority to children 24–35 months old, children who attend group day care centers, children of African-American descent, and children of Alaskan Native or Native American descent not otherwise identified as high risk.

A single dose of pneumococcal polysaccharide vaccine should be given at age 65 years or at the time a high-risk condition is recognized. Children 2–4 years of age with indications for pneumococcal polysaccharide vaccine should receive polysaccharide vaccine at least 2 months after receiving doses of conjugate vaccine. Persons with an indication for polysaccharide vaccine but with unknown vaccination history should receive one dose. A second dose of vaccine should be used for the following groups:

- persons ≥65 years of age who received the vaccine at least 5 years before and were <65 years of age at the time of initial vaccination;
- persons with sickle cell disease, asplenia, renal disease, hematologic or generalized malignancy, or other immunocompromising condition.

For children <10 years of age, the second dose may be given ≥3 years after the first dose; for older persons, revaccination may be given after 5 years. Because of limited data on the safety of multiple doses and on the duration of protection provided by polysaccharide vaccine, recommendations are for a single revaccination 3–5 years after the initial dose. These recommendations have been misinterpreted as suggesting revaccination every 5 years.

Safety/Side Effects
Mild local reactions such as redness, swelling, or tenderness occur in 10%–23% of infants after receipt of conjugate vaccine. Larger areas of redness or swelling or limitations in arm movement may occur in 1%–9%. For pneumococcal polysaccharide vaccine, mild, local side effects occur in approximately half of vaccine recipients and are more common after revaccination. Local reactions usually resolve by 48 hours after vaccination. More severe local reactions are rare. After conjugate vaccine, low-grade fever can occur in up to 24% of children and fever >102.2° F may occur in up to 2.5%. Systemic symptoms, including myalgias and fever, are rare after polysaccharide vaccine.

Precautions and contraindications
Conjugate vaccine is contraindicated for children known to have a hypersensitivity to any component of the vaccine. Health-care providers may delay vaccination of children with moderate or severe illness until the child has recovered, although minor illnesses, such as mild upper-respiratory tract infection with or without low-grade fever, are not

contraindications. Revaccination with pneumococcal polysaccharide vaccine is contraindicated for persons who had a severe reaction (e.g., anaphylactic reaction or localized arthus-type reaction) to the initial dose. Data are limited on the safety of pneumococcal polysaccharide vaccine during the first trimester of pregnancy.

Additional Preventive Measures

Persons who smoke cigarettes can reduce their risk of pneumococcal disease by stopping smoking. In addition, improving control of chronic conditions that are predisposing factors for pneumococcal disease, such as diabetes and HIV, may reduce risk. Chemoprophylaxis is not routinely recommended. Daily penicillin prophylaxis for children with sickle-cell hemoglobinopathy is recommended beginning before 4 months of age. How long to continue prophylaxis is somewhat controversial. However, children with sickle-cell anemia who had taken prophylactic penicillin for prolonged intervals but who had not had a severe pneumococcal infection or a splenectomy have stopped prophylactic penicillin therapy at 5 years of age without increased incidence of pneumococcal bacteremia or meningitis. Penicillin prophylaxis is also used for asplenic persons.

TREATMENT

Pneumococcal disease of all types is usually treated with antibiotics. Mild forms such as uncomplicated ear or sinus infections in healthy persons may resolve without treatment. More serious forms of pneumococcal disease, such as bloodstream infections and pneumonia, require antibiotics and often require hospitalization and intravenous antiobiotics. Pneumococcal meningitis always requires hospitalization and intravenous antibiotics. Because pneumococcal disease is endemic worldwide, care from a physician specializing in travel or tropical medicine is not required.

Bibliography

American Academy of Pediatrics. Pneumococcal infections. In: Pickering LK, ed. Red Book: 2003 Report of the Committee on Infectious Diseases. 26th ed. Elk Grove Village, IL: American Academy of Pediatrics, 2003:490–500.

CDC. Prevention of pneumococcal disease: recommendations of the Advisory Committee on Immunization Practices (ACIP). MMWR Morbid Mortal Wkly Rep 1997;46(No. RR-8):1–24.

CDC. Prevention of pneumococcal disease among infants and young children: recommendations of the Advisory Committee on Immunization Practices. MMWR Morbid Mortal Wkly Rep 2000;49 (No. RR-9):1–35.

Fedson DS, Scott JA, Scott G. The burden of pneumococcal disease among adults in developed and developing countries: what is and is not known. Vaccine 1999;17 Supp 1:S11–8.

Greenwood B. The epidemiology of pneumococcal infection in children in the developing world. Philos Trans R Soc Lond B Biol Sci 1999;354:777–85.

Mandell LA, Bartlett JG, Dowell SF, File Jr. TM, Musher DM, Whitney C. Update of practice guidelines for the management of community-acquired pneumonia in immunocompetent adults. Clin Infect Dis 2003;37:1405–1433.

Robinson KA, Baughman W, Rothrock G, Barrett NL, Pass M, Lexau C, et al. Epidemiology of invasive *Streptococcus pneumoniae* infections in the United States, 1995-1998: opportunities for prevention in the conjugate vaccine era. JAMA 2001;285:1729–35.

Whitney CG, Farley MM, Hadler J, Harrison KH, Bennett NM, Lynfield R, et al. Decline in invasive pneumococcal disease following the introduction of protein-polysaccharide conjugate vaccine. N Engl J Med 2003;348:1737–46.

Whitney C, Schaffner W, Butler J. Rethinking recommendations for use of pneumococcal vaccines in adults. Clin Infect Dis 2001;33:662–75.

–CYNTHIA WHITNEY AND JOHN MORAN

>>Poliomyelitis

DESCRIPTION

Poliomyelitis is an acute viral infection that involves the gastrointestinal tract and occasionally the central nervous system. It is acquired by fecal-oral or oral transmission.

OCCURRENCE

In the pre-vaccine era, infection with poliovirus was common, with epidemics occurring in the summer and fall in temperate areas. The incidence of poliomyelitis declined rapidly after the licensure of inactivated polio vaccine in 1955 and oral polio vaccine in the 1960s. The last cases of indigenously acquired polio in the United States occurred in 1979. Although a polio eradication program led to elimination of polio in the Western Hemisphere, where the last case associated with wild poliovirus was detected in 1991, outbreaks of vaccine-derived poliovirus type 1 occurred in the Dominican Republic and Haiti in 2000–01, in the Philippines in 2001, and a type 2 outbreak occurred in Madagascar in 2002. During 2003–04, poliomyelitis outbreaks occurred in a number of countries in West and Central Africa, following importation of wild polioviruses types 1 and 3 from Nigeria. In spite of these recent outbreaks, the global polio eradication initiative has reduced the number of reported polio cases worldwide by >99% since the mid-1980s, and worldwide eradication of the disease appears feasible in the future.

RISK FOR TRAVELERS

Travelers to countries where poliomyelitis cases still occur should be fully immunized. Because of polio eradication efforts, the number of countries where travelers are at risk for polio has decreased dramatically. Most of the world's population resides in areas now considered free of wild poliovirus circulation, including the Western Hemisphere, the Western Pacific Region (which encompasses China), and the European region.

As of September 2004, poliovirus remains endemic in six countries: Afghanistan, India, Pakistan, Nigeria, Niger, and Egypt. During 2003–2004, an epidemic of poliomyelitis spread from Nigeria to a number of countries in sub-Saharan Africa, including Benin, Burkina Faso, Côte d'Ivoire, Ghana, Guinea, Mali, Togo, Cameroon, Central African Republic, Chad, and the Darfur region of Sudan, as well as Botswana in southern Africa.

CLINICAL DESCRIPTION

Clinical manifestations of poliovirus infection range from asymptomatic (most of infections) to symptomatic, including acute flaccid paralysis of a single limb to quadriplegia, respiratory failure, and, rarely, death.

PREVENTION

A person is considered to be fully immunized if he or she has received a primary series of at least three doses of inactivated poliovirus vaccine (IPV), live oral poliovirus (OPV), or four doses of any combination of IPV and OPV. To eliminate the risk of vaccine-associated paralytic poliomyelitis, OPV is no longer recommended for routine immunization in the United States as of January 1, 2000. OPV is no longer available in this country, although it continues to be used in the majority of countries and for global polio eradication activities.

Infants and Children

Because OPV is no longer recommended for routine immunization in the United States, all infants and children should receive four doses of IPV at 2, 4, and 6–18 months of age, and 4–6 years of age. If accelerated protection is needed, the minimum interval between doses is 4 weeks, although the preferred interval between the second and third doses is 2 months. The minimum age for IPV administration is 6 weeks. Infants and children who have initiated the poliovirus vaccination series with one or more doses of OPV should receive IPV to complete the series.

Adults

Adults who are traveling to areas where poliomyelitis cases are still occurring and who are unvaccinated, incompletely vaccinated, or whose vaccination status is unknown, should receive IPV. Two doses of IPV should be administered at intervals of 4-8 weeks; a third dose should be administered 6–12 months after the second. If three doses of IPV cannot be administered within the recommended intervals before protection is needed, the following alternatives are recommended:

- If >8 weeks is available before protection is needed, three doses of IPV should be administered at least 4 weeks apart.
- If <8 weeks but >4 weeks is available before protection is needed, two doses of IPV should be administered at least 4 weeks apart.
- If <4 weeks is available before protection is needed, a single dose of IPV is recommended.

The remaining doses of vaccine should be administered later, at the intervals recommended above, if the person remains at increased risk for poliovirus exposure. Adults who are traveling to areas where poliomyelitis cases are occurring and who have received a primary series with either IPV or OPV should receive another dose of IPV before departure. For adults, available data do not indicate the need for more than a single lifetime booster dose with IPV.

Allergy to Vaccine

Minor local reactions (pain and redness) can occur following IPV. No serious adverse reactions to IPV have been documented. IPV should not be administered to persons who have experienced a severe allergic (anaphylactic) reaction after a previous dose of IPV or to streptomycin, polymyxin B, or neomycin. Because IPV contains trace amounts of these three antibiotics, hypersensitivity reactions can occur among persons sensitive to them.

Pregnancy

Although no adverse events of IPV have been documented among pregnant women or their fetuses, vaccination of pregnant women should be avoided on theoretical grounds. However, if a pregnant woman is unvaccinated or incompletely vaccinated and requires immediate protection against polio because of planned travel to a country or area where polio cases are occurring, IPV can be administered as recommended in the adult schedule. Breastfeeding is not a contraindication to immunization against polio.

Precautions and Contraindications

IPV may be administered to persons with diarrhea. Minor upper respiratory illnesses with or without fever, mild to moderate local reactions to a previous dose of IPV, current antimicrobial therapy, and the convalescent phase of acute illness are not contraindications for vaccination.

Immunosuppression

IPV may be administered safely to immunodeficient travelers and their household contacts. Although a protective immune response cannot be ensured, IPV may confer some protection to the immunodeficient person. Persons with certain primary immunodeficiency diseases should avoid contact with excreted oral polio vaccine virus (e.g., as may occur with a child vaccinated with OPV within the previous 6 weeks); however, this situation no longer occurs in the United States unless a child receives OPV overseas.

Bibliography

CDC. Poliomyelitis. In: Atkinson W, Hamborsky J, Wolfe S, eds. Epidemiology and prevention of vaccine-preventable diseases. 8th ed. Washington, DC: Public Health Foundation; 2004. p. 89–100.

CDC. Wild Poliovirus Importations — West and Central Africa, January 2003–March 2004. MMWR Morbid Mortal Wkly Rep. 2004;53;433–5.

CDC. Progress toward global eradication of poliomyelitis, January 2003–April 2004. MMWR Morbid Mortal Wkly Rep. 2004;53:532–5.

CDC. Poliomyelitis — Madagascar, 2002. MMWR Morbid Mortal Wkly Rep. 2002;51:622.

CDC. Acute flaccid paralysis associated with circulating vaccine-derived poliovirus — Philippines, 2001. MMWR Morbid Mortal Wkly Rep. 2001;50:874–5.

CDC. Outbreak of poliomyelitis — Dominican Republic and Haiti, 2000–2001. MMWR Morbid Mortal Wkly Rep. 2001;50:855–6.

CDC. Poliomyelitis prevention in the United States — updated recommendations of the Advisory Committee on Immunization Practices (ACIP). MMWR Morbid Mortal Wkly Rep. 2000;49(RR-5):1–22.

CDC. Poliomyelitis — United States, 1975–1984. MMWR Morbid Mortal Wkly Rep. 1986;35:180–2.

World Health Organization. The global poliomyelitis eradication initiative: number of endemic countries at lowest ever. Wkly Epidemiol Rec. 2002;77:414–5.

–LORRAINE ALEXANDER, MARGARET WATKINS, AND JIM ALEXANDER

>>Rabies

DESCRIPTION

Rabies is an acute, fatal encephalomyelitis caused by neurotropic viruses in the family Rhabdoviridae, genus Lyssavirus. It is almost always transmitted by an animal bite that inoculates the virus into wounds. Very rarely, rabies has been transmitted by exposures other than bites that introduce the virus into open wounds or mucous membranes. All mammals are believed to be susceptible, but reservoirs are carnivores and bats. Although dogs are the main reservoir in developing countries, the epidemiology of the disease differs sufficiently from one region or country to another to warrant the medical evaluation of all mammal bites.

OCCURRENCE

Rabies is found on all continents except Antarctica. In certain areas of the world, canine rabies remains highly endemic, including (but not limited to) parts of Afghanistan, Bangladesh, Brazil, Bolivia, China, Colombia, Ecuador, El Salvador, Guatemala, Haiti, India, Indonesia, Mexico, Myanmar (Burma), Nepal, Pakistan, Peru, the Philippines, Sri Lanka, Thailand, Vietnam, and Yemen. The disease is also found in dogs in many of the other countries of Africa, Asia, and Central and South America, except as noted in Table 4–14, which lists countries that have reported no cases of rabies during the most recent period for which information is available (formerly referred to as "rabies-free countries").

Additional information can be obtained from the World Health Organization (http://www.who.int/GlobalAtlas/DataQuery/browse.asp?catID= 011500000000&lev=3), the Pan American Health Organization, local health authorities of the country, the embassy, or the local consulate's office in the United States. Lists are provided only as a guide, because status can change suddenly as a result of disease re-introduction.

RISK FOR TRAVELERS

Travelers to rabies-endemic countries should be warned about the risk of acquiring rabies, although rabies vaccination is not a requirement for entry into any country. Travelers with extensive unprotected outdoor exposure in rural areas, such as might be experienced while bicycling, camping, hiking, or engaging in certain occupational activities, might be

TABLE 4-14. COUNTRIES AND POLITICAL UNITS REPORTING NO INDIGENOUS CASES OF RABIES DURING 2003[1]

REGION	COUNTRIES
Africa	Cape Verde, Libya, Mauritius, Réunion, São Tome and Principe, and Seychelles
Americas	North: Bermuda, St. Pierre and Miquelon
	Caribbean: Antigua and Barbuda, Aruba, Bahamas, Barbados, Cayman Islands, Dominica, Guadeloupe, Jamaica, Martinique, Montserrat, Netherlands Antilles, Saint Kitts (Saint Christopher) and Nevis, Saint Lucia, Saint Martin, Saint Vincent and Grenadines, Turks and Caicos, and Virgin Islands (UK and US)
	South: Uruguay
Asia	Armenia, Cyprus, Hong Kong, Japan, Kuwait, Lebanon, Malaysia (Sabah), Qatar, and Singapore
Europe	Belgium, Denmark,[2] Finland, France,[2] Gibraltar, Greece, Iceland, Ireland, Isle of Man, Italy, Luxemburg, Malta, Netherlands,[2] Norway (mainland), Portugal, Spain[2] (except Ceuta/Melilla), Sweden, Switzerland, and United Kingdom[2]
Oceania[3]	Australia,[2] Cook Islands, Fiji, French Polynesia, Guam, Hawaii, Kiribati, Micronesia, New Caledonia, New Zealand, Palau, Papua New Guinea, Samoa, and Vanuatu

[1]Bat rabies exists in some areas that are reportedly free of rabies in other animals.
[2]Bat lyssaviruses are known to exist in these areas that are reportedly free of rabies in other animals.
[3]Most of Pacific Oceania is reportedly rabies-free.

at high risk even if their trip is brief. Casual exposure to cave air is not a concern, but cavers should be warned not to handle bats.

CLINICAL DESCRIPTION

The disease progresses from a nonspecific prodromal phase to paresis or paralysis; spasms of swallowing muscles can be stimulated by the sight, sound, or perception of water (hydrophobia); delirium and convulsions can develop, followed by coma and death.

PREVENTION

Preexposure vaccination with human diploid cell rabies vaccine (HDCV), purified chick embryo cell (PCEC) vaccine, or rabies vaccine adsorbed (RVA) may be recommended for international travelers based on the local incidence of rabies in the country to be visited, the availability of appropriate antirabies biologicals, and the intended activity and duration of stay of the traveler. Preexposure vaccination may be recommended for veterinarians, animal handlers, field biologists, spelunkers, missionaries, and certain laboratory workers. Table 4–15 provides criteria for preexposure vaccination. Preexposure vaccination does not eliminate the need for additional medical attention after a rabies exposure but simplifies postexposure prophylaxis in populations at risk by eliminating the need for rabies immune globulin (RIG) and by decreasing the number of doses of vaccine required. Preexposure vaccination is of particular importance for travelers at risk of exposure to rabies in countries where biologicals are in short supply and locally available rabies vaccines might carry a high risk of adverse reactions. Preexposure vaccination may also provide some degree of protection when there is an unapparent or unrecognized exposure to rabies and when postexposure prophylaxis might be delayed.

Purified equine rabies immune globulin (ERIG) has been used effectively in some developing countries where human rabies immune globulin (RIG) might not have been available. If necessary, such heterologous product is preferable to no RIG administration in human rabies postexposure prophylaxis. The incidence of adverse reactions after the use of these products has been low (0.8%–6.0%), and most of those that occurred were minor. However, such products are neither evaluated by U.S. standards nor regulated by the U.S. Food and Drug Administration, and their use cannot be unequivocally recommended at this time. In addition, unpurified antirabies serum of equine origin might still be used in some countries where neither human RIG nor ERIG are available. The use of this antirabies serum is associated with higher rates of serious adverse reactions, including anaphylaxis.

Travelers should be advised that any animal bite or scratch should receive prompt local treatment by thorough cleansing of the wound with copious amounts of soap and water and a povidone-iodine solution if available; this local treatment will susbstantially reduce the risk of rabies. Travelers who might have been exposed to rabies should be advised to always contact local health authorities immediately for advice about postexposure prophylaxis and should also contact their personal physician or state health department as soon as possible thereafter.

TABLE 4-15. CRITERIA FOR PREEXPOSURE IMMUNIZATION FOR RABIES

RISK CATEGORY	NATURE OF RISK	TYPICAL POPULATIONS	PREEXPOSURE REGIMEN
Continuous	Virus present continuously, often in high concentrations Specific exposures likely to go unrecognized Bite, nonbite, or aerosol exposure	Rabies research laboratory workers,[1] rabies biologics production workers	Primary course: Serologic testing every 6 months; booster vaccination if antibody titer is below acceptable level[2]
Frequent	Exposure usually episodic with source recognized, but exposure might also be unrecognized Bite, nonbite, or aerosol exposure possible	Rabies diagnostic laboratory workers,[1] cavers, veterinarians and staff, and animal control and wildlife workers in rabies-epizootic areas	Primary course: Serologic testing every 2 years; booster vaccination if antibody titer is below acceptable level[2]
Infrequent (greater than general population)	Exposure nearly always episodic with source recognized Bite or nonbite exposure	Veterinarians, animal control and wildlife workers in areas with low rabies rates; veterinary students; and travelers visiting areas where rabies is enzootic and immediate access to appropriate medical care, including biologics, is limited.	Primary course: No serologic testing or booster vaccination
Rare (general population)	Exposure always episodic, with source recognized Bite or nonbite exposure	U.S. population at large, including individuals in rabies-epizootic areas	No preexposure immunization necessary

[1]Judgment of relative risk and extra monitoring of vaccination status of laboratory workers is the responsibility of the laboratory supervisor (see U.S. Department of Health and Human Service's Biosafety in Microbiological and Biomedical Laboratories, 1999).

[2]Preexposure booster immunization consists of one dose of human diploid cell [rabies] vaccine (HDCV), purified chick embryo cell (PCEC) vaccine, or rabies vaccine adsorbed (RVA), 1.0 mL dose, intramuscular (IM) (deltoid area). Minimum acceptable antibody level is complete virus neutralization at a 1:5 serum dilution by the rapid fluorescent focus inhibition test. A booster dose should be administered if titer falls below this level.

Tables 4–16 and 4–17 provide information on preexposure and postexposure prophylaxis. Routine serologic testing is not necessary for travelers who receive the recommended preeexposure or postexposure regimen with HDCV, PCEC, or RVA vaccines. Exposed travelers previously vaccinated with vaccines other than those produced by cell culture should receive the complete postexposure regimen unless they have developed a laboratory-confirmed antibody response to the primary vaccination. Serologic testing is still recommended for travelers whose immune response might be diminished by drug therapy or by diseases. Rabies preexposure prophylaxis may not be indicated for travelers to the countries in Table 4–14, and postexposure prophylaxis is rarely necessary after exposures to terrestrial animals in these countries.

Adverse Reactions

Travelers should be advised that they may experience local reactions, such as pain, erythema, and swelling or itching at the injection site, or mild systemic reactions, such as headache, nausea, abdominal pain, muscle aches, and dizziness. Approximately 6% of persons receiving booster vaccinations with HDCV can experience an immune complex-like reaction characterized by urticaria, pruritus, and malaise. Once initiated, rabies postexposure prophylaxis should not be interrupted or discontinued because of local or mild systemic reactions to rabies vaccine.

Precautions and Contraindications

Pregnancy

Pregnancy is not a contraindication to postexposure prophylaxis.

Age

In infants and children, the dose of HDCV, PCEC, or RVA for preexposure or postexposure prophylaxis is the same as that recommended for adults. The dose of RIG for postexposure prophylaxis is based on body weight (Table 4–17).

Bibliography

Arguin PM, Krebs JW, Mandel E, et al. Survey of rabies preexposure and postexposure prophylaxis among missionary personnel stationed outside the United States. J Travel Med. 2000;7:10–4.

TABLE 4-16. PREEXPOSURE IMMUNIZATION FOR RABIES[1]

VACCINE	DOSE (mL)	NO. OF DOSES	SCHEDULE (DAYS)	ROUTE
HDCV	1.0	3	0, 7, 21 or 28	Intramuscular
PCEC	1.0	3	0, 7, 21 or 28	Intramuscular
RVA	1.0	3	0, 7, 21 or 28	Intramuscular

HDCV, human diploid cell vaccine; PCEC, purified chick embryo cell; RVA, rabies vaccine adsorbed.

[1]Patients who are immunosuppressed by disease or medications should postpone preexposure vaccinations and consider avoiding activities for which rabies preexposure prophylaxis is indicated. When this course is not possible, immunosuppressed persons who are at risk for rabies should have their antibody titers checked after vaccination. Thus, preexposure immunization of immunosuppressed travelers is not recommended.

TABLE 4-17. POSTEXPOSURE IMMUNIZATION FOR RABIES[1]

IMMUNIZATION STATUS	VACCINE/ PRODUCT	DOSE	NO. OF DOSES	SCHEDULE (DAYS)	ROUTE
Not previously immunized	RIG plus	20 IU/kg body weight	1	0	Infiltrated at bite site (if possible); remainder intramuscular.
	HDCV or PCEC or RVA	1.0 mL	5	0, 3, 7, 14, 28	Intramuscular
Previously immunized[2, 3]	HDCV or PCEC or RVA	1.0 mL	2	0, 3	Intramuscular

RIG, rabies immune globulin; HDCV, human diploid cell (rabies) vaccine; PCEC, purified chick embryo cell; RVA, rabies vaccine adsorbed.

[1]All postexposure prophylaxis should begin with immediate thorough cleansing of all wounds with soap and water.
[2]Preexposure immunization with HDCV, PCEC, or RVA; prior postexposure prophylaxis with HDCV, PCEC, or RVA; or persons previously immunized with any other type of rabies vaccine and a documented history of positive antibody response to the prior vaccination.
[3]RIG should not be administered.

CDC. Human rabies prevention — United States, 1999. Recommendations of the Advisory Committee on Immunization Practices (ACIP). MMWR Morbid Mortal Wkly Rep. 1999;48(RR-1):1–21.

Fooks AR, McElhinney LM, Pounder DJ, et al. Case report: isolation of a European bat lyssavirus type 2a from a fatal human case of rabies encephalitis. J Med Virol. 2003;71:281–9.

Gibbons RV. Cryptogenic rabies, bats, and the question of aerosol transmission. Ann Emerg Med. 2002;39:528–36.

Jerrard DA. The use of rabies immune globulin by emergency physicians. J Emerg Med. 2004;27:15–9.

Moran GJ, Talan DA, Mower W, et al. Appropriateness of rabies postexposure prophylaxis treatment for animal exposures. Emergency ID Net Study Group. JAMA. 2000;284:1001–7.

Rupprecht CE, Hanlon CA, Hemachudha T. Rabies re-examined. Lancet Infect Dis. 2002;2:327–43.

Taplitz RA. Managing bite wounds. Currently recommended antibiotics for treatment and prophylaxis. Postgrad Med. 2004;116:49–52, 55–6, 59.

Warrell MJ, Warrell DA. Rabies and other lyssavirus diseases. Lancet. 2004;363:959–69.

Wilde H, Briggs DJ, Meslin FX, et al. Rabies update for travel medicine advisors. Clin Infect Dis. 2003;37:96–100.

–CHARLES E. RUPPRECHT

>>Rickettsial Infections

DESCRIPTION

Several species of *Rickettsia* can cause illnesses in humans (Table 4–18). The term "rickettsiae" conventionally embraces a polyphyletic group of microorganisms in the class Proteobacteria, comprising species belonging to the genera *Rickettsia*, *Orientia*, *Ehrlichia*, *Anaplasma*, *Neorickettsia*, *Coxiella*, and *Bartonella*. These agents are usually not transmissible directly from person to person except by blood transfusion or organ transplantation, although sexual and placental transmission has been hypothesized for *Coxiella*. Transmission generally occurs via an infected arthropod vector or through exposure to an infected animal reservoir host. Rickettsial agents that cause human disease are typically categorized not by disease manifestation but according to antigenic similarity. The clinical severity and duration of illnesses associated with different rickettsial infections vary considerably, even within a given antigenic group. Rickettsioses range in severity from diseases that are usually relatively mild (rickettsialpox, cat scratch disease, and African tick-bite fever) to those that can be life-threatening (epidemic typhus, Rocky Mountain spotted fever, and Oroya fever), and they vary in duration from those that can be self-limiting to chronic (Q fever and bartonelloses) or recrudescent (Brill-Zinsser disease). Most patients with rickettsial infections recover with timely use of appropriate antibiotic therapy.

Travelers may be at risk for exposure to agents of rickettsial diseases if they engage in occupational or recreational activities that bring them into contact with habitats that support the vectors or animal reservoir species associated with these pathogens.

OCCURRENCE AND RISK FOR TRAVELERS

The geographic distribution and the risks for exposure to rickettsial agents are described below, by disease.

Epidemic Typhus and Trench Fever

Epidemic typhus and trench fever, which are caused by *Rickettsia prowazkeii* and *Bartonella quintanta*, respectively, are transmitted from one person to another by the human body louse. Contemporary outbreaks of both diseases are rare in most developed countries and generally occur only in communities and populations in which body louse infestations are frequent (typically seen in refugee and prisoner populations, particularly during wars or famine). These diseases also occur sporadically in cooler mountainous regions of Africa, South America, Asia, and Mexico, especially during the colder months when louse-infested clothing is not laundered and person-to-person spread of lice is more frequent. Additional foci of trench fever among homeless populations in urban centers of industrialized countries have been recognized recently. Travelers who are not at risk of exposure to lice or to persons with lice are unlikely to acquire these illnesses. However, health-care workers who

Text continued on p. 259

TABLE 4-18. EPIDEMIOLOGIC FEATURES AND SYMPTOMS OF RICKETTSIAL DISEASES

ANTIGENIC GROUP	DISEASE	AGENT	PREDOMINANT SYMPTOMS[1]	VECTOR OR ACQUISITION MECHANISM	ANIMAL RESERVOIR	GEOGRAPHIC DISTRIBUTION OUTSIDE THE US
Typhus fevers	Epidemic typhus, Sylvatic typhus	Rickettsia prowazekii	Headache, chills, fever, prostration, confusion, photophobia, vomiting, rash (generally starting on trunk)	Human body louse, squirrel flea and louse	Humans, flying squirrels (US)	Cool mountainous regions of Africa, Asia, and Central and South America
	Murine typhus	R. typhi	As above, generally less severe	Rat flea	Rats, mice	Worldwide
Spotted fevers	Rocky Mountain spotted fever	R. rickettsii	Headache, fever, abdominal pain, rash (generally starting on extremities)	Tick	Rodents	Mexico, Central and South America
	Mediterranean spotted fever[2]	R. conorii	Fever, eschar, regional adenopathy, rash on extremities	Tick	Rodents	Africa, India, Europe, Middle East, Mediterranean
	African tick-bite fever	R. africae	Fever, eschar(s), regional adenopathy, rash subtle or absent	Tick	Rodents	Sub-Saharan Africa
	North Asian tick typhus	R. sibirica	As above	Tick	Rodents	Russia, China, Mongolia

[1]This represents only a partial list of symptoms. Patients may have different symptoms or only a few of those listed.
[2]Includes 4 different subspecies that can be distinguished serologically and by PCR assay, and respectively are the etiologic agents of Boutonneuse fever and Mediterranean tick fever in Southern Europe and Africa (R. conorii subsp. conorii), Indian tick typhus on Indian subcontinent (R. conorii subsp. indica), Israeli tick typhus in Southern Europe and Middle East (R. conorii subsp. israelensis), and Astrakhan spotted fever in the North Caspian region of Russia (R. conorii subsp. caspiae).

ANTIGENIC GROUP	DISEASE	AGENT	PREDOMINANT SYMPTOMS[1]	VECTOR OR ACQUISITION MECHANISM	ANIMAL RESERVOIR	GEOGRAPHIC DISTRIBUTION OUTSIDE THE US
Spotted fevers–cont'd	Oriental spotted fever	R. japonica	As above	Tick	Rodents	Japan
	Rickettsialpox	R. akari	Fever, eschar, adenopathy, disseminated vesicular rash	Mite	House mice	Russia, South Africa, Korea
	Tick-borne disease	R. slovaca	Necrosis erythema, lymphadenopathy	Tick	Lagomorphs, rodents	Europe
	Aneruptive fever	R. helvetica	Fever, headache, myalgia	Tick	Rodents	Old World
	Cat flea rickettsiosis	R. felis	As murine typhus, generally less severe	Cat and dog flea	Domestic cats, opossums	Europe, South America
	Queensland tick typhus	R. australis	Fever, eschar, regional adenopathy, rash on extremities	Tick	Rodents	Australia, Tasmania
	Flinders Island spotted fever, Thai tick typhus	R. honei	As above but milder, eschar and adenopathy are rare	Tick	Not defined	Australia, Thailand

TABLE 4-18. EPIDEMIOLOGIC FEATURES AND SYMPTOMS OF RICKETTSIAL DISEASES-CONT'D

ANTIGENIC GROUP	DISEASE	AGENT	PREDOMINANT SYMPTOMS[1]	VECTOR OR ACQUISITION MECHANISM	ANIMAL RESERVOIR	GEOGRAPHIC DISTRIBUTION OUTSIDE THE US
Orientia	Scrub typhus	Orientia tsutsugamushi	Fever, headache, sweating, conjunctival injection, adenopathy, eschar, rash (starting on trunk), respiratory distress	Mite	Rodents	Indian Subcontinent, Central, Eastern, and Southeast Asia and Australia
Coxiella	Q fever	Coxiella burnetii	Fever, headache, chills, sweating, pneumonia, hepatitis, endocarditis	Most human infections are acquired by inhalation of infectious aerosols. Tick[3]	Goats, sheep, cattle, domestic cats, other	Worldwide
Bartonella	Cat-scratch disease	Bartonella henselae	Fever, adenopathy, neuroretinitis, encephalitis	Cat flea	Domestic cats	Worldwide
	Trench fever	B. quintana	Fever, headache, pain in the shins, splenomegaly, disseminated rash	Human body louse	Humans	Worldwide
	Oroya fever	B. bacilliformis	Fever, headache, anemia, shifting joint and muscle pain, nodular dermal eruption	Sand fly	Unknown	Peru, Ecuador, Colombia

[3]These arthropods can transmit the pathogen from one animal to another, but are less frequently involved in transmission to humans.

ANTIGENIC GROUP	DISEASE	AGENT	PREDOMINANT SYMPTOMS[1]	VECTOR OR ACQUISITION MECHANISM	ANIMAL RESERVOIR	GEOGRAPHIC DISTRIBUTION OUTSIDE THE US
Ehrlichia	Ehrlichiosis	Ehrlichia chaffeensis[4]	Fever, headache, nausea, occasionally rash	Tick	Various large and small mammals, including deer and rodents	Worldwide
Anaplasma	Anaplasmosis	Anaplasma phagocytophilum[4]	Fever, headache, nausea, occasionally rash	Tick	Small mammals, and rodents	Europe, Asia, Africa
Neorickettsia	Sennetsu fever	Neorickettsia sennetsu	Fever, chills, headache, sore throat, insomnia	Fish fluke	Fish	Japan, Malaysia

[4]Organisms antigenically related to these species are associated with ehrlichial diseases outside the continental United States.

care for these patients may be at risk of acquiring louse-borne illnesses through inhalation or inoculation into the skin of infectious louse feces. In the eastern United States, campers and wildlife workers can acquire typhus if they come in contact with flying squirrels, their ectoparasites, or their nests, which can be made in houses and tree-holes.

Murine Typhus and Cat-Flea Rickettsiosis

Murine typhus, which is caused by infection with R. typhi, occurs worldwide and is transmitted to humans by rat fleas. Flea-infested rats can be found throughout the year in humid tropical environments, but in temperate regions, they are most common during the warm summer months. Travelers who visit rat-infested buildings and homes, especially in harbor or riverine environments, can be at risk for exposure to the agent of murine typhus. Similarly, cat-flea rickettsiosis, which is caused by infection with R. felis, occurs worldwide and is responsible for a murine typhus-like febrile disease in humans. The infection may result from exposure to flea-infested domestic cats and dogs or peridomestic animals.

Scrub Typhus

Mites ("chiggers") transmit Orientia tsutsugamushi, the agent of scrub typhus, to humans. These mites occur year-round in a large area from the Indian subcontinent to Australia and in much of Asia, including Japan, China, Korea, Maritime Provinces and Sakhalin Island of Russia, and Tajikistan. Their prevalence, however, fluctuates with temperature and rainfall. Infection may occur on coral atolls in both the Indian and Pacific Oceans, in rice paddies, on oil palm plantations, and in tropical to desert habitats and elevated river valleys. Humans typically encounter the arthropod vector of scrub typhus in recently disturbed terrain (e.g., forest clearings) or other persisting rat-mite foci with rats and other rodents.

Tick-Borne Rickettsioses

Tick-borne rickettsial diseases have a worldwide distribution but are most common in temperate and subtropical regions. These diseases include Rocky Mountain spotted fever (caused by R. rickettsii), Mediterranean spotted fever (caused by R. conorii), African tick-bite fever (caused by R. africae), Queensland tick typhus (caused by R. australis), North Asian tick spotted fever (caused by R. sibirica), Flinders Island spotted fever and Thai tick typhus (caused by R. honei), and ehrlichioses (caused by Ehrlichia spp. and Anaplasma phagocytophilum) (Table 4–18).

In general, peak transmission of tick-borne rickettsial pathogens occurs seasonally during spring and summer months. Travelers who participate in outdoor activities in grassy or wooded areas (e.g., trekking, camping, or going on safari) may be at risk for acquiring tick-borne illnesses, including those caused by *Rickettsia*, *Anaplasma*, and *Ehrlichia* species.

Rickettsialpox

Rickettsialpox is generally an urban, mite-vectored disease associated with *R. akari*-infected house mice, although feral rodent-mite reservoirs also have been described. Outbreaks of this illness have occurred shortly after rodent extermination programs, since the mites seek new hosts. *R. akari*-infected rodents have been found in urban centers in the former Soviet Union, South Africa, Korea, Croatia, and the United States. Travelers may be at risk for exposure to rodent mites when staying in old urban hostels and cabins.

Q Fever

Q fever occurs worldwide, most often in persons who have frequent contact with goat, sheep, and cattle carcasses and parturient animals (especially farmers, veterinarians, butchers, meat packers, and seasonal workers). Travelers who visit farms or rural communities can be exposed to *Coxiella burnetii*, the agent of Q fever, through airborne transmission (via contaminated soil and dust) or possibly through consumption of unpasteurized milk products or by exposure to infected ticks. These infections may initially result in only mild and self-limiting influenza-like illnesses, but if untreated, they may become chronic, particularly in persons with preexisting heart valve abnormalities or prosthetic valves. Such persons can develop chronic and potentially fatal endocarditis.

Cat-Scratch Disease and Oroya Fever

Cat-scratch disease is contracted through scratches and bites from domestic cats, particularly kittens, infected with *Bartonella henselae*, and possibly from their fleas. Exposure can therefore occur wherever cats are found. Oroya fever is transmitted by sand flies infected with *B. bacilliformis*, which is endemic in the Andean highlands.

CLINICAL PRESENTATION AND DIAGNOSIS

Clinical presentations of rickettsial illnesses differ (Table 4–18), but early symptoms, including fever, headache, and malaise, are generally nonspecific. Rashes are often associated with rickettsioses, and an eschar (thick blackened scab) is seen in scrub typhus and several spotted fever rickettsioses. Illnesses resulting from infection with rickettsial agents often go unrecognized or are attributed to other causes. Atypical presentations are common and may be expected with poorly characterized nonindigenous agents, so appropriate samples should be obtained for examination by specialized reference laboratories. A diagnosis of rickettsial disease is based on two or more of the following: 1) compatible clinical symptoms and epidemiologic history, 2) the development of specific convalescent-phase antibodies reactive with a given pathogen or antigenic group, 3) a positive polymerase chain reaction test result, 4) immunohistologic detection of a microorganism, or 5) isolation of a rickettsial agent. Ascertaining the place and the nature of potential exposures is particularly important for accurate diagnosis, as many rickettsial diseases have strong geographic links or are associated with exposure to specific animal reservoir species or arthropod vectors.

PREVENTION

With the exception of the louse-borne diseases described above, for which contact with infectious arthropod feces is the primary mode of transmission (through autoinoculation into a wound or inhalation), travelers and health-care providers are generally not at risk of becoming infected via exposure to an ill person. Infections result primarily from exposure to an infected vector or animal reservoir. Limiting these exposures remains the best means for reducing the risk for disease. Travelers should be advised that prevention is based on avoidance of vector-infested habitats, use of repellents and protective clothing (see *Protection against Mosquitoes and Other Arthropods*), prompt detection and removal of arthropods from clothing and skin, and attention to hygiene. Disease management should focus on early detection and proper treatment to prevent severe complications of these illnesses.

TREATMENT

Treatments for most rickettsial illnesses are similar and include administration of appropriate antibiotics (most often tetracycline class or chloramphenicol) and supportive care. Treatment should be initiated on the basis of clinical and epidemiologic clues, without waiting for laboratory confirmation. It is advisable to seek specialized infectious disease advice in travel and tropical medicine. No commercially licensed vaccines are available in the United States, and vaccinations to prevent rickettsial infections are not required by any country as a condition for entry.

Bibliography

Comer JA, Paddock CD, Childs JE. Urban zoonoses caused by *Bartonella, Coxiella, Ehrlichia*, and *Rickettsia* species. Vector Borne and Zoonotic Diseases. 2001;1:91–116.

Fournier PE, Allombert C, Supputamongkol Y, et al. Aneruptive fever associated with antibodies to *Rickettsia helvetica* in Europe and Thailand. J Clin Microbiol. 2004;42:816–8.

Isaksson HJ, Hrafnkelsson J, Hilmarsdottir I. Acute Q fever: a cause of fatal hepatitis in an Icelandic traveler. Scand J Infect Dis. 2001;33:314–5.

Jensenius M, Fournier PE, Raoult D. Tick-borne rickettsioses in international travelers. Int J Infect Dis. 2004;8:139–46.

Lewin MR, Bouyer DH, Walker DH, Musher DM. *Rickettsia sibirica* infection in members of scientific expeditions to northern Asia. Lancet. 2003;362:1201–2.

Oteo A, Ibarra V, Blanco JR, et al. *Dermacentor*-borne necrosis erythema and lymphadenopathy: clinical and epidemiological features of a new tick-borne disease. Clin Microbiol Infect. 2004;10:327–31.

Raoult D, Roux V. Rickettsioses as paradigms of new or emerging infectious diseases. Clin Microbiol Rev 1999;10:649–719.

Watt G, Parola P. Scrub typhus and tropical rickettsioses. Curr Opin Infect Dis. 2003;16:429–36.

Weber DJ, Rutala WA. Risks and prevention of nosocomial transmission of rare zoonotic diseases. Clin Infect Dis. 2001;32:446–56.

Zaidi SA, Siger C. Gastrointestinal and hepatic manifestations of tick-borne diseases in the United States. Clin Infect Dis. 2002;34:1397–8.

−MARINA EREMEEVA AND GREGORY DASCH

>>Rubella

DESCRIPTION

Rubella is an acute viral disease that can affect susceptible persons of any age. Although rubella is generally a mild rash illness, if contracted in the early months of pregnancy it is associated with a high rate of fetal loss or a constellation of birth defects, known as congenital rubella syndrome (CRS).

OCCURRENCE

The last major epidemic of rubella in the United States occurred in 1964 and 1965 when millions of rubella cases led to 20,000 cases of infants born with CRS. Following vaccine licensure in 1969, rubella incidence declined rapidly. Each year from 1992 through 2000, <500 cases were reported; each year since 2001, <100 cases have been reported—a 99% decline compared with the pre-vaccine era. Although rubella incidence has decreased in all age groups, the decreases have been greatest among children. Therefore, adults account for an increasing proportion of the few cases that still occur; more than 70% of rubella cases since 2000 have been among adults, compared with 29% in 1991. In 1995–2000, an average of five CRS cases was reported annually; since 2001, an average of one CRS case has been reported annually. From 1997 through 2000, most persons with rubella were born outside the United States. Moreover, since 1997, most women whose infants were reported to have CRS were born outside the United States in countries where routine rubella vaccination programs are not used or have only recently been implemented. During 1997–1999, 21 (81%) of 26 infants reported with CRS were Hispanic, and 24 (92%) of 26 were born to foreign-born mothers.

RISK FOR TRAVELERS

Rubella occurs worldwide, and the risk of exposure to rubella outside the United States can be high. Although more than half of all countries now use rubella vaccine, rubella still remains a common disease in many parts of the world.

CLINICAL PRESENTATION

Rubella usually presents as a nonspecific maculopapular rash lasting 3 days or fewer (hence the term "3-day measles") with generalized lymphadenopathy, particularly of the postauricular, suboccipital and posterior cervical lymph nodes. However, asymptomatic infections are common: up to 50% of infections occur without rash. In adults or adolescents, the rash may be preceded by a 1- to 5-day prodrome of low-grade fever, headache, malaise, anorexia, mild conjunctivitis, coryza, sore throat, and lymphadenopathy.

PREVENTION

Rubella vaccine, which contains live, attenuated rubella virus, is available as a single-antigen preparation or combined with live, attenuated measles or mumps vaccines, or both. Combined measles, mumps, and rubella (MMR) vaccine is recommended whenever one or more of the individual components is indicated and is the most common vaccine formulation available in the United States.

Although vaccination against measles, mumps, or rubella is not a requirement for entry into any country (including the United States), persons traveling or living abroad should ensure that they are immune to all three diseases. Immunity to rubella is particularly important for health-care providers and women of childbearing age. Persons can be considered immune to rubella if they have documentation of receipt of one or more doses of a rubella-containing vaccine on or after their first birthday, or laboratory evidence of rubella immunity. Birth before 1957 provides only presumptive evidence of rubella immunity and does not guarantee that a person is immune. Rubella can occur in susceptible persons born before 1957, and CRS can occur in the offspring of women born before 1957 infected with rubella during pregnancy. The Advisory Committee on Immunization Practices (ACIP) recommends that birth before 1957 not be accepted as evidence of rubella immunity for women who might become pregnant. A clinical diagnosis of rubella is unreliable and should not be considered in assessing immune status. Because many rash illnesses can mimic rubella infection and many rubella infections are unrecognized, the only reliable evidence of previous rubella infection is the presence of serum rubella IgG.

According to the routine childhood immunization schedule (Table 8–2), the first dose of MMR should be routinely administered to infants 12–15 months of age. A single dose of MMR vaccine induces antibody formation to all three viruses in at least 95% of susceptible persons vaccinated at ≥12 months of age. The second dose should be separated from the first dose by a minimum of 28 days. (See Vaccine Recommendations for Infants and Children, for a discussion of the rubella immunization schedule modifications for infants who will be traveling.)

Health-care providers who treat women of childbearing age should routinely determine their rubella immunity status and vaccinate those who are susceptible and not pregnant. Proof of immunity can be either a verified record of vaccination or a positive IgG antibody serologic test. Rubella-susceptible women who 1) do not report being pregnant, 2) are not likely to become pregnant within 1 month, and 3) have no other contraindicating conditions should be vaccinated. Before vaccination, each patient should be counseled to avoid pregnancy for 1 month after vaccination because of the theoretical risk for vaccine virus affecting the fetus. Because routine pregnancy screening is not recommended before rubella vaccination, patients should be counseled regarding the theoretical risk to the fetus from inadvertent vaccination of a pregnant woman.

Adverse Reactions, Precautions, and Contraindications to Rubella Vaccine

Refer to Travelers' Health Information on Measles (Rubeola) for information about adverse reactions, precautions, and contraindications following MMR vaccine.

Bibliography

Reef SE, Frey TK, Theall K, et al. The changing epidemiology of rubella in the 1990s: on the verge of elimination and new challenges for control and prevention. JAMA. 2002;287:464–72.

Robertson SE, Featherstone DA, Gacic-Dobo M, et al. Rubella and congenital rubella syndrome: global update. Rev Panam Salud Pública. 2003;14:306–15.

Watson JC, Hadler SC, Dykewicz CA, et al. Measles, mumps, and rubella—vaccine use and strategies for elimination of measles, rubella, and congenital rubella syndrome and control of mumps: recommendations of the Advisory Committee on Immunization Practices (ACIP). Morbid Mortal Wkly Rep MMWR 1998;47(RR-8):1–57.

–SUSAN REEF

>>Schistosomiasis

DESCRIPTION

Schistosomiasis (also known as bilharzia) is a parasitic infection caused by *Schistosoma* flukes that have complex life cycles involving specific freshwater snail species as intermediate hosts. Infected snails release large numbers of minute, free-swimming larvae (cercariae) that are capable of penetrating the unbroken skin of the human host. Even brief exposure to contaminated freshwater, such as wading, swimming, or bathing, can result in infection. Human schistosomiasis cannot be acquired by contact with salt water (oceans or seas). However, the cercariae of birds and aquatic mammals can penetrate the skin of human beings who enter infested fresh or salt water in many parts of the world, including cool temperate areas. These cercariae die in the skin but may elicit a pruritic rash ("swimmer's itch" or "clam-digger's itch").

OCCURRENCE

This infection occurs widely throughout the tropics and subtropics, affecting some 200 million persons. Schistosomiasis is most prevalent in sub-Saharan Africa. In highly endemic areas, prevalence rates can exceed 50% among the local population, and high rates have been reported among expatriates living in such areas.

RISK FOR TRAVELERS

Exposure to schistosomiasis is a health hazard for persons who travel to endemic areas (see Map 4–10). Outbreaks of schistosomiasis have occurred among adventure travelers on river trips in Africa, as well as among resident expatriates, such as Peace Corps volunteers in high-risk areas. Those at greatest risk are travelers who wade, swim, or bathe in fresh water in areas where sanitation is poor and the snail hosts are present.

CLINICAL PRESENTATION

Clinical manifestations of acute infection can occur within 2-12 weeks of exposure to cercariae-infested water, but most acute infections are asymptomatic. The most common acute syndrome is Katayama fever. Symptoms include fever, loss of appetite, weight loss, abdominal pain, hematuria, weakness, headaches, joint and muscle pain, diarrhea,

MAP 4-10. GEOGRAPHIC DISTRIBUTION OF SCHISTOSOMIASIS

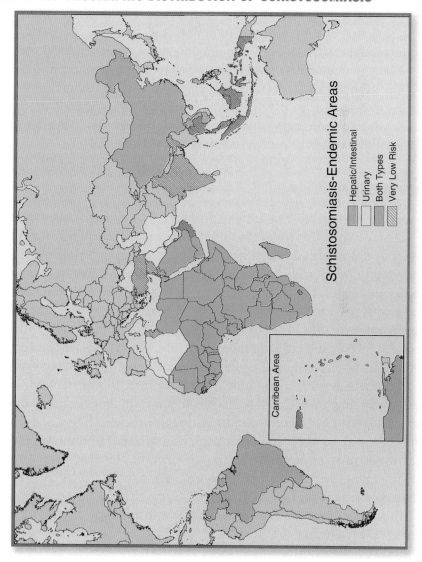

Note that the prevalence of schistosomiasis is changing rapidly. Control programs have eliminated or greatly reduced transmission of schistosomiasis in most countries in Asia and the Americas. On the other hand, the prevalence of schistosomiasis has increased in sub-Saharan Africa, and water resource development projects and population movements have led to introduction of schistosomiasis into regions and countries that were not endemic previously. Japan and Monteserrat have eliminated schistosomiasis. At present, there is believed to be extremely low (or no risk) of schistosomiasis in the shaded countries as indicated on the map. In Brazil, China, Egypt, Philippines, Iran, Morocco, Venezuela, and elsewhere national control programs have reduced morbidity due to schistosomiasis. Organisms causing hepatic or intestinal schistosomiasis include S. mansoni, S. mekongi, S. intercalatum, and S. malayanensis. S. haematobium causes urinary schistosomiasis.

nausea, and cough. Rarely, the central nervous system can be involved, producing seizures or transverse myelitis as a result of mass lesions of the brain or spinal cord. Chronic infections can cause disease in the liver, intestinal tract, bladder (including bladder cancer), kidneys, or lung. Many persons with chronic infections recall no symptoms of acute infection. Diagnosis of infection is usually confirmed by serologic studies or by finding schistosome eggs on microscopic examination of stool or urine. Schistosome eggs can be found as soon as 6-8 weeks after exposure, but are not always detectable.

PREVENTION

No vaccine is available, nor are any drugs recommended as chemoprophylactic agents at this time. Because there is no practical way for the traveler to distinguish infested from noninfested water, travelers should be advised to avoid wading, swimming or other fresh-water contact in endemic countries. Untreated piped water coming directly from canals, lakes, rivers, streams or springs may contain cercariae, but heating bathing water to 50° C (122° F) for 5 minutes or filtering water with fine-mesh filters can eliminate the risk of infection. If such measures are not feasible, travelers should be advised to allow bathing water to stand for 2 days because cercariae rarely remain infective longer than 24 hours. Swimming in adequately chlorinated swimming pools is virtually always safe, even in endemic countries. Vigorous towel drying after accidental exposure to water has been suggested as a way to remove cercariae in the process of skin penetration; however, this may prevent only some infections and should not be recommended to travelers as a preventive measure. Although topical application of the insect repellent DEET can block penetrating cercariae, the effect is short lived and cannot reliably prevent infection.

Upon return from foreign travel, those who may have been exposed to schistosome-infested freshwater should be advised to undergo screening tests. Because serologic tests are more sensitive than microscopic examination of stool and urine for eggs, previously uninfected but potentially exposed travelers should be tested for antibodies to schistosomes if microscopic examination of stool and urine for eggs is negative or not available. CDC performs a screening ELISA that is 99%, 90%, and 50% sensitive for *Schistosoma mansoni*, *S. haematobium*, and *S. japonicum*, respectively, and a confirmatory, species-specific immunoblot that is at least 95% sensitive and 99% specific for all three species. Serologic tests performed in commercial laboratories may not be as sensitive or specific.

TREATMENT

Safe and effective oral drugs are available for the treatment of schistosomiasis. Praziquantel is the drug of choice for all species of *Schistosoma*. Oxamniquine has been effective in treating infections caused by *S. mansoni*. Travelers who suspect they may have schistosomiasis should be advised to contact an infectious disease or tropical medicine specialist.

Bibliography

CDC. Schistosomiasis in U.S. Peace Corps volunteers—Malawi, 1992. MMWR. 1993;42:565–70.

Cetron MS, Chitsulo L, Sullivan JJ, et al. Schistosomiasis in Lake Malawi. Lancet. 1996;348:1274–8.

Corachan M. Schistosomiasis and international travel. Clin Infect Dis. 2002;35:446–50.

Cioli D, Pica-Mattoccia L. Praziquantel. Parasitol Res. 2003;90 Suppl 1:S3–S9.

Jordan P, Webbe G, Sturrock RF, editors. Human schistosomiasis. Wallingford: CAB International; 1993.

Ross AG, Bartley PG, Sleigh AC, et al. Schistosomiasis. N Engl J Med. 2002;346:1212-20.

Savioli L, Albonico M, Engels D, et al. Progress in the prevention and control of schistosomiasis and soil-transmitted helminthiasis. Parasitol Int. 2004;53:103–13.

Tsang VC, Wilkins PP. Immunodiagnosis of schistosomiasis. Screen with FAST-ELISA and confirm with immunoblot. Clin Lab Med. 1991;11:1029–39.

World Health Organization. The control of schistosomiasis. Second report of the WHO Expert Committee. World Health Organ Tech Rep Ser. 1993;830:1–86.

WHO Expert Committee. Prevention and control of schistosomiasis and soil-transmitted helminthiasis. World Health Organ Tech Rep Ser. 2002;912:1–57.

–JAMES MAGUIRE AND BRIAN BLACKBURN

>>Severe Acute Respiratory Syndrome

DESCRIPTION

Severe acute respiratory syndrome (SARS) is a febrile respiratory illness caused by a novel coronavirus, SARS-associated coronavirus (SARS-CoV), which emerged in southern China in November 2002. SARS-CoV is believed to be of zoonotic origin; although several animal species (e.g., civet cats, raccoon dogs) sold for human consumption in markets in southern China have demonstrated evidence of SARS-CoV infection, the natural reservoir of SARS-CoV is unknown.

OCCURRENCE

During November 2002–July 2003, more than 8,000 probable SARS cases, 774 of them fatal, were reported from 29 countries, with most cases in China, Hong Kong, Taiwan, Singapore, and Canada. In the United States, only 8 patients were confirmed to have laboratory evidence of SARS-CoV infection.

From July 2003 through September 2004, 17 laboratory-confirmed SARS cases were reported. Six persons were infected through laboratory exposures: one in Singapore, one in Taiwan, and four in China. One of these six cases initiated a chain of transmission that ultimately resulted in seven additional cases and one death. All the laboratory-acquired infections resulted from lapses in appropriate biosafety procedures.

In addition, in December 2003 and January 2004, four unlinked cases of community-acquired SARS were reported in Guangdong, the province in China where SARS first emerged. The source of infection for these cases was not conclusively determined but is presumed to have been wild animals, possibly those in live-food markets.

CLINICAL PRESENTATION

Following an incubation period of 2–10 days (median 5), the illness typically begins with fever, which is often high (>38°C) and is associated with other constitutional symptoms, such as headache, malaise, myalgia, chills, and rigors. After 3–7 days, lower respiratory symptoms, such as a dry, nonproductive cough or dyspnea, develop and may be accompanied by or progress to hypoxemia. By day 7 of illness, most SARS patients demonstrate abnormalities on chest radiographs. These abnormalities typically appear as focal interstitial infiltrates and progress to more generalized, patchy, interstitial infiltrates, sometimes appearing as areas of consolidation. Diarrhea has been reported in 20% to >60% of patients, depending, in part, on when during the course of illness symptoms were assessed. The overall case-fatality rate of SARS is approximately 10%, but fatality rates exceed 50% in persons >60 years of age.

RISK FOR TRAVELERS

During the spring 2003 outbreak, most travelers were at low risk for acquiring SARS. Those who did become infected usually had another risk factor for SARS infection, such as close contact with a SARS patient in a health-care or household setting, and occasionally they had exposure outside these settings in communities with active SARS transmission. In addition, a few SARS patients may have acquired infection during airplane flights on which an undiagnosed, symptomatic SARS patient was also traveling. When there is no evidence of SARS transmission anywhere in the world, there is essentially no risk of acquiring SARS. In case of a re-emergence of SARS, travelers can get up-to-date information on locations with SARS transmission and ways to decrease their risk of acquiring SARS at CDC's Travelers' Health website: http://www.cdc.gov/travel/.

Although there is no conclusive evidence that direct contact with civets or other wild animals from live-food markets has led to cases of SARS, SARS-CoV has been found in these animals. In addition, some persons working with these animals have had evidence of infection with SARS-CoV or a very similar virus. Therefore, it remains theoretically possible that travelers to China who come in contact with these animals may acquire SARS-CoV infection.

PREVENTION

On the basis of limited available data, prudent travelers to China will avoid visiting live food markets and having direct contact with civets and other wildlife from these markets.

In case of a re-emergence of SARS, travelers to areas reporting SARS cases should avoid settings where transmission is most likely to occur, such as health-care facilities caring for SARS patients and residences of SARS patients. CDC does not recommend the routine use of masks or other personal protective equipment while in public areas, but it does recommend frequent hand-washing to reduce the risk of transmission.

TREATMENT

Because the clinical presentation of SARS is compatible with that of other causes of atypical pneumonia, empiric treatment regimens have included several antibiotics to presumptively treat known bacterial agents of atypical pneumonia. No specific treatment with proven efficacy is available for SARS-CoV illness.

For more information about SARS, see the CDC SARS site at http://www.cdc.gov/ncidod/sars.

Bibliography

CDC. Public health guidance for community-level preparedness and response to severe acute respiratory syndrome (SARS): Version 2 [monograph on the internet]. Atlanta: CDC; 2004 [cited 2004 Oct 11]. Available from: http://www.cdc.gov/ncidod/sars/guidance/index.htm.

Guan Y, Zheng BJ, He YQ, et al. Isolation and characterization of viruses related to the SARS coronavirus from animals in southern China. Science. 2003;302:276–8.

Jernigan JA, Low DE, Helfand RF. Combining clinical and epidemiologic features for early recognition of SARS. Emerg Infect Dis. 2004;10:327–33.

Olsen SJ, Chang HL, Cheung TY, et al. Transmission of the severe acute respiratory syndrome on aircraft. N Engl J Med. 2003;349:2416–22.

Pang X, Zhu Z, Xu F, et al. Evaluation of control measures implemented in the severe acute respiratory syndrome outbreak in Beijing, 2003. JAMA. 2003;290:3215–21.

Peiris JS, Yuen KY, Osterhaus AD, et al. The severe acute respiratory syndrome. N Engl J Med. 2003;349:2431–41.

Xu RH, He JF, Evans MR, et al. Epidemiologic clues to SARS origin in China. Emerg Infect Dis. 2004;10:1030–7.

–UMESH D. PARASHAR, MEHRAN S. MASSOUDI, AND LARRY J. ANDERSON

>>Sexually Transmitted Diseases (STDs)

DESCRIPTION

Sexually transmitted diseases (STDs) are the infections and resulting clinical syndromes caused by more than 25 infectious organisms transmitted through sexual activity. Because STDs are communicable diseases with far-reaching public health consequences, early detection and treatment are important for the sexual and reproductive health of the individual as well as the community. STDs can often result in serious long-term complications, including pelvic inflammatory disease, infertility, stillbirths and neonatal infections, genital cancers, and an increased risk for HIV acquisition and transmission.

OCCURRENCE

Sexually transmitted diseases are among the most common infections with an estimated 18.9 million new infections annually in the United States and 340 million infections worldwide. Travelers who have sexual interactions with core groups of efficient STD transmitters (commercial sex workers) in endemic areas may have high rates of acquisition of an STD, such as gonorrhea. Some STDs are more prevalent in developing countries (e.g., chancroid, lymphogranuloma venereum, and granuloma inguinale) and may be more likely to be exported into developed countries by travelers.

RISK FOR TRAVELERS

International travelers are at risk of contracting STDs, including HIV, if they have sexual contact with partners in locales with high STD prevalence. Increased sexual promiscuity and casual sexual relationships tend to occur during travel abroad to foreign countries and are frequently reported in long-term overseas travelers. Commercial sexual service in various destinations (e.g., Southeast Asia) attracts many foreign travelers. Worldwide, increased rates of infectious syphilis and quinolone-resistant gonorrhea have recently been reported among men who have sex with men (MSM).

CLINICAL PRESENTATION

Any traveler who might have been exposed to an STD and who develops a vaginal or urethral discharge, an unexplained rash or genital lesion, or genital or pelvic pain should be advised to cease sexual activity and promptly seek medical care. Screening for asymptomatic infection should be encouraged among travelers who have had casual sexual activity.

PREVENTION

The prevention and control of STDs are based on education and counseling; specific measures the traveler can take to avoid acquiring or transmitting STDs should be part of the health advice given to travelers. Abstinence or mutual monogamy is the most reliable way to avoid acquisition and transmission of STDs. For persons whose sexual behaviors place them at risk for STDs, correct and consistent use of the male latex condom can reduce the risk of HIV infection and STD transmission during sexual contact. Only water-based lubricants (e.g., K-Y Jelly or glycerine) should be used with latex condoms, because oil-based lubricants (e.g., petroleum jelly, shortening, mineral oil, or massage oils) can weaken latex condoms. Vaginal spermicides containing nonoxynol-9 are not recommended in STD/HIV prevention.

Preexposure vaccination is an effective method for prevention of sexually acquired hepatitis A and B infections. Hepatitis A vaccine is recommended for all unvaccinated persons using injection drugs and MSM. Hepatitis B vaccine is recommended for all unvaccinated persons with a history of STD, multiple sexual partners, use of injection drugs or partner who uses them, or MSM. Vaccines for herpes simplex virus and human papillomavirus are currently in clinical trials and may become available in the next several years.

TREATMENT

Knowledge of the clinical presentation, frequency of infection, and antimicrobial resistance patterns (e.g., quinolone-resistant *Neisseria gonorrhoeae*) are important in the management of STDs that occur in travelers to specific destinations. Treatment directed toward a specific pathogen is the historical norm for most STDs in industrialized countries. Syndromic management, of interest in developing countries, requires only broad clinical manifestations with risk assessment, followed by treatment of the main causes of the syndrome without identification of a specific pathogen. Evaluation and management of STDs should be based on standard guidelines (CDC, WHO) with consideration of the high frequency of antimicrobial resistance in different geographic areas.

Bibliography

Abdullah AM, Ebrahim SH, Fielding R, et al. Sexually transmitted infections in travelers: implications for prevention and control. Clin Infect Dis. 2004;39:533–8.

CDC. Sexually transmitted diseases treatment guidelines 2002. MMWR Morbid Mortal Wkly Rep 2002;51(RR-6):1–78.

CDC. Increases in fluoroquinolone-resistant *Neisseria gonorrhoeae* among men who have sex with men- United States, 2003, and revised recommendations for gonorrhea treatment, 2004. MMWR Morbid Mortal Wkly Rep. 2004;53:335–8.

Memish ZA, Osoba AO. Sexually transmitted diseases and travel. Int J Antimicrob Agents. 2003;21:131–4.

Matteelli A, Carosi G. Sexually transmitted diseases in travelers. Clin Infect Dis. 2001;32:1063–7.

Mulhall BP. Sexual behavior in travellers. Lancet. 1999;353:595–6.

Workowski KA, Levine WC, Wasserheit JN. U.S. Centers for Disease Control and Prevention guidelines for the treatment of sexually

transmitted diseases: an opportunity to unify clinical and public
health practice. Ann Intern Med. 2002;137:255–62.

–KIMBERLY WORKOWSKI

>>Smallpox

In May 1980, WHO declared the global eradication of smallpox. Currently, there is no evidence of smallpox transmission anywhere in the
world. The last reported case of endemic smallpox occurred in Somalia
in October 1977, and the last reported case of laboratory-acquired
smallpox occurred in the United Kingdom in 1978. WHO amended the
International Health Regulations on January 1, 1982, deleting smallpox
from the diseases subject to the regulations. Today, concerns about the
reemergence of smallpox involve its potential use as a biological
weapon.

**Smallpox vaccination should not be given for international
travel.** The currently licensed smallpox vaccine is a live-virus vaccine
containing vaccinia virus, an orthopoxvirus related to smallpox virus
that can provide cross-protection. Smallpox vaccination of civilians is
currently recommended for laboratory workers directly involved with
smallpox or closely related orthopoxviruses (e.g., monkeypox, vaccinia,
and others) and public health, medical, and other designated response
personnel who may be involved as first responders to an intentional
release of smallpox virus. In addition, U.S. military personnel may be
required to have smallpox vaccination as a part of military force protection policies. Health-care workers whose contact with vaccinia virus is
limited to contaminated materials (e.g., dressings) are at a lower risk of
inadvertent infection than laboratory workers, but may be considered
for vaccination.

In response to a confirmed smallpox outbreak within the United States
or internationally, rapid voluntary vaccination **may** be initiated to 1)
supplement priority surveillance and containment control strategies in
areas with smallpox cases, 2) reduce the population at risk for additional intentional releases of smallpox virus if the probability of such
occurrences is considered substantial, or 3) address heightened public
or political concerns regarding access to voluntary vaccination. Large-

scale voluntary smallpox vaccination would be considered part of an overall national vaccination strategy and would be initiated following the approval of the Secretary of Health and Human Services.

MISUSE OF SMALLPOX VACCINE

Smallpox vaccine should never be used for medical reasons other than for the prevention of smallpox or a related orthopoxvirus infection. There is no evidence that smallpox vaccination has therapeutic value in the treatment of recurrent herpes simplex infection, warts, or any other disease.

Bibliography

CDC. Emergency Preparedness and Response website. Available at URL: http://www.bt.cdc.gov/agent/smallpox/index.asp.

CDC. Recommendations for using smallpox vaccine in a pre-event vaccination program: supplemental recommendations of the Advisory Committee on Immunization Practices (ACIP) and the Healthcare Infection Control Practices Advisory Committee (HICPAC). MMWR Morb Mortal Wkly Rep 2003; 52(RR-07):1–16.

CDC. Smallpox vaccination and adverse reactions; guidance for clinicians. MMWR Morb Mortal Wkly Rep 2003; 52(RR04):1–28.

CDC. Cardiac adverse events following smallpox vaccination — United States, 2003. MMWR Morb Mortal Wkly Rep 2003; 52(12):248–250.

Henderson DA. Smallpox: clinical and epidemiological features. Emerg Infect Dis 1999;5:537–9.

Henderson D, Inglesby T, Bartlett J, Ascher MS, Eitzen E, Jahrling PB. Consensus statement: smallpox as a biological weapon: medical and public health management. JAMA 1999; 281:2127-37.

—LISA ROTZ

>>Travelers' Diarrhea

DESCRIPTION

Travelers' diarrhea (TD) is a clinical syndrome resulting from microbial contamination of ingested food and water; it occurs during or shortly after travel, most commonly affecting persons traveling from an area of more highly developed hygiene and sanitation infrastructure to a less developed one. Thus, TD is defined more by circumstances of acquisition than by a specific microbial agent. In fact, there is considerable diversity in etiologic agents, which include bacteria, parasites, or viruses. A similar but less common syndrome is toxic gastroenteritis, caused by ingestion of pre-formed toxins. In this syndrome, vomiting may predominate, and symptoms usually resolve within 12-18 hours.

Pathogen isolation rates among TD studies vary from 30% to 60%. Most cases in which no pathogen is identified respond to antibiotics, suggesting that most of these are bacterial in origin.

Bacterial Enteric Pathogens
Bacteria are the most common cause of TD. In studies of etiologic agents at various destinations, bacteria are responsible for approximately 85% of TD cases, parasites about 10%, and viruses 5%.

Enterotoxigenic Escherichia coli *(ETEC)*
The most common cause of TD worldwide is ETEC. Ingestion of a large inoculum of this organism is necessary to produce disease. These high inoculums occur when there is a breakdown in sanitation, which is often the case in developing countries where ETEC infections are common. ETEC typically produces a watery diarrhea associated with cramps. Fever may be low or absent.

Enteroaggregative E. coli *(EAEC)*
EAEC are increasingly recognized as a cause of TD and may be responsible for up to 25% of cases. EAEC resemble ETEC in clinical presentation and response to antibiotics.

Campylobacter jejuni
Campylobacter jejuni is a common cause of diarrhea in developed countries but is many times more prevalent in developing countries. The risk

of acquiring infection with *Campylobacter* appears to vary by destination, with travel to Asia posing a higher risk in most studies. *Campylobacter* infections may be associated with bloody diarrhea as well as fever.

Salmonella *spp.*
Although nontyphoidal *Salmonella* infections are frequently associated with foodborne outbreaks in industrialized countries, they are an infrequent cause of TD worldwide.

Shigella *spp.*
The low infectious dose of this organism makes it one of the more commonly reported bacteria associated with TD. *Shigella* may cause a bloody diarrhea with constitutional symptoms and fever.

Vibrio *spp.*
Diarrhea caused by *Vibrio parahaemolyticus* and non-O-group 1 *Vibrio cholerae* may be associated with eating raw or partially cooked seafood. *Vibrio cholerae* O-group 1 has in general been a rare cause of TD, but recent reports suggest this organism may be associated with the typical TD clinical picture in Western travelers to developing countries.

Other Bacteria
Other organisms that have been isolated from patients with TD include *Aeromonas hydrophila, Plesiomonas shigelloides,* and *Yersinia enterocolitica.*

Parasitic Enteric Pathogens
Parasitic protozoan pathogens account for about 10% of cases of TD and usually present with a more insidious onset. Travelers often complain of persistent symptoms, and the likelihood of recovery of a parasite rather than bacteria from stool specimens increases proportionately with duration of symptoms. The most common organisms in this category include *Giardia intestinalis, Cryptosporidium parvum, Cyclospora cayetanensis, Entamoeba histolytica,* and *Dientamoeba fragilis.*

Viral Enteric Pathogens
The contribution of viruses to the burden of TD appears to be quite small, although they can cause substantial morbidity from gastroenteritis, with primarily nausea and vomiting. Sporadic viral infections account for 5%–10% of cases of TD. Enteric viruses such as rotavirus and norovirus, which infect children in developing countries, may also

infect travelers to developing countries. Outbreaks of norovirus have been reported on cruise ships. In such outbreaks, a high percentage of susceptible people are likely to become ill.

OCCURRENCE

The most important determinant of risk is travel destination, and there are regional differences in both the risk and etiology of diarrhea. The world map is generally divided into three grades of risk: high, intermediate, and low. (See Map 4–11). Low-risk countries include the USA, Canada, Australia, New Zealand, Japan, and countries in Northern and Western Europe. Intermediate-risk countries include those in Eastern Europe, South Africa, and some of the Caribbean islands. High-risk areas include most of Asia, the Middle East, Africa, and Central and South America. Some destinations that were previously considered high risk have now been classified as low or intermediate risk, including parts of Southern Europe and some of the Caribbean islands. On average, 30%–50% of travelers to high-risk areas will develop TD during a 1- to 2-week stay. Based on the annual figure of 50 million travelers to developing countries, this estimate translates to approximately 50,000 cases of TD each day. In more temperate regions, there may be seasonal variations in diarrhea risk. In South Asia, for example, during the hot months preceding the monsoon, much higher TD attack rates are commonly reported.

RISK FOR TRAVELERS

Travelers' diarrhea occurs equally in males and females and is more common in young adults than in older people. In short-term travelers, bouts of TD do not appear to protect against future attacks, and more than one episode of TD may occur during a single trip.

CLINICAL PRESENTATION

Definitions of TD that rely on rigid criteria for frequency of loose stools in a 24-hour period are commonly used in clinical research studies but are not relevant to the clinical syndrome as it affects travelers. Travelers' diarrhea is characterized by the fairly abrupt onset of loose, watery or semi-formed stools associated with abdominal cramps and rectal urgency. Symptoms may be preceded by a prodrome of gaseousness and abdominal cramping and additional symptoms may be associated, such as nausea, bloating, and fever. Vomiting may occur in up to 15% of

MAP 4-11. AREAS OF RISK FOR TRAVELERS' DIARRHEA

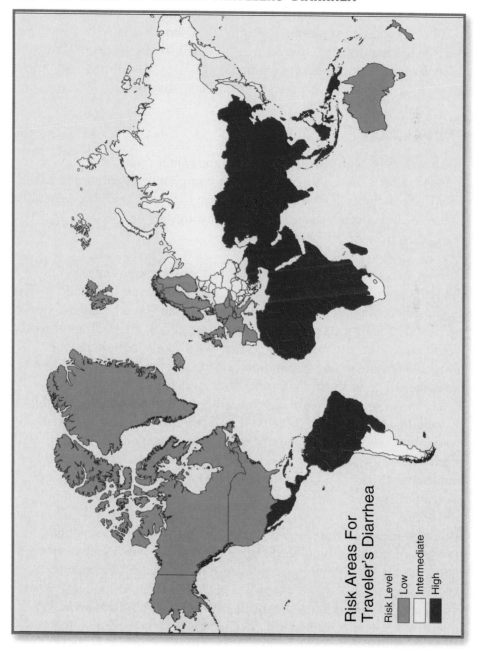

Risk Areas For
Traveler's Diarrhea

Risk Level
Low
Intermediate
High

those affected. Travelers' diarrhea is generally self-limited and lasts 3–4 days even without treatment, but persistent symptoms may occur in a small percentage of travelers. Postinfectious sequelae have been described, including reactive arthritis, Guillain-Barré syndrome, and postinfectious irritable bowel syndrome (PI-IBS). PI-IBS may occur in up to 3% of persons who contracted travelers' diarrhea.

PREVENTION

For travelers to high-risk areas, several approaches may be recommended, which can minimize but never completely eliminate the risk of TD. These include 1) instruction regarding food and beverage selection, 2) use of agents other than antimicrobial drugs for prophylaxis, and 3) use of prophylactic antibiotics.

Care in selecting food and beverages for consumption may minimize the risk for acquiring TD. Travelers should be advised to eat foods that are freshly cooked and served piping hot and to avoid water and beverages diluted with water (reconstituted fruit juices, ice, milk) and foods washed in water, such as salads. Other risky foods include raw or undercooked meat and seafood and raw fruits and vegetables. Safe beverages include those that are bottled and sealed or carbonated. Boiled beverages and those appropriately treated with iodine or chlorine might also be safely consumed. Studies of TD risk at high-risk destinations show that consumption of food or beverages from street vendors poses a particularly high risk, and some studies suggest certain food items such as reheated prepared foods or buffet items are also high risk.

Although food and water precautions continue to be recommended, travelers may have difficulty following this advice. Furthermore, many of the factors that ensure food safety are out of the traveler's control.

The primary agent other than antimicrobial drugs studied for prevention of TD is bismuth subsalicylate (BSS), which is the active ingredient in Pepto-Bismol. Studies from Mexico have shown this agent (taken as either 2 oz of liquid or two chewable tablets four times per day) to reduce the incidence of TD from 40% to 14%. BSS commonly causes blackening of the tongue and stool and may cause nausea, constipation, and rarely tinnitus. BSS should be avoided by travelers with aspirin allergy, renal insufficiency, and gout and by those taking anti-coagulants, probenecid, or methotrexate. In travelers taking aspirin or salicylates for other reasons, the use of BSS may result in salicylate toxicity. Caution should be used in administering BSS to children with viral infections, such as chickenpox or influenza, because of the risk of Reye syndrome. BSS is not recommended for children <3 years of age. Studies have not established the safety of BSS use for periods of greater than 3 weeks.

The use of probiotics, such as *Lactobacillus* GG and *Saccharomyces boulardii*, has been studied in the prevention of TD in limited numbers of subjects. Results are inconclusive.

Travelers should be cautioned that other nonantimicrobial agents, such as enterovioform and related halogenated hydroxyquinoline derivatives, are sometimes available to travelers at their destination. These substances are not useful in preventing TD, may cause serious neurologic adverse events, and should never be used for prophylaxis.

Prophylactic antibiotics have been demonstrated to be quite effective in the prevention of TD. Controlled studies have shown that diarrhea attack rates are reduced from 40% to 4% by the use of antibiotics. The ideal antibiotic is one to which the pathogenic bacteria are sensitive, which has changed over the past few decades as resistance patterns have evolved. Agents such as TMP-SMX and doxycycline are no longer considered effective antimicrobials against enteric bacterial pathogens. The fluoroquinolones have been the most popular and effective antibiotics for the prophylaxis and treatment of bacterial TD pathogens, but increasing resistance to these agents, initially among *Campylobacter* species and now among other TD pathogens, may limit their benefit in the future. A newly approved nonabsorbable antibiotic, rifaximin, is being investigated for its potential use in TD prophylaxis. Prophylactic antibiotics should not be recommended for most travelers. In addition to affording no protection against nonbacterial pathogens, they may also give the traveler a false sense of security, leading to neglect of the food and water precautions that might protect against other enteric diseases. In addition, the use of antibiotics may be associated with allergic or adverse reactions in a certain percentage of travelers, an unnecessary occurrence, as early self-treatment with antibiotics for established TD is quite effective.

Prophylactic antibiotics may be considered for short-term travelers who are high-risk hosts (such as those who are immunosuppressed) or are taking critical trips during which even a short bout of diarrhea could impact the purpose of their trip.

TREATMENT

Antibiotics are the principal element in the treatment of TD. Adjunctive agents used for symptomatic control may also be recommended.

Antibiotics

As bacterial causes of TD far outnumber other microbial etiologies, empiric treatment with an antibiotic directed at enteric bacterial pathogens remains the best therapy for TD. The benefit of treatment of TD with antibiotics has been proven in a number of studies. The effectiveness of a particular antimicrobial depends on the etiologic agent and its antibiotic sensitivity. Both as empiric therapy or for treatment of a specific bacterial pathogen, first-line antibiotics include those of the fluoroquinolone class, such as ciprofloxacin or levofloxacin. Increasing microbial resistance to the fluoroquinolones, especially among *Campylobacter* isolates, may limit their usefulness in some destinations such as Thailand and Nepal. An alternative to the fluoroquinolones in this situation is azithromycin. Rifaximin has been approved for the treatment of TD caused by noninvasive strains of *E. coli*.

The standard treatment regimens consist of 3 days of antibiotic, although when treatment is initiated promptly shorter courses, including single-dose therapy, may reduce the duration of the illness to a few hours.

Nonspecific Agents

Bismuth subsalicylate (Pepto-Bismol), taken as 1 oz of liquid or two chewable tablets every 30 minutes for eight doses, has been shown to decrease stool frequency and shorten the duration of illness in several placebo-controlled studies. This agent has both antisecretory and antimicrobial properties. BSS should be used with caution in travelers on aspirin therapy or anticoagulants or those who have renal insufficiency. In addition, BSS should be avoided in children with viral infections, such as varicella or influenza, because of the risk of Reye syndrome.

Other nonspecific agents, such as kaolin pectin, activated charcoal, and probiotics, have had a limited role in the treatment of TD.

Antimotility Agents

Antimotility agents provide symptomatic relief and serve as useful adjuncts to antibiotic therapy in TD. Synthetic opiates, such as loperamide and diphenoxylate, can reduce bowel movement frequency and enable travelers to resume their activities while awaiting the effects of antibiotics. Loperamide appears to have antisecretory properties as well. Although earlier studies suggest these agents should not be used in diarrheal illness associated with high fever or blood in the stool, more recent studies suggest these medications may be used in such instances as long as antibiotics are administered concurrently. Loperamide and diphenoxylate are not recommended for children <2 years of age.

Oral Rehydration Therapy

Fluid and electrolytes are lost in cases of TD, and replenishment is important, especially in young children or adults with chronic medical illness. In adult travelers who are otherwise healthy, severe dehydration resulting from TD is unusual unless vomiting is present. Nonetheless, replacement of fluid losses remains an important adjunct to other therapy. Travelers should remember to use only beverages that are sealed or carbonated. For more severe fluid loss, replacement is best accomplished with oral rehydration solutions (ORS), such as World Health Organization ORS solutions, which are widely available at stores and pharmacies in most developing countries. (See Table 4–19 for details.) ORS is prepared by adding one packet to the appropriate volume of boiled or treated water. Once prepared, solutions should be consumed or discarded within 12 hours (24 hours if refrigerated).

Treatment of Protozoan Etiologies

The most common parasitic cause of TD is *Giardia intestinalis,* and treatment options include metronidazole, tinidazole, and nitazoxanide. Although cryptosporidiosis is usually a self-limited illness in immunocompetent persons, nitazoxanide can be considered as a treatment option. Cyclosporiasis is treated with TMP-SMX. Treatment of amebia-

TABLE 4-19. COMPOSITION OF WHO ORAL REHYDRATION SOLUTION (ORS) FOR DIARRHEAL ILLNESS

INGREDIENT	AMOUNT	MEASUREMENT
Sodium chloride	3.5 g/L	$\frac{1}{2}$ tsp
Potassium chloride	1.5 g/L	$1\frac{1}{4}$ tsp
Glucose	20.0 g/L	2 tbsp
Trisodium citrate (or sodium bicarbonate)	2.9 g/L (or 2.5 g/L)	$\frac{1}{2}$ tsp
Water	1,000 g	1 liter

sis is with metronidazole or tinidazole, followed by treatment with a luminal agent such as iodoquinol or paromomycin.

Treatment for Children

Children who accompany their parents on trips to high-risk destinations may be expected to have TD as well. There is no reason to withhold antibiotics from children who contract TD. In older children and teenagers, treatment recommendations for TD follow those for adults, with possible adjustments in dose of medication. Macrolides such as azithromycin are considered first-line antibiotic therapy in children, although some experts are using short-course fluoroquinolone therapy with caution for travelers <18 years of age. Rifaximin is approved for use starting at age 12.

Infants and younger children are at higher risk for developing dehydration from TD, which is best prevented by the early use of ORS solutions. Breastfed infants should continue to nurse on demand, and bottle-fed infants should be offered full strength lactose-free or -reduced formula. Older infants and children should continue their regular diets during the illness.

Bibliography

Adachi JA, Jiang ZD, Mathewson JJ, et al. Enteroaggregative *Escherichia coli* as a major etiologic agent in travelers' diarrhea in 3 regions of the world. Clin Infect Dis. 2001;32:1706–9.

DuPont HL, Ericsson CD. Prevention and treatment of travelers' diarrhea. N Engl J Med. 1993;328:1821–7.

DuPont HL, Jiang ZD, Ericsson CD, et al. Rifaximin versus ciprofloxacin for the treatment of travelers' diarrhea: a randomized, double blind clinical trial. Clin Infect Dis 2001;33:1807–15.

Gorbach SL, Kean BH, Evans DG, et al. Travelers' diarrhea and toxigenic *Escherichia coli*. N Engl J Med. 1975;292:933–6.

Hoge CW, Shlim DR, Echeverria P, et al. Epidemiology of diarrhea among expatriate residents living in a highly endemic environment. JAMA. 1996;275:533-8.

Hoge CW, Gambel JM, Srijan A, et al. Trends in antibiotic resistance among diarrheal pathogens isolated in Thailand over 15 years. Clin Infect Dis. 1998;26:341–45.

Shlim, DR. Update in travelers' diarrhea. Infect Dis Clin North Am. In press 2004.

Steffen R, van der Linde F, Gyr K, et al. Epidemiology of diarrhea in travelers. JAMA. 1983;249:1176–80.

Taylor DN, Connor BA, Shlim DR. Chronic diarrhea in the returned traveler. Med Clin North Am. 1999;83:1033–52.

Taylor DN, Sanchez JL, Chandler W, et al. Treatment of travelers' diarrhea: ciprofloxacin plus loperamide compared with ciprofloxacin alone. A placebo-controlled, randomized trial. Ann Intern Med. 1991;114:731–4.

Von Sonnenburg F, Tornieporth N, Waiyaki P, et al. Risk and aetiology of diarrhea at various tourist destinations. Lancet. 2000;356:133–4.

–BRADLEY A. CONNOR

>>Tuberculosis

DESCRIPTION

Mycobacterium tuberculosis is a rod-shaped bacterium that can cause disseminated disease but is most frequently associated with pulmonary infections. The bacilli are transmitted by the airborne route and, depending on host factors, may lead to latent tuberculosis infection (sometimes abbreviated LTBI) or tuberculosis disease (TB). Both conditions can usually be treated successfully with medications.

OCCURRENCE

In many other countries, tuberculosis is much more common than in the United States, and it is an increasingly serious public health problem.

RISK FOR TRAVELERS

To become infected, a person usually has to spend a relatively long time in a closed environment where the air was contaminated by a person with untreated tuberculosis who was coughing and who had numerous *M. tuberculosis* organisms (or tubercle bacilli) in secretions from the lungs or voice box (larynx). Infection is generally transmitted through the air; therefore, there is virtually no danger of its being spread by dishes, linens, and items that are touched, or by most food products. However, it can be transmitted through unpasteurized milk or milk products obtained from infected cattle.

Travelers who anticipate possible prolonged exposure to tuberculosis (e.g., those who could be expected to come in contact routinely with hospital, prison, or homeless shelter populations) should be advised to have a tuberculin skin test before leaving the United States. If the reaction is negative, they should have a repeat test approximately 12 weeks after returning. Because persons with HIV infection are more likely to have an impaired response to the tuberculin skin test, travelers who are HIV positive should be advised to inform their physicians about their HIV infection status. Except for travelers with impaired immunity, travelers who already have a positive tuberculin reaction are unlikely to be reinfected.

Travelers who anticipate repeated travel with possible prolonged exposure or an extended stay over a period of years in an endemic country should be advised to have two-step baseline testing and, if the reaction is negative, annual screening, including a tuberculin skin test.

CDC and state and local health departments have published the results of six investigations of possible tuberculosis transmission on commercial aircraft. In these six instances, a passenger or a member of a flight crew traveled on commercial airplanes while infectious with tuberculosis. In all six instances, the airlines were unaware that the passengers or crew members were infected with tuberculosis. In two of the instances, CDC concluded that tuberculosis was probably transmitted to others on the airplane. The findings suggested that the risk of tuberculosis transmission from an infectious person to others on an airplane was greater on long flights (8 hours or more). The risk of exposure to tuberculosis was higher for passengers and flight crew members sitting or working near an infectious person because they might inhale droplets containing *M. tuberculosis* bacteria.

Based on these studies and findings, WHO issued recommendations to prevent the transmission of tuberculosis in aircraft and to guide potential investigations. The risk of tuberculosis transmission on an airplane does not appear to be greater than in any other enclosed space. To prevent the possibility of exposure to tuberculosis on airplanes, CDC and WHO recommend that persons known to have infectious tuberculosis travel by private transportation (that is, not by commercial airplanes or other commercial carriers), if travel is required. CDC and WHO have issued guidelines for notifying passengers who might have been exposed to tuberculosis aboard airplanes. Passengers concerned about possible exposure to tuberculosis should be advised to see their primary healthcare provider for a tuberculosis skin test.

PREVENTION

Vaccine

Based on WHO recommendations, the Bacille Calmette-Guérin (BCG) vaccine is used in most developing countries to reduce the severe consequences of tuberculosis in infants and children. However, BCG vaccine has variable efficacy in preventing the adult forms of tuberculosis and interferes with testing for latent tuberculosis infection. Therefore, it not routinely recommended for use in the United States.

Other

Travelers should be advised to avoid exposure to known tuberculosis patients in crowded environments (e.g., hospitals, prisons, or homeless shelters). Travelers who will be working in hospitals or health-care settings where tuberculosis patients are likely to be encountered should be advised to consult infection control or occupational health experts about procedures for obtaining personal respiratory protective devices (e.g., N-95 respirators), along with appropriate fitting and training. Additionally, tuberculosis patients should be educated and trained to cover coughs and sneezes with their hands or tissues to reduce spread. Otherwise, no specific preventive measures can be taken or are routinely recommended for travelers.

TREATMENT

Persons who are infected or who become infected with *M. tuberculosis* can be treated to prevent progression to tuberculosis disease. Updated American Thoracic Society (ATS)/CDC recommendations for treatment of latent tuberculosis infection recommend 9 months of isoniazid as the preferred treatment and suggest that 4 months of rifampin is a reasonable alternative. Travelers who suspect that they have been exposed to tuberculosis should be advised to inform their physicians of the possible exposure and receive appropriate medical evaluation. CDC and ATS have published updated guidelines for targeted tuberculin skin testing and treatment of latent tuberculosis infection. Recent data from the WHO suggest that resistance is relatively common in some parts of the world. Travelers who have tuberculin skin test conversion associated with international travel should consult experts in infectious diseases or pulmonary medicine.

Bibliography

American Thoracic Society/Centers for Disease Control and Prevention. Targeted Tuberculin Testing and Treatment of Latent Tuberculosis Infection. Am J Respir & Critical Care Med. 2000;161:S221–47.

American Thoracic Society/Centers for Disease Control and Prevention. Update: Adverse Event Data and Revised American Thoracic Society/CDC Recommendations Against the Use of Rifampin and

Pyrazinamide for Treatment of Latent Tuberculosis Infection—
United States, 2003. MMWR Morbid Mortal Wkly Rep.
2003;52:735–9.

–MICHAEL IADEMARCO

>>Typhoid Fever

DESCRIPTION

Typhoid fever is an acute, life-threatening febrile illness caused by the
bacterium *Salmonella enterica* Typhi.

OCCURRENCE

An estimated 22 million cases of typhoid fever and 200,000 related
deaths occur worldwide each year. Approximately 400 cases of typhoid
fever, mostly among travelers, are reported to the Centers for Disease
Control and Prevention each year.

RISK FOR TRAVELERS

Typhoid vaccination is not required for international travel, but CDC
recommends it for travelers to areas where there is a recognized risk of
exposure to S. Typhi. Risk is greatest for travelers to the Indian Subcontinent and other developing countries in Asia, Africa, the Caribbean,
and Central and South America. Travelers who are visiting relatives or
friends and who may be less likely to eat only safe foods (cooked and
served hot) and beverages (carbonated beverages or those made from
water that has been boiled) are at greater risk. Vaccination is particularly recommended for those who will be traveling in smaller cities, villages, and rural areas off the usual tourist itineraries, where food and
beverage choices may be more limited. Travelers have acquired typhoid
fever even during brief visits of <1 week to countries where the disease
is endemic. While immunization is recommended, travelers should be
cautioned that none of the available typhoid vaccines is 100% effective,
nor do they provide cross protection against other common causes of
gastrointestinal infections. Typhoid vaccination is not a substitute for
careful selection of food and drink.

CLINICAL PRESENTATION

The hallmark of typhoid infection is persistent, high fevers. Other common symptoms and signs include headache, malaise, anorexia, splenomegaly, and relative bradycardia. Many mild and atypical infections occur.

PREVENTION

Vaccine

Two typhoid vaccines are currently available for use in the United States: an oral live, attenuated vaccine (Vivotif Berna vaccine, manufactured from the Ty21a strain of S. Typhi by the Swiss Serum and Vaccine Institute) and a Vi capsular polysaccharide vaccine (ViCPS) (Typhim Vi, manufactured by Aventis Pasteur) for intramuscular use. Both vaccines have been shown to protect 50%–80% of recipients. The intramuscular heat-phenol-inactivated vaccine (manufactured by Wyeth-Ayerst) has been discontinued. Table 4–20 provides information on vaccine dosage and administration. The time required for primary vaccination differs for the two vaccines, as do the lower age limits for use in children.

Primary vaccination with oral Ty21a vaccine consists of a total of four capsules, one taken every other day. The capsules should be kept refrigerated (not frozen), and all four doses must be taken to achieve maximum efficacy. Each capsule should be taken with cool liquid no warmer than 37° C (98.6° F), approximately 1 hour before a meal. This regimen should be completed 1 week before potential exposure. The vaccine manufacturer recommends that Ty21a not be administered to infants or children <6 years of age.

Primary vaccination with ViCPS consists of one 0.5-mL (25-μg) dose administered intramuscularly. One dose of this vaccine should be given at least 2 weeks before expected exposure. The manufacturer does not recommend the vaccine for infants <2 years of age. (See *Vaccine Recommendations for Infants and Children, Typhoid Vaccine,* for a discussion of typhoid immunization for infants who will be traveling.) Current recommendations for revaccination with either vaccine are provided in Table 4–20.

Adverse Reactions

Information on adverse reactions is presented in Table 4–21. Information is not available on the safety of these vaccines when they are used during pregnancy; it is prudent on theoretical grounds to avoid vaccinating pregnant women. (See Chapter 9.) Live, attenuated Ty21a vaccine should not be given to immunocompromised travelers, including those infected with HIV. The intramuscular vaccine presents theoretically safer alternatives for this group. The only contraindication to vaccination with ViCPS vaccine is a history of severe local or systemic reactions after a previous dose. Neither of the available vaccines should be given to travelers with an acute febrile illness.

Precautions and Contraindications

Theoretical concerns have been raised about the immunogenicity of live, attenuated Ty21a vaccine in persons concurrently receiving antibiotics, immune globulin, or viral vaccines. The growth of the live Ty21a strain is inhibited in vitro by various antibacterial agents. Vaccination with Ty21a should be delayed for >24 hours after the administration of any antibacterial agent. Available data do not suggest that simultaneous administration of oral polio or yellow fever vaccine decreases the immunogenicity of Ty21a. If typhoid vaccination is warranted, it should not be delayed because of administration of viral vaccines. Simultaneous administration of Ty21a and immune globulin does not appear to pose a problem.

Other Prevention

See *Risks From Food and Water.*

TREATMENT

Specific antimicrobial therapy shortens the clinical course of typhoid fever and reduces the risk of death. Persons who are potentially exposed to *S.* Typhi and who develop symptoms of typhoid fever should seek appropriate medical care. Antimicrobial therapy should be guided by local data on antimicrobial sensitivity.

Bibliography

Crump JA, Luby SP, Mintz ED. The global burden of typhoid fever. Bull World Health Organ. 2004;82:346–53.

TABLE 4-20. DOSAGE AND SCHEDULE FOR TYPHOID FEVER VACCINATION

VACCINATION	AGE (YRS)	DOSE/MODE OF ADMINISTRATION	NO. OF DOSES	DOSING INTERVAL	BOOSTING INTERVAL
Oral, live, attenuated TY21a vaccine					
Primary series	≥6	1 capsule[1]/oral	4	48 hours	Not applicable
Booster	≥6	1 capsule[1]/oral	4	48 hours	Every 5 years
Vi Capsular polysaccharide vaccine					
Primary series	≥2	0.50 mL/ intramuscular	1	Not applicable	Not applicable
Booster	≥2	0.50 mL/ intramuscular	1	Not applicable	Every 2 years

[1]Administer with cool liquid no warmer than 37° C (98.6° F).

TABLE 4-21. COMMON ADVERSE REACTIONS TO TYPHOID FEVER VACCINES

VACCINE	REACTIONS		
	FEVER	HEADACHE	LOCAL REACTIONS
Ty21a[1]	0%–5%	0%–5%	Not applicable
Vi Capsular polysaccharide	0%–1%	16%–20%	7% erythema or induration ≤1 cm

[1]The side effects of Ty21a are rare and mainly consist of abdominal discomfort, nausea, vomiting, and rash or urticaria.

Klugman KP, Gilbertson IT, Koornhof HJ, et al. Protective activity of Vi capsular polysaccharide vaccine against typhoid fever. Lancet. 1987;2:1165–9.

Levine MM, Ferreccio C, Black RE, et al. Large-scale field trial of Ty21a live oral typhoid vaccine in enteric-coated capsule formulation. Lancet. 1987;1:1049–52.

Mermin JH, Townes JM, Gerber M, et al. Typhoid fever in the United States, 1985–1994: changing risks of international travel and increasing antimicrobial resistance. Arch Intern Med. 1998;158:633-8.

Parry CM, Hien TT, Dougan G, et al. Typhoid fever. N Engl J Med. 2002;347:1770–82.

Simanjuntak CH, Paleologo FP, Punjabi NH, et al. Oral immunization against typhoid fever in Indonesia with Ty21a vaccine. Lancet. 1991;338:1055–9.

Steinberg EB, Bishop RB, Dempsey AF, et al. Typhoid fever in travelers: who should be targeted for prevention? Clin Infect Dis. 2004; 39:186–91.

World Health Organization. Background document: the diagnosis, treatment and prevention of typhoid fever. Geneva, Switzerland: World Health Organization; 2003.

—STEVE LUBY AND ERIC MINTZ

>>Varicella (Chickenpox)

DESCRIPTION

Varicella (chickenpox) is the primary infection with the varicella-zoster virus (VZV). It is a highly contagious rash illness transmitted by airborne or droplet pathways. The usual incubation period is 14–16 days (range 10–21 days). Second cases of varicella have been reported in immunocompetent persons but are rare. Following varicella, VZV establishes latency in sensory nerve ganglia. The virus can reactivate later in life causing herpes zoster (shingles), usually localized to one to three dermatomes. Transmission of VZV to a susceptible person occurs through contact with either a person with varicella or, less commonly, a person with herpes zoster.

Varicella is generally a mild disease in children. It usually lasts 4–7 days and is characterized by a short (1- to 2-day) or absent prodromal period (low-grade fever, malaise) and by a pruritic rash consisting of crops of macules, papules, vesicles, and eventual crusting, which appear in three or more successive waves. Serious complications are the exception but can occur mainly in infants, adolescents, adults, and immunocompromised persons. They include secondary bacterial infections of skin lesions, pneumonia, cerebellar ataxia, and encephalitis. Because the vaccine is 70%–90% effective, a modified varicella, known as breakthrough disease, can occur in some vaccinated persons. Breakthrough disease is almost always mild with rash with fewer than 50 skin lesions, which may be atypical in appearance.

OCCURRENCE

Before introduction of varicella vaccine in the United States in 1995, varicella was endemic with virtually all persons being infected by adulthood. Since implementation of the varicella vaccination program, incidence has declined in all age groups, with the greatest decline among children aged 1–4 years. Data from passive and active surveillance have indicated a decline in varicella cases of 70%–84% between 1995 and 2001, in areas with vaccine coverage of 73%–84% among children aged 19–35 months.

RISK FOR TRAVELERS

Varicella and herpes zoster occur worldwide, but varicella vaccine is routinely used for vaccination of children in only few countries such as the United States, Uruguay, and Quatar. The risk of varicella infection for travelers coming to the United States is lower than for travel anywhere else in the world. However, VZV is still widely circulating in the United States. Additionally, exposure to herpes zoster, while less common than varicella, poses a risk for varicella infection. In temperate climates, in the absence of vaccination, most of varicella cases are reported among preschool and school-aged children during winter and spring. Data suggest that in tropical areas VZV infection occurs more commonly among adults than among children. Reasons for this difference in disease epidemiology are unclear. They may relate to the agent's heat lability and/or to factors such as the tendency for less indoor crowding in tropical regions.

PREVENTION

Varicella vaccine contains live, attenuated VZV. It is currently available only as a single-antigen formulation. Varicella vaccine is recommended for routine immunization of all children without contraindications at 12–18 months of age and for susceptible older children, adolescents, and adults. Those who have a reliable or uncertain history of varicella are considered susceptible. Children 1–12 years of age should receive one dose of vaccine. Persons ≥13 years of age should receive two doses, 4-8 weeks apart. The vaccine should be administered routinely to children 12–18 months of age, regardless of their prior history of varicella. Children ≥19 months of age, adolescents, and adults with reliable parental or personal histories of varicella are considered immune and do not need to be vaccinated. Epidemiologic and serologic studies indicated that >95% of American adults are immune to varicella. In addition, 71%–93% of adults without a reliable history of varicella are actually immune. As a result, serologic testing prior to vaccination is likely to be cost effective for adults. In case of uncertainty, prior varicella disease is not a contraindication to varicella vaccination. Although vaccination against varicella is not a requirement for entry into any country (including the United States), persons traveling or living abroad should ensure that they are immune.

After one dose of varicella vaccine, 97% of children 1–12 years of age develop detectable antibody titers. Vaccine-induced immunity is believed to be long lasting. Vaccine efficacy is estimated to be 70%–90% against disease of any severity and 95% against severe disease. Among healthy adolescents and adults, an average of 78% develop antibody after one dose and 99% develop antibody after a second dose administered 4–8 weeks later.

Varicella vaccine may be administered simultaneously (but at a different site) with any other live or inactivated vaccine. Inactivated vaccines and typhoid vaccines may be administered at any time before or after varicella vaccine. However, if varicella vaccine or live MMR and yellow fever vaccines are not administered simultaneously, their administration should be separated by an interval of at least 28 days. (See Table 1–2 for more details.)

Adverse Reactions

The most common adverse reactions following varicella vaccine are injection site complaints such as pain, soreness, redness, and swelling that are self-limited. Fever occurs in 15% of children and 10% of adolescents and adults. A macular or accine rash usually consisting of a few lesions at the injection site is reported in 3% of children and 1% of adolescents and adults after the second dose. A generalized rash with a small number of lesions may rarely occur as well within 3 weeks of vaccination.

Varicella vaccine is a live virus vaccine and results in a latent infection similar to that caused by wild VZV. Consequently, zoster caused by the vaccine virus has been reported, but appears to occur at a much lower rate than following natural infection. Not all reported cases have been confirmed as having been caused by vaccine virus; many were caused by the wild virus.

Precautions and Contraindications

Allergy

Persons with severe allergy (hives, swelling of the mouth or throat, difficulty breathing, hypotension, and shock) to gelatin or neomycin or who have had a severe allergic reaction to a prior dose should not be vaccinated with varicella vaccine. Varicella vaccine does not contain egg protein or preservative.

Pregnancy

Women known to be pregnant or who are attempting to become pregnant should not receive varicella vaccine. The effects of varicella vaccine on a developing fetus are unknown. Because infection with wild VZV poses only a small risk to the fetus and the vaccine virus is attenuated, the risk to the fetus, if any, should be even lower than from wild VZV. Although the manufacturer's package insert recommends avoiding pregnancy for 3 months following receipt of varicella vaccine, the Advisory Committee on Immunization Practices (ACIP) and the American Academy of Pediatrics (AAP) recommend that pregnancy be avoided for 1 month. Breastfeeding is not a contraindication to the varicella vaccination of either a woman or an infant.

Immunosuppression

Persons with immunosuppression of cellular immune function resulting from leukemia, lymphomas of any type, generalized malignancy, immunodeficiency disease, or immunosuppressive therapy should not be vaccinated. However, vaccine is available to any physician free of charge from the manufacturer through a research protocol for use in patients with leukemia in remission who meet certain eligibility criteria. Treatment with low-dose prednisone (e.g., <2 mg/kg of body weight/day or <20 mg/day) or aerosolized steroid preparations is not a contraindication to varicella vaccination. Persons whose immunosuppressive therapy with steroids has been stopped for 1 month (3 months for chemotherapy) may be vaccinated. In addition, persons with impaired humoral immunity may now be vaccinated. Because children infected with HIV are at greater risk for morbidity from varicella and herpes zoster than are healthy children, the ACIP recommends that, after weighing potential risks and benefits, varicella vaccine should be considered for asymptomatic or mildly symptomatic HIV-infected children in CDC class N1 (no signs or symptoms) or A1 (mild signs or symptoms) with age-specific CD4+ T-lymphocyte percentages of 25%. Eligible children should receive two doses of varicella vaccine, with a 3-month interval between doses. The use of varicella vaccine in other HIV-infected children is being investigated.

Recent Administration of Immune Globulin (IG) or Other Antibody-Containing Blood Products

The effect of the administration of antibody-containing blood products (e.g., IG, whole blood or packed red blood cells, intravenous IG, or varicella zoster IG [VZIG]) on the response to varicella vaccine virus is unknown. Because of the potential inhibition of the response to varicella vaccination by passively transferred antibodies, varicella vaccine should not be administered for at least 5 months after antibody-containing blood products are given. In addition, IG or VZIG should not be administered for 3 weeks following vaccination unless their benefits exceed those of the vaccine. In such cases, the vaccinees should either be revaccinated 5 months later or be tested for immunity 6 months later and revaccinated if seronegative.

No adverse events following varicella vaccination related to the use of salicylates (e.g., aspirin) have been reported to date. However, the manufacturer recommends that vaccine recipients avoid the use of salicylates for 6 weeks after receiving varicella vaccine because of the association between aspirin use and Reye syndrome following varicella.

Although no data exist regarding whether either varicella or live varicella virus vaccine exacerbates tuberculosis, vaccination is not recommended for persons who have untreated active tuberculosis. The effect of varicella vaccine, if any, on tuberculin testing is unknown. However, measles vaccine (and possibly mumps and rubella vaccines) can suppress the response to purified protein derivative (PPD) in a person infected with *Mycobacterium tuberculosis*. Until additional information is available, it is prudent to apply the same procedures for PPD and measles vaccination to varicella vaccine. If PPD testing is needed, it should be done before MMR or varicella vaccination. PPD testing should be delayed for 4–6 weeks after MMR or varicella vaccination. The PPD may be applied at the same time that MMR or varicella, or both, is administered.

Postexposure Prophylaxis
Use of Vaccine
Administration of varicella vaccine to susceptible children within 72 hours and possibly up to 120 hours after varicella exposure may prevent or significantly modify disease and should be considered in these circumstances. Physicians should advise parents and their children that the vaccine may not protect against disease in all cases. In two controlled studies, protective efficacy was ≥90% when children were vaccinated within 3 days of exposure.

Use of Varicella Zoster Immune Globulin (VZIG)
Under rare circumstances, VZIG may be recommended for postexposure prophylaxis. The decision to administer VZIG to a person exposed to varicella should be based on 1) whether the patient is susceptible, 2) whether the exposure is likely to result in infection, and 3) whether the patient is at greater risk for complications than the general population (immunocompromised persons, pregnant women, neonates whose mothers had signs and symptoms of varicella within 5 days before and 2 days after delivery, premature infants). VZIG provides maximum benefit when it is administered as soon as possible after the presumed exposure, but it may be effective if administered as late as 96 hours after exposure. VZIG is available in the United States through the American Red Cross; in other countries availability may vary.

TREATMENT

Acyclovir is an option for treatment of some individuals with varicella. Oral Acyclovir is not recommended for postexposure prophylaxis.

Bibliography

American Academy of Pediatrics. Pickering LK, editor. 2003 Red Book: report of the Committee on Infectious Diseases. 26th ed. Elk Grove Village, IL: American Academy of Pediatrics; 2003.

Arvin AM, Gershon AA. Varicella-zoster virus. Cambridge, England: University Press; 2000.

CDC. Prevention of varicella: recommendations of the Advisory Committee on Immunization Practices (ACIP). MMWR Recomm Rep. 1996;45(RR-11):1–36.

CDC. Prevention of varicella. Updated recommendations of the Advisory Committee on Immunization Practices (ACIP). MMWR Recomm Rep. 1999;48(RR-6):1–5.

Gershon AA, Takahashi M, Seward J. Varicella vaccine. In: Plotkin SA, Orenstein WA, editors. Vaccines. 4th ed. Philadelphia: Saunders; 2004. p. 783–823.

Kilgore PE, Kruszon-Moran D, Seward JF, et al. Varicella in Americans from NHANES III: implications for control through routine immunization. J Med Virol. 2003;70 Supl 1:S111–8.

Seward JF, Watson BM, Peterson CL, et al. Varicella disease after introduction of varicella vaccine in the United States, 1995-2000. JAMA. 2002;287:606–11.

Whitley RJ. Varicella-zoster virus. In: Mandell GL, Bennett JE, Dolin R, editors. Principles and practice of infectious diseases. 5th ed. New York: Churchill Livingstone; 2000. p. 1580–6.

—MONA MARIN, DALYA GURIS, AND AISHA JUMAAN

>>Viral Hemorrhagic Fevers

DESCRIPTION

Viral hemorrhagic fevers are a group of febrile illnesses caused by several distinct families of viruses, all of which are enveloped and have RNA genomes. These groups include Ebola and Marburg viruses, Lassa fever virus, the New World arenaviruses (Guaranito, Machupo, Junin, and Sabia), and Rift Valley fever and Crimean Congo hemorrhagic fever viruses. Although some types cause relatively mild illnesses, many of these viruses can cause severe, life-threatening disease. Severe illness is characterized by vascular damage and increased permeability, multi-organ failure, and shock. (See also Dengue, and Yellow Fever.)

Ebola and Marburg: Filoviral Diseases

Ebola and Marburg are filoviruses that belong to the family Filoviridae and can cause severe hemorrhagic fever in humans and nonhuman primates. Four species of Ebola virus have been identified: Côte d'Ivoire, Sudan, Zaire, and Reston. Ebola-Reston infection is fatal in monkeys but seems not to cause disease in humans. Confirmed cases of Ebola hemorrhagic fever have been reported in the Congo, Côte d'Ivoire, Democratic Republic of Congo, Gabon, Sudan, and Uganda. Occupational infection of a laboratory worker resulting from a needlestick injury has been documented in England and Russia. Marburg virus also is indigenous to Africa. Although the precise geographic range for Marburg virus is unknown, it includes at least parts of Uganda and western Kenya, Democratic Republic of Congo, and possibly Zimbabwe. The reservoir host for Ebola and Marburg viruses is not known. Outbreaks can occur when an index case-patient who has been exposed to that unknown reservoir species returns to a community. Within that community, the outbreak often becomes amplified in the health-care setting.

Lassa Fever: Arenaviral Diseases

Lassa fever is caused by a virus transmitted from asymptomatically infected rodents to humans. Most infections are mild, but some are severe, causing a hemorrhagic fever that is often fatal. The virus, a member of the virus family Arenaviridae, is a single-stranded RNA virus. Arenaviruses are transmitted by animal hosts and can be divided into two groups: the New World or Tacaribe complex and the Old World or lymphocytic choriomeningitis virus (LCMV)/Lassa complex. Viruses causing human illness are Lassa virus, Lassa fever; Junin virus, Argentine hemorrhagic fever; Machupo virus, Bolivian hemorrhagic fever; Guanarito virus, Venezuelan hemorrhagic fever; Sabia virus, Brazilian hemorrhagic fever; LCMV, meningitis, encephalitis, meningo-encephalitis; and Flexal virus, an influenza-like illness that has caused deaths among laboratory personnel handling rodents in Brazil.

Each virus is associated with one or more closely related rodent species that constitute its natural reservoir. Tacaribe complex viruses are generally associated with the New World rats and mice (family Muridae, subfamily Sigmodontinae). The LCM/Lassa complex viruses are associated with the Old World rats and mice (family Muridae, subfamily Murinae). Taken together, these types of rodents are located across most of the earth's land mass, including Europe, Asia, Africa, and the Americas. An exception is Tacaribe virus, found in Trinidad, which was isolated from bats.

Lassa fever is limited to rural areas of West Africa, with areas of hyper-endemicity in eastern Sierra Leone, Guinea, Liberia, and Nigeria. Peridomestic exposure to infected rodents is the most likely source of human infection. Transmission of arenaviruses to humans can occur via inhalation of primary aerosols from rodent urine, by ingestion of contaminated food, or by direct contact of broken skin with rodent excreta. Rodent infestation and inappropriate food storage increase the risk of human infection. Person-to-person spread of Lassa and Machupo viruses has also been described, most notably by large droplet and contact transmission in the hospital setting. Despite one anecdotal report of possible airborne transmission, this mode is not believed to be an important route of infection from person to person. Laboratory handling of infectious specimens and contact with contaminated medical equipment are also associated with transmission.

Rift Valley Fever and Related Bunyaviral Diseases
Rift Valley fever (RVF) is caused by a member of the Bunyaviridae family; it affects primarily livestock and may also infect humans. It is transmitted by several means, including the bites of mosquitoes, percutaneous inoculation, or exposure to aerosols from contaminated blood or fluids of infected animals. Other diseases caused by viruses of the

family Bunyaviridae include hantavirus pulmonary syndrome (HPS), hemorrhagic fever with renal syndrome (HFRS), and Crimean-Congo hemorrhagic fever. Both HPS and HFRS are transmitted to humans through contact with urine, feces, or saliva of infected rodents. Crimean-Congo virus is transmitted to humans by infected ticks or direct handling and preparation of fresh carcasses of infected animals, usually domestic livestock. Nosocomial transmission of Crimean-Congo virus has been frequently reported.

RVF virus is endemic to sub-Saharan Africa, where sporadic outbreaks occur in humans, for example, in the Nile Delta, Egypt (1978 and 1993), Madagascar (1991), and the lower Senegal River basin of Mauritania (1987). A large epidemic also occurred in Kenya and Tanzania during 1997–1998. A recent outbreak (2000) of RVF occurred in southwestern Saudi Arabia and Yemen with a strain of RVF closely related to that of the 1997–1998 East African strain. This outbreak represented the first spread of the virus outside Africa, demonstrating its potential for spread to unaffected regions elsewhere in the tropics. Crimean-Congo hemorrhagic fever (CCHF) is endemic where ticks of the genus *Hyalomma* are found in Africa and Eurasia, including the Balkans, the Middle East, Russia, and western China. Recent cases of CCHF have been confirmed in Oman (1995), United Arab Emirates (1979 and 1994), Saudi Arabia (1990), and Turkey (2004); and antibody to CCHF has been reported in Kuwait. The viruses that cause HPS are present in the New World; those that cause HFRS occur worldwide.

OCCURRENCE

Taken together, the viruses that cause VHF are distributed over much of the globe. Each virus is associated with one or more nonhuman host or vector species, restricting the virus and the disease it causes to the areas inhabited by these species. Viruses causing hemorrhagic fever are initially transmitted to humans when the habitats of infected reservoir hosts or vectors and humans overlap. Risk of VHF is associated with human incursion into such areas. In general, humans are incidental, "dead-end" hosts for these enzootic diseases.

RISK FOR TRAVELERS

The risk for international travelers is generally considered to be low. The viruses carried in rodent reservoirs are transmitted when humans have contact with urine, fecal matter, saliva, or other excreta of infected rodents. The viruses associated with arthropod vectors are usually spread when the vector mosquito or tick bites a human or when a human crushes an infected tick. Some of these vectors may spread the virus to animals, including livestock. Humans may become infected through contact with infected animals (e.g., during birthing, veterinary care, or slaughter). Travelers engaging in animal research, including ecologists, mammalogists, and primatologists, may be at increased risk for exposure to these zoonoses.

During recorded outbreaks of hemorrhagic fever caused by filovirus infections (e.g., Ebola), persons who cared for (fed, washed, or medicated) or worked very closely with infected persons were at highest risk for infection. Health care-associated transmission through contact with infectious body fluids has been an important factor in the spread of this disease.

Several cases of Lassa fever have been confirmed in international travelers. These travelers were staying or living in traditional dwellings in the countryside or in small villages; no risk has been associated with travelers who stay in hotels. Travel involving patient contact or rodent exposure is associated with increased risk. Medical personnel, researchers, and relief workers involved in the management of patients or working in disease-endemic areas should be aware of their risk and should minimize rodent exposure and use personal protective equipment appropriately to prevent health care-associated exposure.

Travelers exposed to the blood or tissues of sick animals or to infected mosquitoes in RVF-endemic areas are at risk for infection. Among travelers to Bunyavirus-endemic regions, those staying in rodent-infested dwellings may be at increased risk for HPS and HFRS.

PREVENTION

Prevention efforts should concentrate on avoiding contact with host or vector species. Investigational vaccines have been developed for Argentine hemorrhagic fever, used extensively for community vaccination in the endemic region, and for Rift Valley fever; however, neither has been approved by the FDA. For the other viruses that cause VHF, no vaccine is available. If prevention methods fail and a traveler becomes ill with

VHF, efforts should focus on supportive care and preventing further transmission from person to person, e.g., through occupational injury among health-care personnel, by re-use of injection needles or syringes, or splashes of infectious body fluids reaching unprotected mucous membranes.

Travelers should not visit locations where an outbreak is occurring. Contact with rodents should be avoided, particularly in Lassa or Bunyavirus-endemic areas. Where RVF is endemic, travelers should avoid direct contact with livestock and minimize their exposure to arthropod bites by using permethrin-impregnated bed nets and insect repellents.

Strict compliance with infection control precautions (i.e., use of disposable gloves, face shields, and disposable gowns to prevent direct contact with body fluids and splashes to mucous membranes when caring for patients or handling clinical specimens; and appropriate use and disposal of sharp instruments) is recommended to avoid health care-associated infections.

Direct contact with the remains of anyone suspected of having died of Ebola or Marburg infection should be avoided. Remains should be buried promptly by trained, specially organized teams using appropriate safety equipment. Contact with or consumption of dead primates should be avoided in areas where outbreaks of filoviral infection have occurred.

TREATMENT

Patients should receive supportive care, including balancing fluids and electrolytes, maintaining oxygenation status and blood pressure, and preventing or providing treatment for any secondary infections. In general, no specific treatments or established cures have proven benefit for patients with VHF. Ribavirin, an antiviral drug, has been effective in treating some patients with Lassa fever, New World arenaviruses, and Crimean-Congo hemorrhagic fever; however, it is not FDA licensed for these indications. Treatment with convalescent-phase plasma has been used with success in some patients with Argentine hemorrhagic fever.

Bibliography

Bausch DG, Borchert M, Grein T, et al. Risk factors for Marburg hemorrhagic fever, Democratic Republic of the Congo. Emerg Infect Dis. 2003;9:1531–7.

Bausch DG, Demby AH, Coulibaly M, et al. Lassa fever in Guinea: I. Epidemiology of human disease and clinical observations. Vector Borne Zoonotic Dis. 2001;1:269–81.

Bausch DG, Ksiazek TG. Viral hemorrhagic fevers including hantavirus pulmonary syndrome in the Americas. Clin Lab Med. 2002;22:981–1020.

De Manzione N, Salas RA, Paredes H, et al. Venezuelan hemorrhagic fever: clinical and epidemiological studies of 165 cases. Clin Infect Dis. 1998;26:308–13.

Francesconi P, Yoti Z, Declich S, et al. Ebola hemorrhagic fever transmission and risk factors of contacts, Uganda. Emerg Infect Dis. 2003;9:1430–7.

Khan AS, Maupin GO, Rollin PE, et al. An outbreak of Crimean-Congo hemorrhagic fever in the United Arab Emirates, 1994-1995. Am J Trop Med Hyg. 1997;57:519–25.

Kilgore PE, Ksiazek TG, Rollin PE, et al. Treatment of Bolivian hemorrhagic fever with intravenous ribavirin. Clin Infect Dis. 1997;24:718–22.

Peters CJ, Jahrling PB, Khan AS. Patients infected with high-hazard viruses: scientific basis for infection control. Arch Virol Suppl. 1996;11:141–68.

Pon E, McKee KT Jr, Diniega BM, et al. Outbreak of hemorrhagic fever with renal syndrome among U.S. Marines in Korea. Am J Trop Med Hyg. 1990;42:612–9.

Woods CW, Karpati AM, Grein T, et al. An outbreak of Rift Valley fever in Northeastern Kenya, 1997–98. Emerg Infect Dis. 2002;8:138–44.

—MICHAEL BELL AND PIERRE ROLLIN

>>Yellow Fever

DESCRIPTION

Yellow fever is a viral disease that is transmitted to humans through the bite of infected mosquitoes. Illness ranges in severity from an influenza-like syndrome to severe hepatitis and hemorrhagic fever. The yellow fever virus is maintained in nature by mosquito-borne transmission between nonhuman primates. Transmission by mosquitoes from one human to another occurs during epidemics of "urban yellow fever."

OCCURRENCE

The disease occurs only in sub-Saharan Africa and tropical South America (see Maps 4–12 and 4–13), where it is endemic and intermittently epidemic. (See Table 4–22 for a list of countries that lie within the endemic zone, which is defined as those areas where there is active yellow fever transmission as well as those in which yellow fever may be more likely to occur because of the presence of the vector and infection in nonhuman primates.) In Africa, where most cases are reported, a variety of vectors are responsible for transmitting the virus. The case-fatality rate is >20%, and infants and children are at greatest risk for infection. In South America, cases occur most frequently in young men who have occupational exposure to forest-dwelling mosquito vectors in forested or transitional areas of Bolivia, Brazil, Colombia, Ecuador, Venezuela, Guyana, French Guiana, and Peru.

RISK FOR TRAVELERS

A traveler's risk of acquiring yellow fever is determined by immunization status, location of travel, season, duration of exposure, occupational and recreational activities while traveling, and the local rate of yellow fever virus transmission at the time. Although reported cases of human disease are the principal indicator of disease risk, they may be absent (because of a high level of immunity in the population) or not detected as a result of poor surveillance. Only a small proportion of yellow fever cases are officially reported because of the occurrence of the disease in remote areas and lack of specific diagnostic facilities.

During interepidemic periods, low-level transmission may not be detected by public health surveillance. Such interepidemic conditions

TABLE 4-22. COUNTRIES IN THE YELLOW FEVER-ENDEMIC ZONE

AFRICA			CENTRAL AND SOUTH AMERICA
Angola	Equatorial Guinea	Rwanda	Argentina[1]
Benin	Ethiopia	Sao Tome and	Bolivia[1]
Burkina Faso	Gabon	Principe	Brazil[1]
Burundi	The Gambia	Senegal	Colombia
Cameroon	Ghana	Sierra Leone	Ecuador[1]
Cape Verde	Guinea	Somalia	French Guiana
Central African	Guinea-Bissau	Sudan	Guyana
Republic	Kenya	Tanzania	Panama[1]
Chad	Liberia	Togo	Paraguay[1]
Congo	Mali	Uganda	Peru[1]
Côte d'Ivoire	Mauritania		Suriname
Democratic Republic	Niger		Trinidad and Tobago
of Congo	Nigeria		Venezuela[1]

[1]These countries are not holo-endemic. Please see Map 4-13 and yellow fever vaccine recommendations for details.

may last years or even decades in certain countries or regions. This "epidemiologic silence" may provide a sense of false security and lead to travel without the benefit of vaccination. Surveys in rural West Africa during "silent" periods have estimated an incidence of yellow fever of 1.1–2.4 cases per 1,000 persons and an incidence of death due to yellow fever of 0.2–0.5 deaths per 1,000 persons; both these ranges are less than the threshold of detection of the surveillance systems in place.

The incidence of yellow fever in South America is lower than that in Africa because the mosquitoes that transmit the virus between monkeys in the forest canopy do not often come in contact with humans and because immunity in the indigenous human population is high. Urban epidemic transmission has not occurred in South America for many years, although the risk of introduction of the virus into towns and cities is ever present. For travelers, the risks of illness and death due to yellow fever are probably 10 times greater in rural West Africa than in South America; these risks vary greatly according to specific location and season. In West Africa, the most dangerous time of year is during the

MAP 4-12. YELLOW FEVER-ENDEMIC ZONES IN AFRICA, 2005

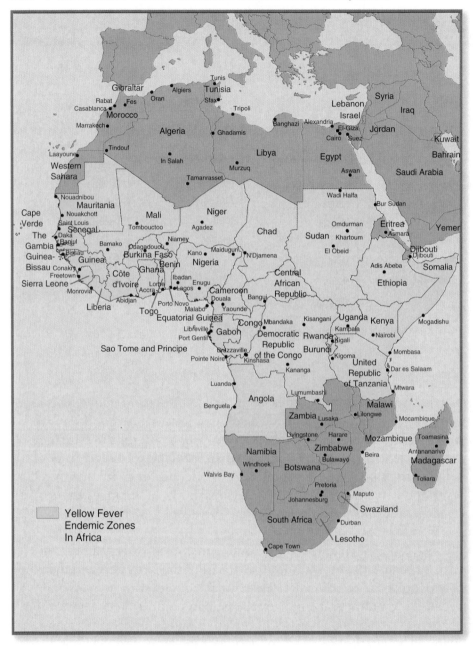

Yellow Fever
Endemic Zones
In Africa

MAP 4-13. YELLOW FEVER-ENDEMIC ZONES IN THE AMERICAS, 2005

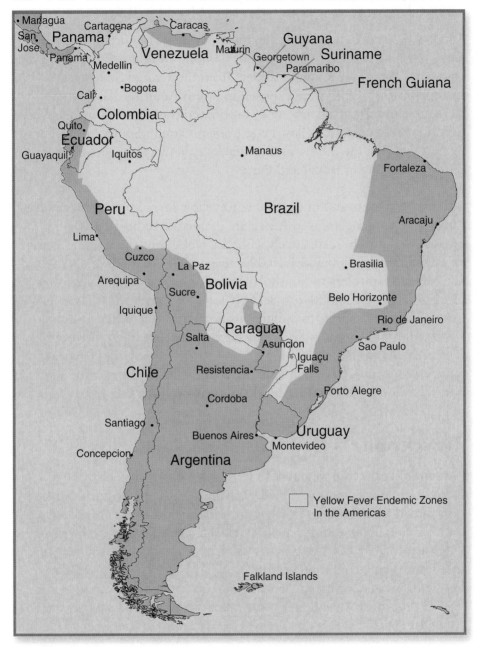

late rainy and early dry seasons (July–October). Virus transmission is highest during the rainy season (January–March) in Brazil.

The low incidence of yellow fever, generally a few hundred reported cases per year, has led to complacency among travelers. Four of the five cases of yellow fever among travelers from the United States and Europe in 1996–2002 were exposed in South America. All five cases were fatal and occurred among unvaccinated travelers. An increase in enzootic and epizootic yellow fever transmission in South America was detected during the 1990s, and yellow fever activity appears to be currently expanding in Brazil and Peru.

The risks of illness and of death due to yellow fever in an unvaccinated traveler in endemic areas in Africa are estimated to be 1:1,000 and 1:5,000 per month, respectively. (For a 2-week stay, the risks of illness and death are 1:2,000 and 1:10,000, respectively.) The risks of illness and death to travelers to South America are probably 10 times lower (1:20,000 and 1:100,000, respectively for a two week trip). These estimates are based on risk to indigenous populations and may overestimate the risk to travelers, who may have a different immunity profile, take precautions against getting bitten by mosquitoes, and have less outdoor exposure. Based on data for U.S. travelers, the risk for illness in a traveler due to yellow fever has been estimated to be 0.4–4.3 cases per million travelers to yellow fever-endemic areas.

PREVENTION

Personal Protection Measures

In addition to vaccination, travelers to areas with yellow fever transmission should be advised to take precautions against exposure to mosquitoes. Staying in air-conditioned or well-screened quarters and wearing long-sleeved shirts and long pants will help to prevent mosquito bites. Insect repellents containing DEET should be used on exposed skin. Permethrin-containing repellents should be applied to clothing. (For further prevention information, see *Protection against Mosquitoes and Other Arthropods*.)

Vaccine

Yellow fever is preventable by a relatively safe, effective vaccine. To meet international vaccination requirements, yellow fever vaccines must be manufactured under approval by the World Health Organization and administered at an approved yellow fever vaccination center. For all eligible persons, a single injection of 0.5 mL of reconstituted vaccine should be administered subcutaneously. Authorized U.S. vaccination centers can be identified by contacting state or local health departments or by visiting CDC's Travelers' Health website, where there is a listing of current authorized yellow fever vaccination providers in the United States (http://www2.ncid.cdc.gov/travel/yellowfever/).

Adverse Reactions
General Events
Reactions to yellow fever vaccine are generally mild. Vaccine recipients have reported mild headaches, myalgia, low-grade fevers, or other minor symptoms that may begin within days after vaccination and last 5–10 days after vaccination. In clinical trials, the incidence of mild adverse events has been ~25%, but many events may have been unrelated, as the trials were not placebo-controlled. Approximately 1% of vaccinees find it necessary to curtail regular activities. Immediate hypersensitivity reactions, characterized by rash, urticaria, or asthma or a combination of these, are uncommon (incidence <1 case per 131,000 vaccinees). Unrecognized allergy to eggs or chicken or to the hydrolyzed gelatin used to stabilize the vaccine may be responsible for hypersensitivity reactions. Persons who have allergies to egg, chicken, or gelatin should be evaluated by an allergist to determine whether they can safely receive yellow fever vaccine.

Yellow Fever Vaccine-Associated Neurologic Disease
Historically, yellow fever vaccine-associated adverse events were seen primarily among infants, and presented as encephalitis. Since 1992, five cases of encephalitis among adult recipients of yellow fever vaccine have been reported to the U.S. Vaccine Adverse Event Reporting System (VAERS). In addition, ten cases of autoimmune neurologic disease have been reported to VAERS, including patients with Guillain-Barré syndrome and acute disseminated encephalomyelits. All patients with yellow fever vaccine-associated neurologic disease (YEL-AND) had an onset of illness 4–23 days after vaccination. All cases were in first-time vaccine recipients. The risk for vaccine-associated neurologic disease does not appear to be limited to infants, and crude estimates in the United States of the reported frequency range from 4 to 6 cases per 1,000,000 doses distributed.

Yellow Fever Vaccine-Associated Viscerotropic Disease

A serious adverse reaction syndrome has recently been described among recipients of yellow fever vaccines produced by several different manufacturers. This syndrome was previously reported as febrile multiple organ system failure and is now called yellow fever vaccine-associated viscerotropic disease (YEL-AVD). Since 1996, nine cases of yellow fever vaccine-associated viscerotropic disease, a disease clinically and pathologically resembling naturally acquired yellow fever, have been reported in the U.S.; an additional 17 cases have been identified worldwide as of October 2004. All U.S. cases required intensive care after experiencing fever, hypotension, respiratory failure, elevated hepatocellular enzymes, hyperbilirubinemia, lymphocytopenia, and thrombocytopenia; eight of the nine also had renal failure, which required hemodialysis. Six (67%) of the U.S. cases have been fatal. In several cases for which tissue samples were available, immunohistochemistry demonstrated viral dissemination throughout the body, including liver, lung, spleen, lymph node, brain, and smooth muscle; however, in many cases, tissue samples were not available for histopathologic review or detection of virus. All cases reported thus far have occurred in primary vaccinees. Yellow fever vaccines must be considered as a possible, but rare, cause of yellow fever vaccine-associated viscerotropic disease that is similar to fulminant yellow fever caused by wild-type yellow fever virus. Accurately measuring the incidence of vaccine-associated viscerotropic disease is currently precluded by lack of adequate prospective data; however, crude estimates in the United States of the reported frequency range from 3 to 5 cases per 1,000,000 doses distributed. This frequency appears to be higher for persons >60 years of age, as much as 19 cases per million doses distributed.

Because of recent reports of deaths from yellow fever among unvaccinated travelers to areas endemic for yellow fever and of these reports of vaccine-associated viscerotropic disease, yellow fever vaccination of travelers to high-risk areas should be encouraged as a key prevention strategy; however, physicians should be careful to administer the vaccine only to persons truly at risk for exposure to yellow fever. Additional surveillance to better monitor and quantify wild-type yellow fever activity, as well as yellow fever vaccine-specific adverse outcomes, should be established. Studies are being conducted to clarify the cause and risk factors for these rare adverse events associated with the yellow fever vaccines.

Precautions and Contraindications
Age
The risk for adverse reactions appears to be age related. Infants <6 months of age should not be vaccinated because they are more suscepti- ble to the serious adverse reaction of yellow fever vaccine-associated neurotropic disease (also known as postvaccinal encephalitis) than are older children. Immunization should be delayed until an infant is at least 9 months of age. (See *Vaccine Recommendations for Infants and Children, Yellow Fever Vaccine,* for a discussion of yellow fever immunization for infants and children.) In unusual circumstances, physicians considering vaccinating infants aged <9 months should contact the Division of Vector-Borne Infectious Diseases (970-221-6400) or the Division of Global Migration and Quarantine (404-498-1600) at CDC for advice.

A recent analysis of adverse events passively reported to the Vaccine Adverse Event Reporting System (VAERS) during 1990-2002 indicates that persons >60 years of age may be at increased risk for systemic adverse events following vaccination compared with younger persons. Travelers aged >60 years should discuss with their physicians the risks and benefits of vaccination in the context of their destination-specific risk for exposure to yellow fever virus.

History of Thymus Disease
Recently, a history of thymus disease has been identified as a contraindi- cation to yellow fever vaccine. Four (15%) of the 26 vaccine recipients with YEL-AVD worldwide have had a history of diseases involving the thymus, all of which are extremely rare, suggesting that compromised thymic function may be another independent risk factor for YEL-AVD. One fatal case in the United States occurred in a 67-year-old woman who had a history of thymectomy for a malignant thymoma approxi- mately 2 years before vaccination. A second case in the United States occurred in a 70-year-old man who had a history of hyperthyroidism, myasthenia gravis, and thymectomy for thymoma 20 years before vacci- nation. This patient survived. A third case was reported from Switzerland and occurred in a 50-year-old man who had a history of thymectomy due to thymoma 8 years prior to vaccination. This patient also survived. Most recently, a fatal case (male, age 44 years) of viscerotropic disease with fulminant hepatic failure temporally associated with yellow fever vaccine was reported from Colombia. This patient had a thymectomy due to benign thymoma 2 years before vaccination.

In addition to concerns about vaccinating elderly travelers, health-care providers should be careful to ask about a history of thymus disorder, including myasthenia gravis, thymoma, or prior thymectomy, when screening a patient before administering yellow fever vaccine. For persons with such a history, alternative means of prevention should be recommended, if travel plans cannot be altered to avoid yellow fever-endemic areas.

Pregnancy
The safety of yellow fever vaccination during pregnancy has not been established, and the vaccine should be administered only if travel to an endemic area is unavoidable and if an increased risk for exposure exists. If international travel requirements, rather than an increased risk for infection, are the only reason to vaccinate a pregnant woman, efforts should be made to obtain a waiver letter from the traveler's physician. Pregnant women who must travel to areas where the risk for yellow fever infection is high should be vaccinated. Despite the apparent safety of this vaccine, infants born to these women should be monitored closely for evidence of congenital infection and other possible adverse effects resulting from yellow fever vaccination. If vaccination of a pregnant woman is deemed necessary, serologic testing to document an immune response to the vaccine can be considered, because the seroconversion rate for pregnant women in a developing nation has been reported to be substantially lower than that observed for other healthy adults and children. To discuss the need for serologic testing, the appropriate state health department or CDC's Division of Vector-Borne Infectious Diseases at 970-221-6400 or Division of Global Migration and Quarantine at 404-498-1600 should be contacted for more information.

Lactation
Whether this vaccine is excreted in breast milk is not known. There have been no reports of adverse events or transmission of the vaccine viruses from nursing mother to infant. As a precautionary measure, vaccination of nursing mothers should be avoided, because of the theoretical risk of the transmission of virus to the breastfed infant. When travel of nursing mothers to high-risk yellow fever endemic areas cannot be avoided or postponed, these women may be vaccinated.

Immunosuppression
Infection with yellow fever vaccine virus poses a theoretical risk for travelers with immunosuppression in association with AIDS or other mani-

festations of HIV infection; leukemia, lymphoma, or generalized malignancy; with a history of thymus disease or thymectomy; or with the administration of corticosteroids, alkylating drugs, antimetabolites, or radiation. There is a single report of a 53 year-old patient with undiagnosed HIV infection who had a low CD4+ count (108 cells/mm^3) and who developed YEL-AND and died of meningoencephalitis. Immunosuppressed patients should not be vaccinated. If travel to a yellow fever-infected zone is necessary, patients should be advised of the risks posed by such travel, instructed in methods for avoiding vector mosquitoes, and supplied with vaccination waiver letters by their physicians. Low-dose (i.e., 20 mg prednisone or equivalent/day), short-term (i.e., <2 weeks) systemic corticosteroid therapy or intra-articular, bursal, or tendon injections with corticosteroids and intranasal corticosteroids should not be sufficiently immunosuppressive to constitute an increased hazard to recipients of yellow fever vaccine.

Persons who are HIV-infected but do not have AIDS or other symptomatic manifestations of HIV infection, who have established laboratory verification of adequate immune system function (e.g. CD4+ T lymphocyte cell counts >200/mm^3), and who cannot avoid potential exposure to yellow fever virus should be offered the choice of vaccination. If international travel requirements are the only reason to vaccinate an asymptomatic HIV-infected person, rather than an increased risk for infection, efforts should be made to obtain a waiver letter from the traveler's physician. Asymptomatic HIV-infected persons who must travel to areas where the risk for yellow fever infection is high should be offered the choice of vaccination and monitored closely for possible adverse effects. Family members of immunosuppressed or HIV-infected persons who themselves have no contraindications can receive yellow fever vaccine.

Data regarding seroconversion rates after yellow fever vaccination among asymptomatic HIV-infected persons are limited, but they do indicate that the seroconversion rate among such persons is reduced. Because vaccination of asymptomatic HIV-infected persons might be less effective than that of persons not infected with HIV, measurement of the neutralizing antibody response to vaccination should be considered before travel. Physicians should consult the applicable state health department or CDC's Division of Vector-Borne Infectious Diseases at 970-221-6400 or Division of Global Migration and Quarantine at 404-498-1600, for more information.

Hypersensitivity

Live yellow fever vaccine is produced in chick embryos and should not be given to persons hypersensitive to eggs. Generally, persons who are able to eat eggs or egg products may receive the vaccine. However, some egg-sensitive persons are not allergic to cooked eggs and may not know they are susceptible to allergic reactions following raw eggs or egg-containing vaccines. If vaccination of a person with a questionable history of egg or chicken hypersensitivity is considered essential because of high risk for exposure, an intradermal test dose may be administered under close medical supervision. Specific directions for skin testing are found in the package insert. In some instances, small test doses for vaccine administered intradermally have led to an antibody response. Gelatin is used as a stabilizer in several vaccines, including yellow fever vaccine, and might be the stimulus for some allergic reactions to yellow fever vaccine. If international travel regulations are the only reason to vaccinate a traveler hypersensitive to eggs or gelatin, efforts should be made to obtain a waiver.

Simultaneous Administration of Other Vaccines and Drugs

Studies have shown that the immune response to yellow fever vaccine is not inhibited by administration of certain other live, attenuated vaccines concurrently or at various intervals of a few days to one month. Smallpox, measles, BCG, and oral (live) typhoid vaccines have been administered in combination with yellow fever vaccines without interference. Additionally, reactions to vaccination are no more severe when these vaccines are administered concurrently. Hepatitis A, hepatitis B, Vi capsular polysaccharide typhoid, meningococcal, inactivated poliovirus, diphtheria-pertussis-tetanus and yellow fever vaccines may be given concurrently. If live-virus vaccines are not given concurrently, 4 weeks should be allowed to elapse between sequential vaccinations.

No data are available on possible interference between yellow fever vaccine and influenza, pneumococcal polysaccharide or conjugate, rabies, or Japanese encephalitis vaccines.

A prospective study of persons given yellow fever vaccine along with 5 mL of commercially available immune globulin showed no alteration of the immunologic response to yellow fever vaccine when compared with controls. Although chloroquine inhibits replication of yellow fever virus in vitro, it does not adversely affect antibody responses to yellow fever vaccine in persons receiving the drug as antimalarial prophylaxis.

International Certificate of Vaccination for Yellow Fever

International regulations require proof of vaccination for travel to and from certain countries. For purposes of international travel, yellow fever vaccine produced by different manufacturers worldwide must be approved by WHO and administered at an approved yellow fever vaccination center. In the United States, state and territorial health departments have authority to designate nonfederal vaccination centers; these can be identified by contacting state or local health departments or by visiting CDC's Travelers' Health website, where there is a listing of current authorized yellow fever vaccination providers (http://www2.ncid. cdc.gov/travel/yellowfever/). Vaccinees should receive a completed International Certificate of Vaccination, signed and validated with the center's stamp where the vaccine was given. This certificate is valid 10 days after vaccination and for a subsequent period of 10 years.

To prevent importation and transmission, a number of countries require a certificate from travelers arriving from infected areas or from countries with infected areas, even if only in transit. Such requirements may be strictly enforced, particularly for persons traveling from Africa or South America to Asia. Some countries in Africa require evidence of vaccination from all entering travelers; others may waive the requirements for travelers coming from nonendemic areas and staying in the country <2 weeks (see *Yellow Fever Vaccine Requirements and Information on Malaria Risk and Prophylaxis, by Country*). Travelers with a specific contraindication to yellow fever vaccine should be advised to obtain a waiver before traveling to countries requiring vaccination.

Vaccination is also recommended for travel to countries that do not officially report the disease but lie in the yellow fever-endemic zone (see Maps 4–12 and 4–13 and Table 4–22). The actual areas of yellow fever virus activity can extend beyond the officially reported endemic zones.

An International Certificate of Vaccination must be complete in every detail; if incomplete or inaccurate, it is not valid. Revisions of this certificate dated 9–66, 9–69, 9–71, 1–74, 9–77, 1–82, or 11–91 are acceptable. A copy of the International Certificate of Vaccination, PHS-731, may be purchased for $1.25 ($15.00 per 100) from the Superintendent of Documents, U.S. Government Printing Office, Washington, D.C. 20402, telephone 1-202-512-1800. The stock number is 017-001-00483-9.

Authorization To Provide Vaccinations and To Validate the International Certificate of Vaccination

A yellow fever vaccination must be given at an official yellow fever vaccination center as designated by respective state health departments or the Division of Global Migration and Quarantine, CDC. The accompanying certificate must be validated by the center that administers the vaccine. The certificate can be validated at most city, county, and state health departments or by vaccinating physicians who possess a "Uniform Stamp." State health departments are responsible for designated nonfederal yellow fever vaccination centers and issuing Uniform Stamps to be used to validate the International Certificate of Vaccination. Information about the location and hours of yellow fever vaccination centers may be obtained by contacting local or state health departments or visiting CDC's Travelers' Health website at http://www2.ncid.cdc.gov/travel/yellowfever/. Health-care providers administering vaccine to travelers should emphasize that an International Certificate of Vaccination must be validated to be acceptable to quarantine authorities. Failure to secure validations can cause a traveler to be revaccinated, quarantined, or denied entry.

The following section should be completed at the time of vaccination:

INTERNATIONAL CERTIFICATE OF VACCINATION OR REVACCINATION AGAINST YELLOW FEVER
CERTIFICAT INTERNATIONAL DE VACCINATION DU DE REVACCINATION CONTRE LA FIEVRE JAUNE

This is to certify that
Je soussigné(e) certifie que _____   sex
                                                      sexe_____

whose signature follows   date of birth
dont la signature suit_____   né(e) _____

has on the date indicated been vaccinated or revaccinated against yellow fever.
A été vacciné(e) ou revacciné (e) contre la fièvre jaune è la date indiquée.

Date	Signature and professional status of vaccinator Signature et titre du vaccinateur	Manufacturer & Batch number of vaccine Fabricant du vaccine Et numero du lot	Official stamp of Vaccinating center Cachet official du Centre de vaccination
1.			
2.			

Persons Authorized To Sign the Certificate

The International Certificate of Vaccination must be signed by a licensed physician or by a person designated by the physician. A signature stamp is not acceptable.

Vaccination Certificate Requirements for Direct Travel from the United States to Other Countries

For direct travel from the United States, only the following countries require an International Certificate of Vaccination against yellow fever.

TABLE 4-23. COUNTRIES THAT REQUIRE PROOF OF VACCINATION AGAINST YELLOW FEVER

Benin	Côte d'Ivoire	Liberia	São Tome and Principe
Burkina Faso	Democratic Republic of Congo	Mali	Togo
Cameroon		Niger	
	French Guiana		
Central African Republic	Gabon	Mauritania (for a stay >2 weeks)	
Congo	Ghana	Rwanda	

For travel to and between other countries, individual country requirements should be checked. No vaccinations are currently required for return to the United States.

Exemption from Vaccination

Travelers who do not have the required vaccinations or appropriate documentation of a vaccination waiver upon entering a country might be subject to vaccination, medical follow-up, isolation, or quarantine, or a combination of these. In a few countries, unvaccinated travelers are denied entry.

Some countries do not require an International Certificate of Vaccination for infants <6 months of age, <9 months of age, or <1 year of age.

Travelers should be advised to check the individual country requirements in *Yellow Fever Vaccine Requirements and Information on Malaria Risk and Prophylaxis, by Country.*

If a physician concludes that a particular vaccination should not be administered for medical reasons, the traveler should be given a signed and dated statement of the reasons on the physician's letterhead stationary.

No other reasons are acceptable for exemption from vaccination.

Waiver Letters from Physicians
A physician's letter clearly stating the contraindications to vaccination is acceptable to some governments. Ideally, it should be written on letterhead stationery and bear the stamp used by health department and official immunization centers to validate the international certificate of vaccination. Under these conditions, it is also useful for the traveler to obtain specific and authoritative advice from the embassy or consulate of the country or countries he or she plans to visit. Waivers of requirements obtained from embassies or consulates should be documented by appropriate letters and retained for presentation with the International Certificate of Vaccination and the section on Medical Contraindication to Vaccination completed.

MEDICAL CONTRAINDICATION TO VACCINATION
Contre-indication médicale á la vaccination

This is to certify that immunization against
Je soussigné(e) certifie que la vaccination contre

_____ for
(Name of disease – Nom de la maladie)   pour

_____ is medically
(Name of traveler – Nom du voyageur)   est médicalement

contraindicated because of the following conditions:
contre-indiquée pour les raisons suivantes:

_____

_____

_____

_____

_____
(Signature and address of physician)
(Signature et adresse du medecin)

Vaccination for Travel on Military Orders

Because military requirements may exceed those indicated in this publication, any person who plans to travel on military orders (civilians and military personnel) should be advised to contact the nearest military medical facility to determine the requirements for the trip.

TREATMENT

Patients should receive supportive care. In general, no specific treatments or established cures have proven benefit for patients with yellow fever or yellow fever vaccine-related illness.

Bibliography

Barwick RS, Marfin AA, Cetron MS. Yellow fever vaccine-associated disease [Chapter 3]. In: Scheld WM, Murray BE, Hughes JM, eds. Emerging Infections. 6th ed. Washington, DC: ASM Press, 2004,25–34.

CDC. Yellow fever Vaccine Information Statement (VIS) http://www.cdc.gov/nip/publications/VIS/vis-yf.pdf

CDC. Adverse events associated with 17D-derived yellow fever vaccination—United States, 2001-2002. MMWR Morbid Mortal Wkly Rep 2002; 51:989.

CDC. Yellow fever vaccine; recommendations of the Advisory Committee on Immunization Practices (ACIP). MMWR Morbid Mortal Wkly Rep 2002; 51(RR-17):1.

Chan RC, Penney DJ, Little D, Carter IW, Roberts JA, Rawlinson WD. Hepatitis and death following vaccination with 17D-204 yellow fever vaccine. Lancet. 2001;358:121–2.

Martin M, Tsai TF, Cropp B, Chang G-JJ, Holmes DA, et al. Fever and Multisystem organ failure associated with 17D-204 yellow fever vaccination: a report of four cases. Lancet. 2001;358:98–104.

Monath TP: Yellow fever [Chapter 34]. In: Plotkin SA, Orenstein WA, eds. Vaccines. 4th ed. Philadelphia, PA: W.B. Saunders, 2004, p. 1095.

Vasconcelos PF, Luna EJ, Galler R, Silva LJ. Coimbra TL, Barros VL et al. Serious adverse events associated with yellow fever 17DD vaccine in Brazil: a report of two cases. Lancet. 2001;358:91-7.

Yellow Fever Vaccine Safety Working Group. History of thymoma and yellow fever vaccination. Lancet. 2004;364(9438):936.

–MICHELLE RUSSELL, RACHEL BARWICK EIDEX, EDWARD HAYES, ANTHONY MARFIN, THOMAS MONATH, DIRK TEUWEN, MEGAN RANNEY, AND MARTIN CETRON

CHAPTER 5

Yellow Fever Vaccine Requirements and Information on Malaria Risk, by Country

| COUNTRY | YELLOW FEVER VACCINE | | MALARIA | | |
	COUNTRY REQUIREMENTS[1]	CDC RECOMMENDATIONS[2]	AREA OF RISK	CHLOROQUINE RESISTANCE	RECOMMENDED PROPHYLAXIS
Afghanistan	If traveling from an endemic zone	None	Risk April-December in all areas at altitudes <2,000 m (<6,561 ft)	Confirmed	Atovaquone/proguanil; doxycycline; or mefloquine
Albania	If traveling from an endemic zone and >1 year of age	None	None	Not applicable	Not applicable
Algeria	If traveling from an endemic zone and >1 year of age	None	Risk is limited to one small focus in Sahara region in Ihrir (Illizi Department). Risk is very limited; therefore, prophylaxis is not recommended.	None	None
Andorra	Not required	None	None	Not applicable	Not applicable
Angola	If traveling from an endemic zone and >1 year of age	For all travelers >9 months of age	All	Confirmed	Atovaquone/proguanil; doxycycline; or mefloquine
Anguilla (U.K.)	If traveling from an endemic zone and >1 year of age	None	None	Not applicable	Not applicable

[1]Yellow fever vaccine entry **requirements** are necessary for travelers to comply with in order to enter the country. In general, these are in place to prevent importation and transmission of yellow fever virus. Countries requiring yellow fever vaccination for entry adhere to the regulations put forth by WHO as stated in the International Health Regulations. Some countries require vaccination for travelers coming from an endemic zone. "Traveling from an endemic zone" is defined as transit through an endemic zone in the previous 6 days.

[2]The information in the section on yellow fever vaccine **recommendations** is advice given by CDC to prevent yellow fever infections among travelers.

COUNTRY	YELLOW FEVER VACCINE			MALARIA		
	COUNTRY REQUIREMENTS[1]	CDC RECOMMENDATIONS[2]	AREA OF RISK	CHLOROQUINE RESISTANCE	RECOMMENDED PROPHYLAXIS
Antigua and Barbuda	If traveling from an endemic zone and >1 year of age	None	None	Not applicable	Not applicable
Argentina	Not required	For all travelers >9 months of age going to the northern and north-eastern forested areas, including Iguaçu Falls (see map 4-13)	Rural areas of Salta and Jujuy province (along Bolivian border) and Misiones and Corrientes province (along border of Paraguay)	None	Chloroquine
Armenia	Not required	None	Risk limited to western border areas: Masis, Ararat, and Artashat regions in Ararat District	None	Chloroquine
Aruba	If traveling from an endemic zone and >6 months of age[3]	None	None	Not applicable	Not applicable
Australia; Including Cocos (Keeling) Islands. Note: Australia is not bound by the International Health Regulations.	All persons >1 year of age who, within 6 days of arrival in Australia, have been in or have passed through an endemic zone	None	None	Not applicable	Not applicable

[3]Please note, the U.S. Advisory Committee for Immunization Practices recommends avoiding vaccination in infants <9 months of age; travel of infants <9 months of age to countries in the yellow fever-endemic zone or to countries experiencing a yellow fever epidemic should be postponed or avoided, whenever possible. If travel is unavoidable, medical waivers may be considered for infants <9 months of age to meet the entry requirements of these countries.

COUNTRY	YELLOW FEVER VACCINE		AREA OF RISK	MALARIA	
	COUNTRY REQUIREMENTS[1]	CDC RECOMMENDATIONS[2]		CHLOROQUINE RESISTANCE	RECOMMENDED PROPHYLAXIS
Austria	Not required	None	None	Not applicable	Not applicable
Azerbaijan	Not required	None	Rural lowlands in the provinces of Agcabadi, Barda, Beylaqan, Bilasuvar, Calilabad, Fuzuli, Imisli, Kurdamir, Saatli, Sabirabad, and Zardab, between the Kura and Arax rivers	None	Chloroquine
Azores (Portugal)	If traveling from an endemic zone and >1 year of age	None	None	Not applicable	Not applicable
Bahamas, The	If traveling from an endemic zone and >1 year of age	None	None	Not applicable	Not applicable
Bahrain	Not required	None	None	Not applicable	Not applicable
Bangladesh	Not If traveling from an endemic zone. Any person (including infants)[3] arriving by air or sea without a certificate within 6 days of departure from or	None	All, except no risk in city of Dhaka	Confirmed	Atovaquone/ proguanil; doxycycline; or mefloquine

| COUNTRY | YELLOW FEVER VACCINE | | | MALARIA | |
	COUNTRY REQUIREMENTS[1]	CDC RECOMMENDATIONS[2]	AREA OF RISK	CHLOROQUINE RESISTANCE	RECOMMENDED PROPHYLAXIS
	transit through an infected area will be quarantined up to 6 days. Required also for travelers arriving from or transiting: **Africa:** Angola, Benin, Burkina Faso, Burundi, Cameroon, Central African Republic, Chad, Congo, Côte d'Ivoire, Democratic Republic of Congo, Equatorial Guinea, Ethiopia, Gabon, The Gambia, Ghana, Guinea, Guinea Bissau, Kenya, Liberia, Malawi, Mali, Mauritania, Niger, Nigeria, Rwanda, São Tomé and Principe, Senegal, Sierra Leone, Somalia, Sudan (south of 15° N), Tanzania, Togo, Uganda, and Zambia **Americas:** Belize, Bolivia, Brazil, Columbia, Costa Rica, Ecuador, French Guiana, Guatemala, Guyana, Honduras, Nicaragua, Panama, Peru, Suriname, and Venezuela **Caribbean:** Trinidad and Tobago				

| | YELLOW FEVER VACCINE | | | MALARIA | |
COUNTRY	COUNTRY REQUIREMENTS[1]	CDC RECOMMENDATIONS[2]	AREA OF RISK	CHLOROQUINE RESISTANCE	RECOMMENDED PROPHYLAXIS
Barbados	If traveling from an endemic zone and >1 year of age	None	None	Not applicable	Not applicable
Belarus	Not required	None	None	Not applicable	Not applicable
Belgium	Not required	None	None	Not applicable	Not applicable
Belize	If traveling from an endemic zone and >1 year of age	None	All, except no risk in Belize City	None	Chloroquine
Benin	Required upon arrival from all countries if traveler is >1 year of age	For all travelers >9 months of age	All	Confirmed	Atovaquone/ proguanil; doxycycline; or mefloquine
Bermuda (U.K.)	Not required	None	None	Not applicable	Not applicable
Bhutan	If traveling from an endemic zone	None	Risk in the southern belt of five districts: Chirang, Samchi, Samdrupjongkhar, Sarpang and Shemgang	Confirmed	Atovaquone/ proguanil; doxycycline; or mefloquine

| COUNTRY | YELLOW FEVER VACCINE | | MALARIA | | |
	COUNTRY REQUIREMENTS[1]	CDC RECOMMENDATIONS[2]	AREA OF RISK	CHLOROQUINE RESISTANCE	RECOMMENDED PROPHYLAXIS
Bolivia	If traveling from an endemic zone	For all travelers >9 months of age traveling to areas east of the Andes Mountains (see map). Does not include the cities of La Paz or Sucre	Risk in areas <2,500 m (<8,202 ft) in the following departments: Beni, Chuquisaca, Cochabamba, La Paz, Pando, Santa Cruz, and Tarija. No risk in city of La Paz	Confirmed	Atovaquone/ proguanil; doxycycline; or mefloquine
Bosnia and Herzegovina	Not required	None	None	Not applicable	Not applicable
Botswana	If traveling from an endemic zone and >1 year of age	None	Risk north of 21° S in the northern districts of Central, Chobe, Ngamiland, North East, and Okavango	Confirmed	Atovaquone/ proguanil; doxycycline; or mefloquine

| COUNTRY | YELLOW FEVER VACCINE | | MALARIA | | |
	COUNTRY REQUIREMENTS[1]	CDC RECOMMENDATIONS[2]	AREA OF RISK	CHLOROQUINE RESISTANCE	RECOMMENDED PROPHYLAXIS
Brazil	If traveling from the endemic zones listed below and >9 months of age: **Africa:** Angola, Benin, Burkina Faso, Burundi, Cameroon, Cape Verde, Central African Republic, Democratic Republic of Congo, Congo, Côte d'Ivoire, Ethiopia, Gabon, The Gambia, Ghana, Guinea, Guinea Bissau, Equatorial Guinea, Liberia, Mali, Mauritania, Niger, Nigeria, Kenya, Rwanda, São Tomé & Principe, Senegal, Sierra Leone, Somalia, Sudan, Tanzania, Togo, Uganda **Americas:** Bolivia, Colombia, Ecuador, Guyana, French Guyana, Peru, Surinam, Venezuela **Central America & Caribbean:** Panama, Trinidad and Tobago	For all travelers >9 months of age going to the endemic zone in Brazil, which includes the states of Acre, Amapá, Amazones, Goias, Maranhaõ, Mato Grosso, Mato Grosso do Sul, Minas Gerais, Pará, Rondônia, Roraima and Tocantins, and areas in the endemic zone of the states of Bahia, Parana, Piaui, Rio Grande do Sul, and Sao Paulo (see map). Vaccination is recommended for travelers visiting Iguaçu Falls. Coastal cities, including Rio de Janeiro, Sao Paulo, Salvador, Recife, and Fortaleza, are NOT within the endemic zone.	States of Acre, Rondônia, Amapá, Amazonas, Roraima, and Tocantins. Parts of states of Maranhaõ (western part), Mato Grosso (northern part), and Pará (except Belem City). There is also transmission in urban areas, including large cities such as Porto Velho, Boa Vista, Macapa, Manaus, Santarem, and Maraba, where the transmission occurs on the periphery of these cities.	Confirmed	Atovaquone/ proguanil; doxycycline; or mefloquine
British Indian Ocean Territory; Includes Diego Garcia (UK)	Not required	None	None	Not applicable	Not applicable

| COUNTRY | YELLOW FEVER VACCINE | | MALARIA | | |
	COUNTRY REQUIREMENTS[1]	CDC RECOMMENDATIONS[2]	AREA OF RISK	CHLOROQUINE RESISTANCE	RECOMMENDED PROPHYLAXIS
Brunei	If traveling from an endemic zone and >1 year of age	None	None	Not applicable	Not applicable
Bulgaria	Not required	None	None	Not applicable	Not applicable
Burkina Faso	Required upon arrival from all countries if traveler is >1 year of age	For all travelers >9 months of age	All	Confirmed	Atovaquone/ proguanil; doxycycline; or mefloquine
Burma (Myanmar)	If traveling from an endemic zone. Required also for nationals and residents of Burma departing for an endemic zone.	None	Rural only. No risk in cities of Rangoon (Yangon) and Mandalay.	Confirmed	Atovaquone/ proguanil; doxycycline; or mefloquine in all areas *except* in the states of Shan, Kayah, and Kayin must take atovaquone/proguanil or doxycyline only
Burundi	If traveling from an endemic zone and >1 year of age	For all travelers >9 months of age	All	Confirmed	Atovaquone/ proguanil; doxycycline; or mefloquine

| COUNTRY | YELLOW FEVER VACCINE | | MALARIA | | |
	COUNTRY REQUIREMENTS[1]	CDC RECOMMENDATIONS[2]	AREA OF RISK	CHLOROQUINE RESISTANCE	RECOMMENDED PROPHYLAXIS
Cambodia	If traveling from an endemic zone	None	All, including risk in the temple complex at Angkor Wat. No risk in Phnom Penh and around Lake Tonle Sap.	Confirmed	Atovaquone/ proguanil or doxycycline must be taken in western provinces bordering Thailand; other areas can use Atovaquone/ proguanil; doxycycline; or mefloquine
Cameroon	Required upon arrival from all countries if traveler is >1 year of age	For all travelers >9 months of age	All	Confirmed	Atovaquone/ proguanil; doxycycline; or mefloquine
Canada	Not required	None	None	Not applicable	Not applicable
Canary Islands (Spain)	Not required	None	None	Not applicable	Not applicable
Cape Verde	If traveling from an endemic zone and >1 year of age	For all travelers >9 months of age	Limited risk on the island of Saõ Tiago only	Confirmed	Atovaquone/ proguanil; doxycycline; or mefloquine

| COUNTRY | YELLOW FEVER VACCINE | | | MALARIA | | |
	COUNTRY REQUIREMENTS[1]	CDC RECOMMENDATIONS[2]	AREA OF RISK	CHLOROQUINE RESISTANCE	RECOMMENDED PROPHYLAXIS
Cayman Islands (U.K.)	Not required	None	None	Not applicable	Not applicable
Central African Republic	Required upon arrival from all countries if traveler is >1 year of age	For all travelers >9 months of age	All	Confirmed	Atovaquone/ proguanil; doxycycline; or mefloquine
Chad	Not required	For all travelers >9 months of age. Chad recommends vaccination for all travelers >1 year of age.	All	Confirmed	Atovaquone/ proguanil; doxycycline; or mefloquine
Chile	Not required	None	None	Not applicable	Not applicable

COUNTRY	YELLOW FEVER VACCINE		MALARIA		
	COUNTRY REQUIREMENTS[1]	CDC RECOMMENDATIONS[2]	AREA OF RISK	CHLOROQUINE RESISTANCE	RECOMMENDED PROPHYLAXIS
China	If traveling from an endemic zone	None	Travelers to cities and popular tourist areas, including Yangtze River cruises, are not at risk and do not need to take chemoprophylaxis. Rural areas only of the following provinces: Hainan, Yunnan, Fujian, Guangdong, Guangxi, Guizhou, Sichuan, Tibet (in the Zangbo River valley only), Anhui, Hubei, Hunan, Jiangsu, Jiangxi, and Shandong. In provinces with risk, transmission exists in rural communities <1,500 m only during warm weather: north of latitude 33° N, July–November; between latitude 25° N and 33° N, May–December. South of latitude 25° N, transmission occurs year-round.	Confirmed in the provinces of Hainin and Yunnan. Other provinces do not have chloroquine-resistant malaria.	Atovaquone/proguanil; doxycycline; or mefloquine in Hainan and Yunnan; Chloroquine in all other areas

| COUNTRY | YELLOW FEVER VACCINE | | | MALARIA | | |
	COUNTRY REQUIREMENTS[1]	CDC RECOMMENDATIONS[2]	AREA OF RISK	CHLOROQUINE RESISTANCE	RECOMMENDED PROPHYLAXIS	
Christmas Island (Australia) Note: Christmas Island is not bound by the International Health Regulations	All travelers >1 year of age, who within the past 6 days have traveled or passed through an endemic area, as listed by WHO	None	None	Not applicable	Not applicable	
Colombia	Not required	Recommended for all travelers >9 months of age. Travelers whose itinerary is limited to the cities of Bogota, Cali, or Medellin are at lower risk and may consider foregoing vaccination.	Risk in all rural areas at altitudes <800 m (2,624 ft). No risk in Bogotá and vicinity.	Confirmed	Atovaquone/ proguanil; doxycycline; or mefloquine	
Comoros	Not required	None	All	Confirmed	Atovaquone/ proguanil; doxycycline; or mefloquine	

COUNTRY	YELLOW FEVER VACCINE		MALARIA		
	COUNTRY REQUIREMENTS[1]	CDC RECOMMENDATIONS[2]	AREA OF RISK	CHLOROQUINE RESISTANCE	RECOMMENDED PROPHYLAXIS
Congo	Required upon arrival from all countries if traveler is >1 year of age	For all travelers >9 months of age	All	Confirmed	Atovaquone/proguanil; doxycycline; or mefloquine
Cook Islands (New Zealand)	Not required	None	None	Not applicable	Not applicable
Costa Rica	Not required	None	Risk in Alajuela, Limón, Guanacaste, and Heredia provinces. No risk in Limón city (Puerto Limon).	None	Chloroquine
Côte d'Ivoire (Ivory Coast)	Required upon arrival from all countries if traveler is >1 year of age	For all travelers >9 months of age	All	Confirmed	Atovaquone/proguanil; doxycycline; or mefloquine
Croatia	Not required	None	None	Not applicable	Not applicable
Cuba	Not required	None	None	Not applicable	Not applicable
Cyprus	Not required	None	None	Not applicable	Not applicable
Czech Republic	Not required	None	None	Not applicable	Not applicable

| | YELLOW FEVER VACCINE | | | MALARIA | |
COUNTRY	COUNTRY REQUIREMENTS[1]	CDC RECOMMENDATIONS[2]	AREA OF RISK	CHLOROQUINE RESISTANCE	RECOMMENDED PROPHYLAXIS
Democratic Republic of the Congo (formerly Zaire)	Required upon arrival from all countries if traveler is >1 year of age	For all travelers >9 months of age	All	Confirmed	Atovaquone/ proguanil; doxycycline; or mefloquine
Denmark	Not required	None	None	Not applicable	Not applicable
Djibouti	If traveling from an endemic zone and >1 year of age	None	All	Confirmed	Atovaquone/ proguanil; doxycycline; or mefloquine
Dominica	If traveling from an endemic zone and >1 year of age	None	None	Not applicable	Not applicable
Dominican Republic	Not required	None	Rural; highest risk in provinces bordering Haiti	None	Chloroquine
Easter Island (Chile)	Not required	None	None	Not applicable	Not applicable
East Timor	Required from travelers coming from an endemic zone	None	All	Confirmed	Atovaquone/ proguanil; doxycycline; or mefloquine

	YELLOW FEVER VACCINE		MALARIA		
COUNTRY	COUNTRY REQUIREMENTS[1]	CDC RECOMMENDATIONS[2]	AREA OF RISK	CHLOROQUINE RESISTANCE	RECOMMENDED PROPHYLAXIS
Ecuador; Including the Galápagos Islands	If traveling from an endemic zone and >1 year of age	For all travelers >9 months of age who are traveling to areas east of the Andes Mountains (see map), NOT including the cities of Quito and Guayaquil or the Galápagos Islands	Risk in all areas at altitudes <1,500 m (<4,921 ft). No risk in the cities of Guayaquil and Quito, the central highland tourist areas, and the Galápagos Islands.	Confirmed	Atovaquone/ proguanil; doxycy- cline; or mefloquine
Egypt	If traveling from an endemic zone and >1 year of age. Air passen- gers in transit but coming from these countries or areas without a certificate will be detained in the precincts of the airport until they resume their journey. All travelers arriving from Sudan are required to have a vaccination certificate or a location certificate issued by a Sudanese official center stating that they have not been in Sudan south of 15° N within the previous 6 days. Required also for travelers arriving from or transiting:	None	Very limited risk in El Faiyûm area only. No risk in tourist areas, including Nile River cruises. Risk is very limited; therefore, prophylaxis is not recommended.	None	None

	YELLOW FEVER VACCINE			MALARIA		
COUNTRY	COUNTRY REQUIREMENTS[1]	CDC RECOMMENDATIONS[2]	AREA OF RISK	CHLOROQUINE RESISTANCE	RECOMMENDED PROPHYLAXIS	
	Africa: Angola, Benin, Burkina Faso, Burundi, Cameroon, Central African Republic, Chad, Congo, Côte d'Ivoire, Democratic Republic of the Congo, Equatorial Guinea, Ethiopia, Gabon, Gambia, Ghana, Guinea, Guinea-Bissau, Kenya, Liberia, Mali, Niger, Nigeria, Rwanda, São Tomé and Principe, Senegal, Sierra Leone, Somalia, Sudan (south of 15°N), Tanzania, Togo, Uganda, Zambia **Americas:** Belize, Bolivia, Brazil, Colombia, Costa Rica, Ecuador, French Guiana, Guyana, Panama, Peru, Suriname, Venezuela **Caribbean:** Trinidad and Tobago					
El Salvador	If traveling from an endemic zone and >6 months of age[3]	None	Rural areas of Santa Ana, Ahuachapán, and La Unión departments	None	Chloroquine	

COUNTRY	YELLOW FEVER VACCINE		AREA OF RISK	MALARIA	
	COUNTRY REQUIREMENTS[1]	CDC RECOMMENDATIONS[2]		CHLOROQUINE RESISTANCE	RECOMMENDED PROPHYLAXIS
Equatorial Guinea	If traveling from an endemic zone	For all travelers >9 months of age	All	Confirmed	Atovaquone/ proguanil; doxycycline; or mefloquine
Eritrea	If traveling from an endemic zone	None	All areas at altitudes <2,200 m (7,218 ft). No risk in Asmara.	Confirmed	Atovaquone/ proguanil; doxycycline; or mefloquine
Estonia	Not required	None	None	Not applicable	Not applicable
Ethiopia	If traveling from an endemic zone and >1 year of age	For all travelers >9 months of age	All areas at altitudes <2,000 m (6,561 ft). No risk in Addis Ababa.	Confirmed	Atovaquone/ proguanil; doxycycline; or mefloquine
Falkland, South Georgia & South Sandwich Islands (U.K.)	Not required	None	None	Not applicable	Not applicable
Faroe Islands (Denmark)	Not required	None	None	Not applicable	Not applicable

| COUNTRY | YELLOW FEVER VACCINE | | MALARIA | | |
	COUNTRY REQUIREMENTS[1]	CDC RECOMMENDATIONS[2]	AREA OF RISK	CHLOROQUINE RESISTANCE	RECOMMENDED PROPHYLAXIS
Fiji	If traveling from an endemic zone and >1 year of age and within 10 days of having stayed overnight or longer in an endemic zone	None	None	Not applicable	Not applicable
Finland	Not required	None	None	Not applicable	Not applicable
France	Not required	None	None	Not applicable	Not applicable
French Guiana	Required upon arrival from all countries if traveler is >1 year of age	For all travelers >9 months of age	All	Confirmed	Atovaquone/proguanil; doxycycline; or mefloquine

| COUNTRY | YELLOW FEVER VACCINE | | MALARIA | | |
	COUNTRY REQUIREMENTS[1]	CDC RECOMMENDATIONS[2]	AREA OF RISK	CHLOROQUINE RESISTANCE	RECOMMENDED PROPHYLAXIS
French Polynesia, includes the island groups of Society Islands (Tahiti, Moorea, and Bora-Bora); Marquesas Islands (Hiva Oa and Ua Huka); and Austral Islands (Tubuai and Rurutu)	If traveling from an endemic zone and >1 year of age	None	None	Not applicable	Not applicable
Gabon	Required upon arrival from all countries if traveler is >1 year of age	For all travelers >9 months of age	All	Confirmed	Atovaquone/ proguanil; doxycycline; or mefloquine
Gambia, The	If traveling from an endemic zone and >1 year of age	For all travelers >9 months of age	All	Confirmed	Atovaquone/ proguanil; doxycycline; or mefloquine
Georgia	Not required	None	Southeastern part of the country in the districts of Lagodekhi, Sighnaghi, Dedophilistskaro, Saraejo,	None	Chloroquine

| COUNTRY | YELLOW FEVER VACCINE | | AREA OF RISK | MALARIA | |
	COUNTRY REQUIREMENTS[1]	CDC RECOMMENDATIONS[2]		CHLOROQUINE RESISTANCE	RECOMMENDED PROPHYLAXIS
Germany	Not required	None	Gardabani, and Marneuli in the Kakheti and Kveno Kartli regions. No risk in Tbilisi.	Not applicable	Not applicable
Ghana	Required upon arrival from all countries	For all travelers >9 months of age	All	Confirmed	Atovaquone/ proguanil; doxycy-cline; or mefloquine
Gibraltar (U.K.)	Not required	None	None	Not applicable	Not applicable
Greece	Not required	None	None	Not applicable	Not applicable
Greenland (Denmark)	Not required	None	None	Not applicable	Not applicable
Grenada	If traveling from an endemic zone and >1 year of age	None	None	Not applicable	Not applicable
Guadeloupe, including St. Barthelemy and Saint Martin (France)	If traveling from an endemic zone and >1 year of age	None	None	Not applicable	Not applicable

| COUNTRY | YELLOW FEVER VACCINE | | MALARIA | | |
	COUNTRY REQUIREMENTS[1]	CDC RECOMMENDATIONS[2]	AREA OF RISK	CHLOROQUINE RESISTANCE	RECOMMENDED PROPHYLAXIS
Guam (U.S.)	Not required	None	None	Not applicable	Not applicable
Guatemala	If traveling from an endemic zone and >1 year of age	None	Rural areas only at altitudes <1,500 m (<4,921 ft). No risk in Antigua or Lake Atitlán.	None	Chloroquine
Guinea	If traveling from an endemic zone and >1 year of age	For all travelers >9 months of age	All	Confirmed	Atovaquone/ proguanil; doxycycline; or mefloquine
Guinea-Bissau	If traveling from an endemic zone and >1 year of age Required also for travelers arriving from: **Africa:** Angola, Benin, Burkina Faso, Burundi, Cape Verde, Central African Republic, Chad, Congo, Côte d'Ivoire, Democratic Republic of the Congo, Djibouti, Equatorial Guinea, Ethiopia, Gabon, Gambia, Ghana, Guinea, Kenya, Liberia, Madagascar, Mali, Mauritania, Mozambique, Niger, Nigeria, Rwanda, São Tomé and Principe, Senegal, Sierra Leone, Somalia,	For all travelers >9 months of age	All	Confirmed	Atovaquone/ proguanil; doxycycline; or mefloquine

	YELLOW FEVER VACCINE			MALARIA		
COUNTRY	COUNTRY REQUIREMENTS[1]	CDC RECOMMENDATIONS[2]	AREA OF RISK	CHLOROQUINE RESISTANCE	RECOMMENDED PROPHYLAXIS
	Tanzania, Togo, Uganda, Zambia **Americas:** Bolivia, Brazil, Colombia, Ecuador, French Guiana, Guyana, Panama, Peru, Suriname, Venezuela				
Guyana	If traveling from an endemic zone Required also for travelers arriving from: **Africa:** Angola, Benin, Burkina Faso, Burundi, Cameroon, Central African Republic, Chad, Congo, Côte d'Ivoire, Democratic Republic of the Congo, Gabon, Gambia, Ghana, Guinea, Guinea-Bissau, Kenya, Liberia, Mali, Niger, Nigeria, Rwanda, São Tomé and Principe, Senegal, Sierra Leone, Somalia, Tanzania, Togo, Uganda **Americas:** Belize, Bolivia, Brazil, Colombia, Costa Rica, Ecuador, French Guiana, Guatemala, Honduras, Nicaragua, Panama, Peru, Suriname, and Venezuela	For all travelers >9 months of age	Risk in all areas of the interior; sporadic cases have also been reported along the coastal region	Confirmed	Atovaquone/proguanil; doxycycline; or mefloquine

| COUNTRY | YELLOW FEVER VACCINE | | MALARIA | | |
	COUNTRY REQUIREMENTS[1]	CDC RECOMMENDATIONS[2]	AREA OF RISK	CHLOROQUINE RESISTANCE	RECOMMENDED PROPHYLAXIS
Haiti	If traveling from an endemic zone	None	All except no risk in cruise port of Labadee	None	Chloroquine
Holy See	Not required	None	None	Not applicable	Not applicable
Honduras	If traveling from an endemic zone	None	Risk in rural areas only and in Roatán and other Bay Islands	None	Chloroquine
Hong Kong SAR (China)	Not required	None	None	Not applicable	Not applicable
Hungary	Not required	None	None	Not applicable	Not applicable
Iceland	Not required	None	None	Not applicable	Not applicable
India	If traveling from an endemic zone Required also for travelers arriving from or transiting: **Africa:** Angola, Benin, Burkina Faso, Burundi, Cameroon, Central African Republic, Chad, Congo, Côte d'Ivoire, Democratic Republic of the Congo, Equatorial Guinea, Ethiopia, Gabon, Gambia, Ghana, Guinea, Guinea-Bissau, Kenya, Liberia, Mali, Niger, Nigeria, Rwanda, São Tomé and Principe,	None	All areas, including the cities of Delhi and Bombay. Risk in areas at altitudes <2,000 m (6,561 ft) in Himachal Pradesh, Jammu, Kashmir, and Sikkim.	Confirmed	Atovaquone/ proguanil; doxycycline; or mefloquine

| COUNTRY | YELLOW FEVER VACCINE | | MALARIA | | |
	COUNTRY REQUIREMENTS[1]	CDC RECOMMENDATIONS[2]	AREA OF RISK	CHLOROQUINE RESISTANCE	RECOMMENDED PROPHYLAXIS
	Senegal, Sierra Leone, Somalia, Sudan, Togo, Uganda, United Republic of Tanzania, Zambia **Americas:** Bolivia, Brazil, Colombia, Ecuador, French Guiana, Guyana, Panama, Peru, Suriname, and Venezuela **Caribbean:** Trinidad and Tobago Any person (except infants ≤6 months) arriving without a certificate within 6 days of departure from or transit through an endemic area will be isolated for up to 6 days.[3]				
Indonesia	If traveling from an endemic zone	None	Risk in all areas of Irian Jaya (western half of the island of New Guinea) and at the temple complex of Borobudur. Risk in rural areas only in other islands. No risk in for the cities of Java and Sumatra or in the main resort areas of Java and Bali.	Confirmed	Atovaquone/ proguanil; doxycycline; or mefloquine

| COUNTRY | YELLOW FEVER VACCINE | | MALARIA | | |
	COUNTRY REQUIREMENTS[1]	CDC RECOMMENDATIONS[2]	AREA OF RISK	CHLOROQUINE RESISTANCE	RECOMMENDED PROPHYLAXIS
Iran	Not required	None	Risk in the provinces of Sistan-Baluchestan, the southern tropical part of Kerman, and Hormozgan	Confirmed	Atovaquone/ proguanil; doxycycline; or mefloquine
Iraq	If traveling from an endemic zone	None	Risk in Basrah province and in areas at altitudes <1500 m (<4,921 ft) in provinces of Duhok, Erbil, Ninawa, Sulaimaniya, and Ta'mim	None	Chloroquine
Ireland	Not required	None	None	Not applicable	Not applicable
Israel	Not required	None	None	Not applicable	Not applicable
Italy	Not required	None	None	Not applicable	Not applicable
Jamaica	If traveling from an endemic zone and >1 year of age	None	None	Not applicable	Not applicable
Japan	Not required	None	None	Not applicable	Not applicable
Jordan	If traveling from an endemic zone and >1 year of age	None	None	Not applicable	Not applicable
Kazakhstan	If traveling from an endemic zone	None	None	Not applicable	Not applicable

| COUNTRY | YELLOW FEVER VACCINE | | | MALARIA | | |
	COUNTRY REQUIREMENTS[1]	CDC RECOMMENDATIONS[2]	AREA OF RISK	CHLOROQUINE RESISTANCE	RECOMMENDED PROPHYLAXIS
Kenya	If traveling from an endemic zone and >1 year of age	For all travelers >9 months of age. The cities of Nairobi and Mombasa have lower risk of transmission than rural areas.	All areas (including game parks) at altitudes <2,500 m (<8,202 ft). No risk in Nairobi.	Confirmed	Atovaquone/ proguanil; doxycycline; or mefloquine
Kiribati (formerly Gilbert Islands) includes these islands: Tarawa, Tabuaeran (Fanning Island), and Banaba (Ocean Island)	If traveling from an endemic zone and >1 year of age	None	None	Not applicable	Not applicable
Korea, North	Not required	None	Limited malaria risk in some southern areas	None	Chloroquine
Korea, South	Not required	None	Risk limited to demilitarized zone (DMZ) and to rural areas in the northern parts of Kyonggi and Kangwon provinces	None	Chloroquine

COUNTRY	YELLOW FEVER VACCINE		MALARIA		
	COUNTRY REQUIREMENTS[1]	CDC RECOMMENDATIONS[2]	AREA OF RISK	CHLOROQUINE RESISTANCE	RECOMMENDED PROPHYLAXIS
Kuwait	Not required	None	None	Not applicable	Not applicable
Kyrgyzstan	Not required	None	Risk in some southern and western parts of the country, mainly in the provinces of Batken, Osh, and Zhele-Abadskaya in the areas bordering Tajikistan and Uzbekistan	None	Chloroquine
Laos	If traveling from an endemic zone	None	All, except no risk in city of Vientiane	Confirmed	Atovaquone/proguanil; doxycycline; or mefloquine
Latvia	Not required	None	None	Not applicable	Not applicable
Lebanon	If traveling from an endemic zone	None	None	Not applicable	Not applicable
Lesotho	If traveling from an endemic zone	None	None	Not applicable	Not applicable
Liberia	Required upon arrival from all countries if traveler is >1 year of age	For all travelers >9 months of age	All	Confirmed	Atovaquone/proguanil; doxycycline; or mefloquine
Libya	If traveling from an endemic zone	None	None	Not applicable	Not applicable
Liechtenstein	Not required	None	None	Not applicable	Not applicable

| | YELLOW FEVER VACCINE | | | MALARIA | | |
COUNTRY	COUNTRY REQUIREMENTS[1]	CDC RECOMMENDATIONS[2]	AREA OF RISK	CHLOROQUINE RESISTANCE	RECOMMENDED PROPHYLAXIS
Lithuania	Not required	None	None	Not applicable	Not applicable
Luxembourg	Not required	None	None	Not applicable	Not applicable
Macao SAR (China)	Not required	None	None	Not applicable	Not applicable
Macedonia, the Former Yugoslav Republic of	Not required	None	None	Not applicable	Not applicable
Madagascar	If traveling from an endemic zone	None	All	Confirmed	Atovaquone/ proguanil; doxycycline; or mefloquine
Madeira Islands (Portugal)	If traveling from an endemic zone and >1 year of age	None	None	Not applicable	Not applicable
Malawi	If traveling from an endemic zone	None	All	Confirmed	Atovaquone/ proguanil; doxycycline; or mefloquine

| COUNTRY | YELLOW FEVER VACCINE | | MALARIA | | |
	COUNTRY REQUIREMENTS[1]	CDC RECOMMENDATIONS[2]	AREA OF RISK	CHLOROQUINE RESISTANCE	RECOMMENDED PROPHYLAXIS
Malaysia	If traveling from an endemic zone and >1 year of age. A certificate is also required from travelers who have transited an endemic area within the preceding 6 days.	None	Risk limited to rural areas. No risk in urban and coastal areas. Note: No risk in Republic of Singapore.	Confirmed	Atovaquone/ proguanil; doxycycline; or mefloquine
Maldives	If traveling from an endemic zone	None	None	Not applicable	Not applicable
Mali	Required upon arrival from all countries if traveler is >1 year of age	For all travelers >9 months of age	All	Confirmed	Atovaquone/ proguanil; doxycycline; or mefloquine
Malta	If traveling from an endemic zone and >9 months of age Children <9 months of age arriving from an endemic zone may be subject to isolation or surveillance	None	None	Not applicable	Not applicable
Marshall Islands	Not required	None	None	Not applicable	Not applicable
Martinique (France)	Not required	None	None	Not applicable	Not applicable

| COUNTRY | YELLOW FEVER VACCINE | | MALARIA | | |
	COUNTRY REQUIREMENTS[1]	CDC RECOMMENDATIONS[2]	AREA OF RISK	CHLOROQUINE RESISTANCE	RECOMMENDED PROPHYLAXIS
Mauritania	Required upon arrival from all countries if traveler is >1 year of age **Exception:** Not required for travelers from a nonendemic zone who stay <2 weeks	For all travelers >9 months of age	All, except no risk in the northern areas of Dakhlet-Nouadhibou and Tiris-Zemmour	Probable	Atovaquone/proguanil; doxycycline; or mefloquine
Mauritius	If traveling from an endemic zone	None	Rural only. No risk on Rodrigues Island.	None	Chloroquine
Mayotte (French territorial collectivity)	Not required	None	All	Confirmed	Atovaquone/proguanil; doxycycline; or mefloquine

| COUNTRY | YELLOW FEVER VACCINE | | MALARIA | | |
	COUNTRY REQUIREMENTS[1]	CDC RECOMMENDATIONS[2]	AREA OF RISK	CHLOROQUINE RESISTANCE	RECOMMENDED PROPHYLAXIS
Mexico	Not required	None	Risk in rural areas, including resorts in rural areas of the following states: Campeche, Chiapas, Guerrero, Michoacán, Nayarit, Oaxaca, Quintana Roo, Sinaloa, and Tabasco. In addition, risk exists in the state of Jalisco (in its mountainous northern area only). Risk also exists in an area between 24° N and 28° N latitude, and 106° W and 110° W longitude, which lies in parts of Sonora, Chihuahua, and Durango. No malaria risk exists along the United States-Mexico border. No malaria risk exists in the major resorts along the Pacific and Gulf coasts.	None	Chloroquine
Micronesia, Federated States of; Includes: Yap Islands, Pohnpei, Chuuk, and Kosrae	Not required	None	None	Not applicable	Not applicable

| COUNTRY | YELLOW FEVER VACCINE | | AREA OF RISK | MALARIA | |
	COUNTRY REQUIREMENTS[1]	CDC RECOMMENDATIONS[2]		CHLOROQUINE RESISTANCE	RECOMMENDED PROPHYLAXIS
Moldova	Not required	None	None	Not applicable	Not applicable
Monaco	Not required	None	None	Not applicable	Not applicable
Mongolia	Not required	None	None	Not applicable	Not applicable
Montserrat (U.K.)	If traveling from an endemic zone and >1 year of age	None	None	Not applicable	Not applicable
Morocco	Not required	None	Risk in rural areas of Chefchaouen province. No risk in Tangier, Rabat, Casablanca, Marrakech, and Fès. Risk is very limited; therefore, prophylaxis is not recommended.	None	None
Mozambique	If traveling from an endemic zone and >1 year of age	None	All	Confirmed	Atovaquone/proguanil; doxycycline; or mefloquine
Namibia	If traveling from an endemic zone and >1 year of age. Required also for travelers on unscheduled flights who have transited an infected area. Children <1 year of age may be subject to surveillance.	None	Risk in the provinces of Kunene, Ohangwena, Okavango, Caprivi, Omaheke, Omusati, Oshana, Oshikoto, and Otjozondjupa	Confirmed	Atovaquone/proguanil; doxycycline; or mefloquine

	YELLOW FEVER VACCINE		AREA OF RISK	MALARIA		
COUNTRY	COUNTRY REQUIREMENTS[1]	CDC RECOMMENDATIONS[2]	AREA OF RISK	CHLOROQUINE RESISTANCE	RECOMMENDED PROPHYLAXIS	
Nauru	If traveling from an endemic zone and >1 year of age	None	None	Not applicable	Not applicable	
Nepal	If traveling from an endemic zone	None	Rural areas in the Terai and Hill districts. Risk at altitudes <1,200 m (3,937 ft). No risk in Kathmandu on typical Himalayan treks.	Confirmed	Atovaquone/ proguanil; doxycycline; or mefloquine	
Netherlands	Not required	None	None	Not applicable	Not applicable	
Netherlands Antilles (Bonaire, Curaçao, Saba, St. Eustasius, and St. Martin)	If traveling from an endemic zone and >6 months of age[3]	None	None	Not applicable	Not applicable	
New Caledonia (France)	If traveling from an endemic zone and >1 year of age. Note: In the event of an epidemic threat to the territory, a specific vaccination certificate may be required.	None	None	Not applicable	Not applicable	
New Zealand	Not required	None	None	Not applicable	Not applicable	

| COUNTRY | YELLOW FEVER VACCINE | | AREA OF RISK | MALARIA | |
	COUNTRY REQUIREMENTS[1]	CDC RECOMMENDATIONS[2]		CHLOROQUINE RESISTANCE	RECOMMENDED PROPHYLAXIS
Nicaragua	If traveling from an endemic zone and >1 year of age	None	Risk in rural areas only and in outskirts of Managua	None	Chloroquine
Niger	Required upon arrival from all countries if traveler is >1 year of age	For all travelers >9 months of age	All	Confirmed	Atovaquone/ proguanil; doxycy- cline; or mefloquine
Nigeria	If traveling from an endemic zone and >1 year of age	For all travelers >9 months of age	All	Confirmed	Atovaquone/ proguanil; doxycy- cline; or mefloquine
Niue (New Zealand)	If traveling from an endemic zone and >1 year of age	None	None	Not applicable	Not applicable
Norfolk Island (Aust)	If traveling from an endemic zone and >1 year of age	None	None	Not applicable	Not applicable
Northern Mariana Islands (U.S.) Includes Saipan, Tinian, and Rota Island	Not required	None	None	Not applicable	Not applicable
Norway	Not required	None	None	Not applicable	Not applicable

| COUNTRY | YELLOW FEVER VACCINE | | MALARIA | | |
	COUNTRY REQUIREMENTS[1]	CDC RECOMMENDATIONS[2]	AREA OF RISK	CHLOROQUINE RESISTANCE	RECOMMENDED PROPHYLAXIS
Oman	If traveling from an endemic zone	None	Limited risk in remote areas of Musandam Province. Risk is very limited; therefore, prophylaxis is not recommended.	Confirmed	None
Pakistan	If traveling from an endemic zone. Not required for infants <6 months of age if the mother's certificate shows she was vaccinated before the child's birth.[3]	None	Risk in all areas (including all cities) at altitudes <2,000 m (6,562 ft)	Confirmed	Atovaquone/ proguanil; doxycycline; or mefloquine
Palau	If traveling from an endemic zone and >1 year of age	None	None	Not applicable	Not applicable
Panama	Not required.	For all travelers >9 months of age traveling to the provinces of Darien, Kunayala (San Blas) and Panama (see map), excluding the Canal Zone	Risk exists in rural areas of Bocas Del Toro, Darién, and San Blas provinces. No risk in Panama City or in the former Canal Zone.	Confirmed in Darién and San Blas provinces, including San Blas Islands	Chloroquine in Bocas Del Toro; Atovaquone/ proguanil; doxycycline; or mefloquine in Darién and San Blas
Papua New Guinea	If traveling from an endemic zone and >1 year of age	None	Risk throughout <1800 m	Confirmed	Atovaquone/ proguanil; doxycycline; or mefloquine

| COUNTRY | YELLOW FEVER VACCINE | | AREA OF RISK | MALARIA | |
	COUNTRY REQUIREMENTS[1]	CDC RECOMMENDATIONS[2]		CHLOROQUINE RESISTANCE	RECOMMENDED PROPHYLAXIS
Paraguay	If traveling from an endemic zone	For all travelers >9 months of age traveling to the forested areas on the east and west (see map)	Risk in the departments of Alto Paraná, Caaguazú, and Canendiyú	None	Chloroquine
Peru	If traveling from an endemic zone and >6 months of age[3]	For all travelers >9 months of age traveling to areas east of the Andes Mountains (see map). Travelers who are limiting travel to the cities of Cuzco and Machu Picchu do not need vaccination. Peru recommends vaccination for those who intend to visit any jungle areas of the country <2,300 m (<7,546 ft).	Risk in all departments *except:* Arequipa, Moquegua, Puno, and Tacna. Risk in Puerto Maldonado. Travelers who will visit only in Lima and its vicinity, coastal areas south of Lima, or the highland tourist areas (Cuzco, Machu Picchu, and Lake Titicaca) are not at risk and need no prophylaxis.	Confirmed	Atovaquone/ proguanil; doxycycline; or mefloquine

| COUNTRY | YELLOW FEVER VACCINE | | MALARIA | | |
	COUNTRY REQUIREMENTS[1]	CDC RECOMMENDATIONS[2]	AREA OF RISK	CHLOROQUINE RESISTANCE	RECOMMENDED PROPHYLAXIS
Philippines	If traveling from an endemic zone and >1 year of age	None	Risk exists in areas below 600 m, except no risk in the provinces of Aklan, Bilaran, Bohol, Camiguin, Capiz, Catanduanes, Cebu, Guimaras, Iloilo, Leyte, Masbate, northern Samar, Sequijor and metropolitan Manila. No risk is considered to exist in urban areas.	Confirmed on islands of Basilan, Luzon, Mindanao, Mindoro, Palawan, and Sulu Archipelago	Atovaquone/ proguanil; doxycycline; or mefloquine on islands of Basilan, Luzon, Mindanao, Mindoro, Palawan, and Sulu Archipelago. All other areas chloroquine.
Pitcairn Islands (U.K.)	If traveling from an endemic zone and >1 year of age	None	None	Not applicable	Not applicable
Poland	Not required	None	None	Not applicable	Not applicable
Portugal	Required only for travelers >1 year of age arriving from an endemic zone and destined for the Azores and Madeira. However, no certificate is required for travelers in transit at Funchal, Santa Maria, and Porto Santo.	None	None	Not applicable	Not applicable
Puerto Rico (U.S.)	Not required	None	None	Not applicable	Not applicable

| COUNTRY | YELLOW FEVER VACCINE | | MALARIA | | |
	COUNTRY REQUIREMENTS[1]	CDC RECOMMENDATIONS[2]	AREA OF RISK	CHLOROQUINE RESISTANCE	RECOMMENDED PROPHYLAXIS
Qatar	Not required	None	None	Not applicable	Not applicable
Réunion (France)	If traveling from an endemic zone and >1 year of age	None	None	Not applicable	Not applicable
Romania	Not required	None	None	Not applicable	Not applicable
Russia	Not required	None	None	Not applicable	Not applicable
Rwanda	Required upon arrival from all countries if traveler is >1 year of age	For all travelers >9 months of age	All	Confirmed	Atovaquone/ proguanil; doxycy- cline; or mefloquine
Saint Helena (U.K.)	If traveling from an endemic zone and >1 year of age	None	None	Not applicable	Not applicable
Saint Kitts (Saint Christopher) and Nevis (U.K.)	If traveling from an endemic zone and >1 year of age	None	None	Not applicable	Not applicable
Saint Lucia	If traveling from an endemic zone and >1 year of age	None	None	Not applicable	Not applicable

| | YELLOW FEVER VACCINE | | | MALARIA | |
COUNTRY	COUNTRY REQUIREMENTS[1]	CDC RECOMMENDATIONS[2]	AREA OF RISK	CHLOROQUINE RESISTANCE	RECOMMENDED PROPHYLAXIS
Saint Pierre and Miquelon (France)	Not required	None	None	Not applicable	Not applicable
Saint Vincent and the Grenadines	If traveling from an endemic zone and >1 year of age	None	None	Not applicable	Not applicable
Samoa (formerly Western Samoa)	If traveling from an endemic zone and >1 year of age	None	None	Not applicable	Not applicable
Samoa, American (U.S.)	Not required	None	None	Not applicable	Not applicable
San Marino	Not required	None	None	Not applicable	Not applicable
São Tomé and Príncipe	Required upon arrival from all countries if traveler is >1 year of age	For all travelers >9 months of age	All	Confirmed	Atovaquone/proguanil; doxycycline; or mefloquine
Saudi Arabia	If traveling from an endemic zone	None	Risk in Al Bahah, Al Madinah, Asir, Jizan, Makkah, Najran, and Tabuk province. No risk in urban areas of Jeddah, Mecca, Medina, and Ta'if.	Confirmed	Atovaquone/proguanil; doxycycline; or mefloquine

| COUNTRY | YELLOW FEVER VACCINE | | MALARIA | | |
	COUNTRY REQUIREMENTS[1]	CDC RECOMMENDATIONS[2]	AREA OF RISK	CHLOROQUINE RESISTANCE	RECOMMENDED PROPHYLAXIS
Senegal	If traveling from an endemic zone	For all travelers >9 months of age	All	Confirmed	Atovaquone/ proguanil; doxycycline; or mefloquine
Serbia and Montenegro	Not required	None	None	Not applicable	Not applicable
Seychelles	If traveling from an endemic zone and >1 year of age	None	None	Not applicable	Not applicable
Sierra Leone	If traveling from an endemic zone	For all travelers >9 months of age	All	Confirmed	Atovaquone/ proguanil; doxycycline; or mefloquine
Singapore	If traveling from an endemic zone and >1 year of age	None	None	Not applicable	Not applicable
Slovakia	Not required	None	None	Not applicable	Not applicable
Slovenia	Not required	None	None	Not applicable	Not applicable

| COUNTRY | YELLOW FEVER VACCINE | | MALARIA | | |
	COUNTRY REQUIREMENTS[1]	CDC RECOMMENDATIONS[2]	AREA OF RISK	CHLOROQUINE RESISTANCE	RECOMMENDED PROPHYLAXIS
Solomon Islands	If traveling from an endemic zone	None	Risk in all areas except for the southern province of Rennell and Bellona, the eastern province of Temotu, and the outer islands of Tikopia, Anuta, and Fatutaka	Confirmed	Atovaquone/ proguanil; doxycycline; or mefloquine
Somalia	If traveling from an endemic zone	For all travelers >9 months of age	All	Confirmed	Atovaquone/ proguanil; doxycycline; or mefloquine
South Africa	If traveling from an endemic zone and >1 year of age	None	Risk exists in the low altitude areas of the Mpumalanga Province, Northern Province, and northeastern KwaZulu-Natal as far south as the Tugela River. Risk in Kruger National Park.	Confirmed	Atovaquone/ proguanil; doxycycline; or mefloquine
Spain	Not required	None	None	Not applicable	Not applicable
Sri Lanka	If traveling from an endemic zone and >1 year of age	None	Risk in all areas, except no risk in the districts of Colombo, Galle, Kalutara, and Nuwara Eliya	Confirmed	Atovaquone/ proguanil; doxycycline; or mefloquine

COUNTRY	YELLOW FEVER VACCINE		AREA OF RISK	MALARIA	
	COUNTRY REQUIREMENTS[1]	CDC RECOMMENDATIONS[2]		CHLOROQUINE RESISTANCE	RECOMMENDED PROPHYLAXIS
Sudan	If traveling from an endemic zone and >1 year of age. May be required for travelers leaving Sudan.	For all travelers >9 months of age	All	Confirmed	Atovaquone/proguanil; doxycycline; or mefloquine
Suriname	If traveling from an endemic zone	For all travelers >9 months of age	Risk in all areas, except no risk in Paramaribo and coastal districts of Nickerie, Coronie, Saramacca, Wanica, Commewijne, Marowijne north of latitude 5° N	Confirmed	Atovaquone/proguanil; doxycycline; or mefloquine
Swaziland	If traveling from an endemic zone	None	All lowlands	Confirmed	Atovaquone/proguanil; doxycycline; or mefloquine
Sweden	Not required	None	None	Not applicable	Not applicable
Switzerland	Not required	None	None	Not applicable	Not applicable
Syria	If traveling from an endemic zone	None	Risk along the northern border in El Hassaka province	None	Chloroquine
Taiwan	If traveling from an endemic zone	None	None	Not applicable	Not applicable

COUNTRY	YELLOW FEVER VACCINE		MALARIA		
	COUNTRY REQUIREMENTS[1]	CDC RECOMMENDATIONS[2]	AREA OF RISK	CHLOROQUINE RESISTANCE	RECOMMENDED PROPHYLAXIS
Tajikistan	Not required	None	Southern border; some central (Dushanbe), western (GornoBadakhshan), and northern (Leninabad) areas	Confirmed	Atovaquone/proguanil; doxycycline; or mefloquine
Tanzania	If traveling from an endemic zone and >1 year of age	For all travelers >9 months of age. The city of Dar es Salaam has a lower risk of transmission than rural areas.	All areas at altitudes <1,800 m (<5,906 ft)	Confirmed	Atovaquone/proguanil; doxycycline; or mefloquine
Thailand	If traveling from an endemic zone and >1 year of age	None	Limited risk in the areas that border Cambodia, Laos, and Burma (Myanmar). No risk in cities and no risk in major tourist resorts. No risk in Bangkok, Chiang Mai, Chiang Rai, Pattaya, Phuket Island, and Ko Samui.	Confirmed	Atovaquone/proguanil or doxycycline in areas of the Thailand/Burma and Thailand/Cambodia borders. All other areas Atovaquone/proguanil; doxycycline; or mefloquine
Togo	Required upon arrival from all countries if traveler is >1 year of age	For all travelers >9 months of age	All	Confirmed	Atovaquone/proguanil; doxycycline; or mefloquine

| COUNTRY | YELLOW FEVER VACCINE | | MALARIA | | |
	COUNTRY REQUIREMENTS[1]	CDC RECOMMENDATIONS[2]	AREA OF RISK	CHLOROQUINE RESISTANCE	RECOMMENDED PROPHYLAXIS
Tokelau (New Zealand)	Not required	None	None	Not applicable	Not applicable
Tonga	If traveling from an endemic zone and >1 year of age	None	None	Not applicable	Not applicable
Trinidad and Tobago	If traveling from an endemic zone and >1 year of age	For all travelers >9 months of age	None	Not applicable	Not applicable
Tunisia	If traveling from an endemic zone and >1 year of age	None	None	Not applicable	Not applicable
Turkey	Not required	None	Risk in the provinces of Icel, Adana, Osmaniyeh, Hatay, Kahraman Maras, Gaziantep, Kilis, Adryaman, Sanliurfa, Elazig, Diyarbakar, Mardin, Bingol, Mus, Batman, Bitlis, Siirt, Sirnak, Van, Hakkari. No risk on the Incerlik U.S. Air Force base and on typical cruise itineraries.	None	Chloroquine
Turkmenistan	Not required	None	Risk in some villages in the Mary district	None	Chloroquine

| COUNTRY | YELLOW FEVER VACCINE | | MALARIA | | |
	COUNTRY REQUIREMENTS[1]	CDC RECOMMENDATIONS[2]	AREA OF RISK	CHLOROQUINE RESISTANCE	RECOMMENDED PROPHYLAXIS
Turks and Caicos Islands (U.K.)	If traveling from an endemic zone and >1 year of age	None	None	Not applicable	Not applicable
Tuvalu	Not required	None	None	Not applicable	Not applicable
Uganda	If traveling from an endemic zone and >1 year of age	For all travelers >9 months of age	All	Confirmed	Atovaquone/ proguanil; doxycycline; or mefloquine
Ukraine	Not required	None	None	Not applicable	Not applicable
United Arab Emirates	Not required	None	None	Not applicable	Not applicable
United Kingdom (with Channel Islands and Isle of Man)	Not required	None		Not applicable	Not applicable
United States	Not required	None	None	Not applicable	Not applicable
Uruguay	Not required	None	None	Not applicable	Not applicable

| COUNTRY | YELLOW FEVER VACCINE | | MALARIA | | |
	COUNTRY REQUIREMENTS[1]	CDC RECOMMENDATIONS[2]	AREA OF RISK	CHLOROQUINE RESISTANCE	RECOMMENDED PROPHYLAXIS
Uzbekistan	Not required	None	Sporadic cases reported in Uzunskiy, Sariassiskiy and Shurchinskiy districts (Surkhanda-Rinskaya Region)	None	Chloroquine
Vanuatu	Not required	None	All	Confirmed	Atovaquone/ proguanil; doxycycline; or mefloquine
Venezuela	Not required	For all travelers >9 months of age traveling to Venezuela, except the northern coastal area (see map). The cities of Caracas and Valencia are not in the endemic zone.	Risk exists in rural areas of the following states: Apure, Amazonas, Barinas, Bolivar, Sucre, Tachira, and Delta Amacuro. Risk in Angel Falls.	Confirmed	Atovaquone/ proguanil; doxycy-cline; or mefloquine
Vietnam	If traveling from an endemic zone and >1 year of age	None	Rural only, except no risk in the Red River delta and the coastal plain north of the Nha Trang. No risk in Hanoi, Ho Chi Minh City (Saigon), Da Nang, Nha Trang, Qui Nhon, and Haiphong.	Confirmed	Atovaquone/ proguanil; doxycycline; or mefloquine

| COUNTRY | YELLOW FEVER VACCINE | | MALARIA | | |
	COUNTRY REQUIREMENTS[1]	CDC RECOMMENDATIONS[2]	AREA OF RISK	CHLOROQUINE RESISTANCE	RECOMMENDED PROPHYLAXIS
Virgin Islands, British	Not required	None	None	Not applicable	Not applicable
Virgin Islands, U.S.	Not required	None	None	Not applicable	Not applicable
Wake Island, U.S.	Not required	None	None	Not applicable	Not applicable
Western Sahara	Not required	None	Risk is very limited; therefore, prophylaxis is not recommended.	None	None
Yemen	If traveling from an endemic zone and >1 year of age	None	All areas at altitudes <2,000 m (<6,561 ft). No risk in Sana'a.	Confirmed	Atovaquone/ proguanil; doxycycline; or mefloquine
Zambia	Not required	None	All	Confirmed	Atovaquone/ proguanil; doxycycline; or mefloquine
Zimbabwe	If traveling from an endemic zone and >1 year of age	None	All, except no risk in cities of Harare and Bulawayo	Confirmed	Atovaquone/ proguanil; doxycycline; or mefloquine

CHAPTER 6

Non-Infectious Risks During Travel

>>Jet Lag

The term "jet lag" is used to describe the symptoms that result from a difference between the internal clock and the external environment when a traveler crosses several time zones rapidly. Physiologic rhythms that are innately synchronized with the day-night cycle have to be reset to match the new time zone. Although incompletely understood, these rhythms include diurnal variation in body temperature and cortisol secretion. The major known mediator of the internal clock is melatonin, which is secreted by the pineal gland and induces sleepiness. Daylight suppresses melatonin secretion; meals and other factors also influence secretion.

Symptoms of jet lag are temporary and include excessive daytime sleepiness, nighttime insomnia, decreased performance, headache, general malaise, and gastrointestinal symptoms. Individual responses to crossing time zones and ability to adapt to the new time zone vary. Increasing age, crossing more time zones, or traveling eastward generally increase the time required for adaptation. Eastward travel is associated with difficulty in falling asleep at the new bedtime and difficulty arising in the morning, while westward travel is associated with early evening sleepiness and predawn awakening.

A variety of nonpharmacologic therapies have been used to attenuate the symptoms of jet lag. In principle, efforts to adjust light exposure, activity, and meal times to the new schedule as soon as possible after arrival promote more rapid resetting of the internal clock. Outside daylight, even on cloudy days, is more intense than interior lighting. Light masks and light boxes are available for purchase and at some hotels. Persons traveling eastward should seek bright light in the morning, while those traveling westward should seek bright light in the afternoon. In general, the more time spent outdoors in the first several days following travel, the faster the adjustment to the new time zone. The Argonne diet, which alternates high- and low-calorie days before departure, is often cited but has not been formally studied. The main benefit of this diet may be the inclusion of high-protein breakfasts, which increase levels of tyrosine and thus epinephrine and dopamine, promoting alertness, and high-carbohydrate dinners, which increase serotonin and melatonin, promoting evening sleepiness.

Over-the-counter and prescription medications have been used to promote sleep on long trips or at the new bedtime after arrival. Melatonin is available in the United States as an herbal supplement, although it is regulated in Canada and prohibited in some European countries. Since it is not under FDA regulation, rigorous studies of safety or standardization of doses are not available. However, melatonin seems to be safe and well tolerated, and doses of 0.5-5 mg promoted sleep and decreased jet lag in travelers crossing five or more time zones. Five-mg doses promoted more rapid sleep than lower doses; doses >5 mg had no additional benefit. Slow-release forms were not effective. Melatonin should be taken at the target bedtime, beginning 3-4 days before departure if possible. Zolpidem, a prescription nonaddictive sedative, has been shown to promote sleep in a small group of travelers; its effect on the internal clock is not known. Benzodiazepines may have a direct effect on neurons mediating the internal clock, as well as a hypnotic effect. Short-acting drugs in this class, such as temazepam, should be used to minimize oversedation the next day.

Agents that promote alertness, such as caffeine, and prescription medications, such as amphetamines and pemoline, may interfere with normal sleep and often have adverse effects and potential for dependence. One small study suggests that NADH (nicotinamide adenine dinucleotide), available as a nutritional supplement, may improve performance on the first post-arrival day; more data regarding its efficacy and safety are needed.

Bibliography

Reid KJ, Chang AM, Zee PC. Circadian rhythm sleep disorders. Med Clin North Am. 2004;88:631–51.

Herxheimer A. Melatonin for the prevention and treatment of jet lag. Cochrane Database Syst Rev. 2002;4:463–6.

Jamieson AO, Zammit GK, Rosenberg RS, et al. Zolpidem reduces the sleep disturbance of jet lag. Sleep Med. 2001;2:423–30.

Virre ES, Kay GG. Assessing the efficacy of pharmaceuticals and nutraceuticals as countermeasures for jet lag. Proceedings of the 7th Conference of the International Society of Travel Medicine; 2001 May 27–31; Innsbruck, Austria.

–TAMARA FISK

>>Motion Sickness

Motion sickness, a common problem in travelers by automobile, train, air, and particularly sea, usually causes mild to moderate discomfort but in severe cases can be incapacitating. It affects up to half of children traveling in automobiles or airplanes and almost 100% of boat passengers in very rough seas. Motion sickness is more common in women, especially during pregnancy or menstruation, children age 2–12, and in persons who have migraine headaches, but little is known about individual susceptibility. Sensation of head position and movement is generated in the semicircular canals (angular acceleration or rotation) and otolith organs (vertical acceleration) in the inner ears and carried to the central nervous system via cranial nerve VIII. The signs and symptoms of motion sickness occur when sensory information about the body's position in or movement through space is contradictory or contrary to prior experience. Resulting signs and symptoms include dizziness, nausea, vomiting, pallor, and cold sweats.

Travelers who are susceptible to motion sickness can minimize symptoms by choosing seats with the smoothest ride (front seat of a car, forward cars of a train, and the seats over the wings in an airplane), focusing on distant objects rather than trying to read or look at something inside the vehicle, minimizing head movement, and if necessary lying supine.

Medications that may ameliorate symptoms of motion sickness include scopolamine (available in both patch and oral form), oral meclizine, dimenhydrinate, diphenhydramine, and promethazine (Table 6–1). Choice of medication is based on trip duration, underlying medical conditions, and concerns about sedation. Scopolamine patches are appropriate for longer voyages and should be applied 4 hours before departure and changed every 3 days if needed. Oral scopolamine is effective for 6–8 hours and can be used for short journeys or for the interval between application of the patch and onset of effectiveness. Other oral medications are efficacious for several hours and can also be used for shorter journeys. Oral medications should be started 1 hour before departure. All these medications can impair alertness and must be used with caution by persons operating vehicles or heavy machinery. This effect is additive with alcohol and is least severe with scopolamine. In addition, because these drugs all have anticholinergic properties, they should be avoided in travelers with narrow-angle glaucoma, pyloric obstruction, or prostatic hyper-

TABLE 6-1. DOSAGES OF ANTI-MOTION SICKNESS MEDICATIONS

MEDICATION	DOSE	CONTRAINDICATIONS	ADVERSE EFFECTS	COMMENTS
Scopolamine	Patch: change every 72 hours. Apply to hairless area behind ear. Oral: 0.4-0.8 mg every 6-8 hrs	Gastrointestinal or bladder neck obstruction (e.g., prostatic hypertrophy), liver or kidney disease, risk for narrow-angle glaucoma	Dry mouth, bradycardia, blurred vision (especially in hyperopic persons), decreased memory for new information, decreased attention and alertness	Useful for longer journeys. Do not touch eyes after applying patch. Contraindicated in children.
Dimenhydrinate	Adult: 25-50 mg up to 4 times per day. Children: 1.25 mg/kg, up to 25 mg. Can be repeated every 6 hrs	Use with caution in persons with asthma, cardiac arrhythmias, pyloric or bladder neck obstruction, narrow-angle glaucoma.	Drowsiness, thickened respiratory secretions, dry mouth, blurred vision, paradoxical excitation in children	
Diphenhydramine	Adult: 25-50 mg up to 4 times per day. Children: 1 mg/kg, up to 25 mg	As for dimenhydrinate	As for dimenhydrinate	
Promethazine	Adult: 25-50 mg up to 4 times per day	As for dimenhydrinate	As for dimenhydrinate; hypotension, abnormal movements	May be combined with ephedrine to help maintain alertness. Primarily controls nausea. Not recommended for children.
Meclizine	25-50 mg daily	Asthma, narrow-angle glaucoma, bladder neck obstruction	Drowsiness, dry mouth, occasional blurred vision	Not recommended for children.

trophy and should be used with caution in those with asthma and cardio-vascular disease. Side effects include dry mouth, blurred vision (especially for persons with hyperopia), and bradycardia. Promethazine primarily decreases nausea and has been combined with ephedrine (25–50 mg) to decrease sedation. Only dimenhydrinate and diphenhydramine are recommended for use in children. They may cause paradoxical excitation and should not be used in children <2 years of age.

Nonpharmacologic methods for motion sickness may benefit some persons but have not been proven consistently effective. High levels of ginger have been helpful in some persons. Pressure on the P6 acupuncture point of the wrist provides relief of nausea in pregnancy and after chemotherapy, but evidence for efficacy in motion sickness is contradictory.

Bibliography

Parrott AC. Transdermal scopolamine: a review of its effects upon motion sickness, psychological performance, and physiological functioning. Aviat Space Environ Med. 1989;60:1–9.

Schmid R, Schick T, Steffen R, et al. Comparison of seven commonly used agents for prophylaxis of seasickness. J Travel Med. 1994;1:203–6.

Takeda N, Morita M, Horii A, et al. Neural mechanisms of motion sickness. J Med Invest. 2001;48:44–59.

–TAMARA FISK

>>Sunburn

DESCRIPTION

Sunlight, exposed skin, and time are all that are needed for sunburn. Sunlight consists of infrared, visible and ultraviolet light, and ultraviolet light consists of UVA, UVB and UVC rays. The UVA rays cause tanning and wrinkling, while UVB rays cause sunburn, aging, wrinkling, and skin cancer. UVC rays do not cause any health effects because they do not reach the earth's surface. Despite these hazards, sun exposure has benefits. UV radiation helps make vitamin D, a key factor for good calcium absorption. However, travelers should be aware of the risks of overexposure to these harmful UV rays.

OCCURRENCE

Exposure to sunlight is influenced by geography, climate, and time of day and year. Countries near the equator and at higher elevation receive more UV rays. Sunlight exposure is highest during the summer and from 10:00 a.m. to 4:00 p.m. Outdoor activities, whether snow skiing or spending the day at the beach, can increase the chances of getting sunburned. Snow and light-colored sand reflect UV light and increase sunburn risks. In these situations, UV rays may reach exposed skin from above and below. Even on cloudy days UV radiation reaches the earth.

Many drugs increase sensitivity to sunlight and the risk of getting sunburn. Some common ones include thiazides, diuretics, tetracycline, doxycycline, sulfa antibiotics, and nonsteroidal anti-inflammatory drugs, such as ibuprofen.

CLINICAL PRESENTATION

Unlike a thermal burn, sunburn is not immediately apparent. Symptoms usually start about 4 hours after sun exposure, worsen in 24–36 hours, and resolve in 3–5 days. In mild sunburn, the skin becomes red, warm, and tender. More serious burns are painful, and the skin becomes swollen and may blister. When a large area is burned, headache, fever, nausea, and fatigue may develop. The pain from sunburn is worse 6–48 hours after sun exposure. Skin peeling usually begins 3–8 days after exposure. Severe sunburns can be serious in babies, small children, and older adults. Years of overexposure to the sun may lead to premature wrinkling, aging of the skin, age spots, and skin cancer.

In addition to the skin, eyes can get burned from sun exposure. Sunburned eyes become red, dry, painful, and feel gritty. Chronic exposure to sunlight may cause pterygium (tissue growth that leads to blindness), cataracts, and perhaps macular degeneration, a leading cause of blindness.

PREVENTION

Several steps can be taken to reduce the risk for sunburn. Dermatologists recommend using a full-spectrum sunscreen that blocks or absorbs all UV rays. Sunscreen comes in creams, gels, lotions, and wax sticks. While the type of sunscreen is a matter of personal choice, travelers may want to choose a water-resistant product that will not be easily removed by sweating or swimming. Sunscreens should be used regularly, even on cloudy days, because most of the UV rays pass through the clouds. Sunscreens can be applied under makeup. Although some cosmetic products contain sunscreens, their sun protection factor (SPF) is usually not high enough to be very protective.

Effective sunscreens should have an SPF of at least 15. SPF refers to the amount of time that a person will be protected from a burn. An SPF of 15 will allow persons to stay out in the sun 15 times longer than they normally would be able to stay without burning. The SPF rating applies only to UVB radiation. While the SPF number represents the most protection under the best conditions, sunscreen performance is affected by wind, humidity, perspiration, and proper application. Sunscreen should be liberally applied (at least one ounce) at least 20 minutes before going out in the sun. Special attention should be given to covering the ears, scalp, lips, neck, tops of feet, and backs of hands. Sunscreen should be reapplied at least every 2 hours and after every time a person gets out of the water or perspires. Some sunscreens may also lose efficacy when applied with insect repellents, necessitating more frequent application when the two products are used together.

Another effective way to prevent sunburn is by wearing appropriate clothing. Dark clothing with a tight weave is more protective than light-colored, loosely woven clothing. High-SPF clothing has been developed to provide more protection for patients with photosensitive skin or a history of skin cancer. This type of clothing contains colorless compounds, fluorescent brighteners, or specially treated resins that absorb UV and often provides an SPF of 30 or higher. Travelers should also wear wide-brimmed hats and sunglasses with almost 100% UV protection and with side panels to prevent excessive sun exposure to the eyes.

The UV index, which indicates how much ultraviolet light exposure will occur, can be found in the weather section of most large daily newspapers, in some television weather forecasts, and on the Internet. The UV index ranges from 1 (low) to 11 or higher (extremely high). Travelers are advised to take extra precautions to prevent sunburn when the UV index is higher.

TREATMENT

There is no quick cure for minor sunburn. Symptomatic treatment can be initiated with aspirin, acetaminophen, or ibuprofen to relieve pain and headache and reduce fever. (Children and teenagers should generally not be given aspirin because of the danger of Reye syndrome.) Drinking plenty of water helps to replace fluid losses. Cool baths or the gentle application of cool wet cloths on the burned area may also provide some comfort. Travelers with sunburns should avoid further exposure until the burn has resolved. Additional symptomatic relief can be achieved through the application of a topical moisturizing cream, aloe, or 1% hydrocortisone cream. A low-dose (0.5%–1%) hydrocortisone cream can be helpful in reducing the burning sensation and swelling and speeding up healing.

If blistering occurs, lightly bandage or cover the area with gauze to prevent infection. The blisters should not be broken, as this will slow the healing process and increase the risk of infection. When the blisters break and the skin peels, dried fragments may be removed and an antiseptic ointment or hydrocortisone cream may be applied.

Indications for medical attention include severe sunburns (covering >15% of the body), dehydration, high fever, or extreme pain.

Bibliography

Glanz K, Saraiya M. Guidelines for school programs to prevent skin cancer. MMWR Morbid Mortal Wkly Rep [serial on the Internet]. 2002 April [cited 2004 Oct 18];51(RR-4):1-18. Available from: http://www.cdc.gov/mmwr/PDF/rr/rr5104.pdf.

Murphy ME, Montemarano AD, Debboun M, et al. The effect of sunscreen on the efficacy of insect repellent: a clinical trial. J Am Acad Dermatol. 2000;43(2 Pt 1):219–22.

–ALDEN HENDERSON

>>Temperature Extremes

Heat and cold can be directly or indirectly responsible for some illnesses and can contribute to exacerbations of additional medical problems. In addition to the actual temperature, environmental factors such as humidity and wind velocity can also contribute to loss of ability to adequately regulate one's body temperature.

HEAT

People have heat-related illness when their bodies are unable to compensate and properly cool themselves. In such cases, the body temperature rises rapidly. Very high body temperatures may damage the brain or other vital organs. Sweating is the normal physiologic mechanisms for the dissipation of excess body heat. When the humidity is high, sweat will not evaporate as quickly, preventing the body from releasing heat quickly. The elderly and persons with existing cardiac disease may be more susceptible to the adverse effects of excessive heat. However, young and healthy individuals can also be affected if they participate in strenuous physical activities while traveling in hot conditions.

Heat Exhaustion

Heat exhaustion is a milder form of heat-related illness that can develop after several days of exposure to high temperatures and inadequate or unbalanced replacement of fluids. Symptoms include headache, fatigue, nausea, a rapid pulse, and heavy sweating.

Heatstroke

Heatstroke is the most serious heat-related illness. It occurs when the body becomes unable to control its temperature: the body's temperature rises rapidly, the body loses its ability to sweat, and it is unable to cool down. Body temperatures rise to 106° F or higher within 10–15 minutes. Heat stroke can cause death or permanent disability if emergency treatment is not provided. Symptoms include an extremely high body temperature (above 103° F); red, hot, and dry skin (no sweating); a rapid, strong pulse; headache; dizziness; and nausea.

Prevention

Travelers should be made aware that acclimatization, which may take days, will be required in tropical regions.

When traveling in hot climates, fluid intake should be increased, particularly during vigorous exercise. To avoid dehydration, travelers should be advised not to wait until they are thirsty to drink. During heavy exertion in a hot environment, consumption of two to four glasses (16–32 ounces) of cool fluids each hour should be the goal; liquids that contain caffeine, alcohol, or large amounts of sugar should be avoided, as they can exacerbate dehydration. A sports beverage or salt tablets can replace the salt and minerals lost in sweat, although in most circumstances plain water will suffice.

Travelers in very hot climates should consider limiting activities to morning and evening hours when it is often cooler, resting as often as needed. Protection can be increased by wearing a hat and by making sure to use sunscreen even on cloudy days. During the warmer hours it is preferable to seek activities in air-conditioned facilities.

Treatment

Persons with symptoms suggestive of heat exhaustion should rest, drink cool nonalcoholic beverages, and try to lower their body temperature with a cool shower, bath, or swim. If symptoms do not start to resolve within an hour or if they progress to those of heatstroke, attempts to lower the body temperature should be continued and medical attention should be sought immediately.

COLD

Excessive cold affects persons who are inadequately dressed or who remain outside for extended periods of time in cold climates. Cold particularly affects two groups of people: the elderly, because they have slower metabolisms, and the young, because infants and children lose body heat more easily than do adults and are unable to generate sufficient body heat by shivering.

Hypothermia

Hypothermia usually occurs at very cold temperatures but can occur at cool temperatures if a person becomes chilled from rain, sweat, submersion in cold water, and during cold windy conditions. The warning signs of hypothermia include shivering, confusion, memory loss, drowsiness, exhaustion, fumbling hands, and slurred speech. If the body temperature of someone with these signs is <95° F, medical attention should be sought immediately.

Frostbite

Frostbite occurs under very cold conditions when tissues actually freeze, meaning that ice crystals form within the cells, causing them to rupture. Frostbitten skin appears white or grayish-yellow and becomes unusually firm or waxy and numb. Frostbite most often affects the nose, ears, cheeks, chin, fingers, and toes.

Prevention

To prevent hypothermia and frostbite, travelers should dress warmly in layers with a hat, scarf, mittens, sweater, and coats. The outer layer of clothing should be tightly woven, preferably wind and water resistant, to reduce body-heat loss caused by wind. Wool, silk, or polypropylene inner layers of clothing will retain more body heat than cotton. Excess perspiration will increase heat loss, so extra layers of clothing can be removed when becoming too warm. Travelers should also wear water-proof shoes to avoid wet cold feet. In cold conditions, drinking warm beverages and avoiding alcohol will also help maintain an appropriate body temperature.

Treatment

First aid for these cold-related conditions includes getting the person warm. Persons with symptoms suggestive of hypothermia or frostbite should seek emergency medical attention.

Bibliography

Biem J, Koehncke N, Classen D, Dosman J. Out of the cold: management of hypothermia and frostbite. CMAJ. 2003;168:305–11.

Bouchama A, Knochel JP. Heat stroke. N Engl J Med. 2002;346:1978–88.

Murphy JV, Banwell PE, Roberts AH, McGrouther DA. Frostbite: pathogenesis and treatment. J Trauma. 2000;48(1):171–8.

Naughton MP, Henderson A, Mirabelli MC, et al. Heat-related mortality during the 1999 heat wave in Chicago. Am J Prev Med 2002;22:221–7.

–PAUL ARGUIN AND PHYLLIS KOZARSKY

>>Altitude Illness

Travelers whose itineraries will take them above an altitude of 1,829–2,438 m (6,000–8,000 ft) should be aware of the risk of altitude illness. Travelers are exposed to higher altitudes in a number of ways: by flying into a high-altitude city, by driving to a high-altitude destination, or by hiking or climbing in high mountains. Examples of high-altitude cities with airports are Cuzco, Peru (3,000 m; 11,000 ft); La Paz, Bolivia (3,444 m; 11,300 ft); and Lhasa, Tibet (3,749 m; 12,500 ft).

Travelers vary considerably in their susceptibility to altitude illness, and no screening tests are available to predict someone's risk for altitude illness. Susceptibility to altitude illness appears to be inherent in some way and is not affected by training or physical fitness. How a traveler has responded in the past to exposure to high altitude is the most reliable guide for future trips but is not infallible.

Travelers with underlying medical conditions, such as congestive heart failure, myocardial ischemia (angina), sickle cell disease, or any form of pulmonary insufficiency, should be advised to consult a doctor familiar with high-altitude illness before undertaking such travel. The risk of new ischemic heart disease in previously healthy travelers does not appear to be increased at high altitudes.

Most people do not have visual problems at high altitude. However, at very high altitudes some persons who had incisional radial keratotomy (a procedure widely performed from the late 1970s to the early 1990s) may develop acute farsightedness. The laser surgery for vision correction that replaced radial keratotomy (e.g., Lasik and other procedures) is not associated with visual disturbances at high altitudes.

Altitude illness is the result of traveling to a higher altitude faster than the body can adapt to that new altitude. Fluid leakage from blood vessels appears to be the main cause of symptoms. Altitude illness is divided into three syndromes: acute mountain sickness (AMS), high-altitude cerebral edema (HACE), and high-altitude pulmonary edema (HAPE). AMS is the most common form of altitude illness and, while it can occur at altitudes as low as 1,219–1,829 m (4,000–6,000 ft), most often it occurs in abrupt ascents to >2,743 meters (>9,000 ft). The symptoms resemble those of an alcohol hangover: headache, fatigue, loss of appetite, nausea, and, occasionally, vomiting. The onset of AMS is delayed, usually beginning 6–12 hours after arrival at a higher altitude, but occasionally ≥24 hours after ascent.

HACE is considered a severe progression of AMS. In addition to the AMS symptoms, lethargy becomes profound, confusion can manifest, and ataxia will be demonstrated during the tandem gait test. A traveler who fails the tandem gait test has HACE by definition, and immediate descent is mandatory.

HAPE can occur by itself or in conjunction with HACE. The initial symptoms are increased breathlessness with exertion, and eventually increased breathlessness at rest. The diagnosis can usually be made when breathlessness fails to resolve after several minutes of rest. At this point, it is critical to descend to a lower altitude. HAPE can be more rapidly fatal than HACE.

Determining an itinerary that will avoid any occurrence of altitude illness is difficult because of variations in individual susceptibility, as well as in starting points and terrain. The main point of instructing travelers about altitude illness is not to prevent any possibility of altitude illness, but to prevent death from altitude illness. The onset of symptoms and clinical course are sufficiently slow and predictable that there is no reason for someone to die from altitude illness unless trapped by weather or geography in a situation in which descent is impossible. The three rules that travelers should be made aware of to prevent death from altitude illness are:

- Learn the early symptoms of altitude illness and be willing to admit that you have them.
- Never ascend to sleep at a higher altitude when experiencing any of the symptoms of altitude illness, no matter how minor they seem.
- Descend if the symptoms become worse while resting at the same altitude.

Studies have shown that travelers who are on organized group treks to high-altitude locations are more likely to die of altitude illness than travelers who are by themselves. This is most likely the result of group pressure (whether perceived or real) and a fixed itinerary. The most important aspect of preventing severe altitude illness is to refrain from further ascent until all symptoms of altitude illness have disappeared.

Children are as susceptible to altitude illness as adults, and young children who cannot talk can show very nonspecific symptoms, such as loss of appetite and irritability. There are no studies or case reports of harm to a fetus if the mother travels briefly to high altitude during pregnancy. However, most authorities recommend that pregnant women stay below 3,658 m (12,000 ft) if possible.

Three medications have been shown to be useful in the prevention and treatment of altitude illness. Acetazolamide (Diamox) can prevent AMS when taken before ascent and can speed recovery if taken after symptoms have developed. The drug appears to work by acidifying the blood, which causes an increase in respiration and thus aids in acclimatization. An effective dose that minimizes the common side effects of increased urination, along with paresthesias of the fingers and toes, is 125 mg every 12 hours, beginning the day of ascent. However, most clinical trials have been done with higher doses of 250 mg two or three times a day. Allergic reactions to acetazolamide are extremely rare, but the drug is related to sulfonamides and should not be used by sulfa-allergic persons, unless a trial dose is taken in a safe environment before travel.

Dexamethasone has been shown to be effective in the prevention and treatment of AMS and HACE. The drug prevents or improves symptoms, but there is no evidence that it aids acclimatization. Thus, there is a risk of a sudden onset or worsening of symptoms if the traveler stops taking the drug while ascending. It is preferable for the traveler to use acetazolamide to prevent AMS while ascending and to reserve the use of dexamethasone to treat symptoms while trying to descend. The adult dosage is 4 mg every 6 hours.

HAPE is always associated with increased pulmonary artery pressure. Drugs that can selectively lower pulmonary artery pressure have been shown to be of benefit in preventing and treating HAPE. Nifedipine has been shown to prevent and ameliorate HAPE in persons who are particularly susceptible to HAPE. The adult dosage is 10–20 mg every 8 hours. Sildenafil citrate (Viagra) can also selectively lower pulmonary artery pressure, with less effect on systemic blood pressure. Preliminary studies suggest that this class of drug may prove useful in prevention and treatment of HAPE.

Newer medications have recently been tried to help prevent AMS and HAPE. When taken before ascent, gingko biloba, an herbal remedy, was shown to reduce the symptoms of AMS in adults in two small trials. Gingko has not yet been compared with acetazolamide, although a study is planned. Inhaled salmeterol (a beta-adrenergic agonist) was demonstrated to help prevent HAPE in a small group of climbers who had previously shown susceptibility to HAPE. Whether salmeterol will prove beneficial in a more general population remains to be seen. The mechanism of action of salmeterol suggests that it could be of benefit in treating already established HAPE, but there are no studies yet to confirm this. Salmeterol was chosen for prophylactic studies because of a longer duration of action. The less expensive albuterol may also be effective, but no studies utilizing this drug at altitude have been done.

For trekking groups and expeditions going into remote high-altitude areas, where descent to a lower altitude could be problematic, a pressurization bag (the Gamow bag) can prove extremely beneficial. Persons with altitude illness can be zipped into the bag, and a foot pump can increase the pressure inside the bag by 2 lbs. per in^2, mimicking a descent of 1,500–1,800 m (5,000–6,000 ft), depending on the starting altitude. The total packed weight of the bag and pump is approximately 6.5 kg.

For most travelers, the best way to avoid altitude illness is to plan a gradual ascent, with extra rest days at intermediate altitudes. If ascent must be rapid, acetazolamide may be used prophylactically, and dexamethasone and pulmonary artery pressure-lowering drugs, such as nifedipine or sildenafil, may be carried for emergencies.

Bibliography

Hackett PH. High altitude and common medical conditions. In: Hornbein TF, Schoene RB, editors. High altitude: an exploration of human adaptation. New York: Marcel Dekker, Inc.; 2001. p. 839–85.

Hackett PH, Roach RC. High-altitude illness. N Engl J Med. 2001;345:107–14.

Pollard AJ, Murdoch DR. The high altitude medicine handbook. 3rd ed. Abingdon, UK: Radcliffe Medical Press; 2003.

Sartori C, Alleman Y, Duplain H, et al. Salmeterol for the prevention of high-altitude pulmonary edema. N Engl J Med 2002;346:1631–6.

Shlim DR, Houston R. Helicopter rescues and deaths among trekkers in Nepal. JAMA 1989;261:1017–9.

–DAVID SHLIM

>>Swimming and Recreational Water Safety

Deaths due to drowning are estimated at 450,000 per year worldwide. Before departure, travelers should be reminded of some basic principles of water safety to reduce their risk of drowning while swimming or boating. Travelers should be advised never to swim alone or when under the influence of alcohol or drugs. Likewise, no one should ever dive or jump into an unfamiliar body of water without first determining the depth (at least 9 feet for jumping and diving) and the terrain, and whether there are any hidden obstacles. Children should always be supervised when swimming or playing in or around the water. Travelers should try to select swimming sites that have lifeguards. A personal flotation device (life jacket) should always be worn when boating, skiing, or using personal watercraft, regardless of the distance to be traveled, the size of the boat, or swimming ability. Travelers should also be advised to learn cardiopulmonary resuscitation (CPR) and basic first aid to assist others in the event of a drowning or near drowning.

Travelers should be aware of local weather conditions and forecasts. They should be advised to be alert for and heed colored beach warning flags. Strong winds and thunderstorms with lightning strikes are dangerous to swimmers and boaters. Travelers should be reminded that open water usually has limited visibility, and conditions can sometimes change from hour to hour. Winds and currents are often unpredictable, moving rapidly and quickly changing direction. Swimmers and boaters should watch for dangerous waves and signs of rip currents (e.g., water that is discolored and unusually choppy, foamy, or filled with debris). A strong water current can carry even expert swimmers far from shore.

Swimmers caught in a rip current should swim parallel to the shore until free of the current and then swim toward the shore.

Biting and stinging fish, corals, and jellyfish can be hazardous if touched. Larger marine animals are generally harmless and unless deliberately or accidentally threatened, injuries seldom result from aggressive action by the animals. Wounds acquired in the marine environment can be contaminated with bacteria, often contain foreign bodies, and occasionally contain venom. Travelers should be advised to wear protective gloves and footwear and avoid contact with corals and other marine animals.

Bibliography

American Academy of Pediatrics Committee on Injury, Violence, and Poison Prevention. Prevention of drowning in infants, children, and adolescents. Pediatrics. 2003;112:437–9.

Browne ML, Lewis-Michl EL, Stark AD. Watercraft-related drownings among New York State residents, 1988–1994. Public Health Rep. 2003;118:459–63.

Browne ML, Lewis-Michl EL, Stark AD. Unintentional drownings among New York State residents, 1988–1994. Public Health Rep. 2003;118:448–58.

CDC. Nonfatal and fatal drownings in recreational water settings— United States, 2001–2002. MMWR Morbid Mortal Wkly Rep. 2004;53:447–52.

Peden MM, McGee K. The epidemiology of drowning worldwide. Inj Control Saf Promot. 2003;10:195–9.

–PAUL ARGUIN

>>Scuba Diving

Scuba diving presents a variety of unique medical challenges for the traveling diver. Because diving injuries are generally rare, few health-care providers are trained in their diagnosis and treatment. Thus, the recreational diver must be able to recognize the signs of injury and ensure the availability of dive medicine help when needed.

FITNESS TO DIVE

Planning for dive-related travel should consider any changes in health status, recent injuries, or surgery. In general, respiratory disorders, as well as any disorders affecting higher function and consciousness (e.g., diabetes mellitus or asthma) and psychological problems (e.g., anxiety) raise concerns about diving fitness.

DIVING DISORDERS

Ear Barotrauma

Ear barotrauma is the most common injury in divers. On descent, failure to equalize pressure changes within the middle ear space creates a pressure gradient across the eardrum, which can cause bleeding or fluid accumulation in the middle ear and stretching or rupture of the eardrum and the membranes covering the windows of the inner ear. Symptoms can include pain, ringing in the ear, vertigo, a sensation of fullness in the ear and decreased hearing. With small pressure differences, symptoms are usually short lived, but will be exacerbated by continued diving. Larger pressure differences, especially with forceful attempts at clearing, tend to cause greater damage.

A diver who may have sustained ear barotrauma should discontinue diving and seek medical attention.

Decompression Illness

Decompression illness (DCI) is an all-inclusive term that comprises dysbaric injuries, arterial gas embolism (AGE), and decompression sickness (DCS). Because the two diseases are considered to result from separate causes, they are described separately. However, from a clinical and practical standpoint, distinguishing them in the field may be impossible and unnecessary, since the initial treatment is the same for both. DCI can occur even in divers who have carefully followed the standard decompression tables and the principles of safe diving.

Arterial Gas Embolism

Overinflation of the lungs can result as a scuba diver ascends toward the surface without exhaling. During ascent, compressed gas trapped in the lung increases in volume until the expansion exceeds the elastic limit of lung tissue, causing damage and allowing gas bubbles to escape into the spaces around the lung. Air entering the pleural space causes lung collapse or pneumothorax. Air can also enter the mediastinum (space around the heart, trachea and esophagus), causing mediastinal emphysema. Air in the mediastinum frequently tracks under the skin (subcutaneous emphysema) or into the tissue around the larynx, precipitating a change in the voice characteristics. While mediastinal or subcutaneous emphysema usually resolves spontaneously, pneumothorax may require specific treatment to remove the air and reinflate the lung.

Air can also enter the arterial blood, where bubbles distribute into the body tissues, including the heart and brain, where they disrupt circulation. AGE may cause minimal neurologic symptoms or symptoms may be dramatic and require immediate attention. These signs and symptoms include numbness, weakness, tingling, dizziness; visual blurring; chest pain; personality change; bloody froth from mouth or nose; paralysis or seizures; loss of consciousness; or death. In general, any scuba diver who surfaces unconscious or loses consciousness within 10 minutes after surfacing should be assumed to have AGE. Institution of basic life support, including the administration of 100% oxygen, is indicated, followed by rapid evacuation to a hyperbaric treatment facility.

Decompression Sickness
Breathing air under pressure causes inert gas (nitrogen) to diffuse into the body's tissues. This diffusion occurs at different rates in various tissues and continues as long as the partial pressure of inspired gas is greater than the absorbed gas in the tissues. Thus, the amount of inert gas absorbed is dependent on the depth and time spent at depth. As the diver ascends to the surface, this process is reversed as the partial pressure of residual gas exceeds that in the circulatory and respiratory systems. Ascent from a dive can cause supersaturation of inert gas (tissue partial pressure exceeding ambient pressure), allowing dissolved gas to form bubbles in tissues and causing signs and symptoms of decompression sickness. These symptoms include joint aches or pain; numbness, tingling, mottling or marbling of skin; coughing spasms, shortness of breath; itching; unusual fatigue; dizziness, weakness; personality changes; loss of bowel or bladder function; staggering, loss of coordination, tremors; or paralysis; and collapse or unconsciousness.

Serious permanent injury may result from both DCS and AGE.

FLYING AFTER DIVING

There is an increased risk of developing decompression sickness when divers are exposed to altitude too soon following a dive. The cabin pressure of commercial aircraft may be the equivalent of 8,000 ft. Thus, divers should avoid flying or altitude exposure >2,000 ft. for a minimum of 12 hours after surfacing from a single no-decompression dive. After repetitive dives or multiple days of diving, a diver should wait a minimum of 18 hours before ascending to altitude, to reduce the risk of decompression sickness. These recommended preflight surface intervals do not guarantee avoidance of DCS. Longer surface intervals will further reduce DCS risk.

PREVENTION OF DIVING DISORDERS

Recreational divers should dive conservatively and well within the safe limits of their dive tables or computers. Risk factors for DCI are primarily dive depth and bottom time; however, factors such as rapid ascent, repetitive dives, strenuous exercise, dives >60 feet, and altitude exposure soon after a dive also increase risk. Divers should be cautioned to stay well hydrated and rested, dive within the limits of their training, and follow established guidelines for dives unique to the travel destination. Diving is a skill that requires training and certification and should be done with a companion.

TREATMENT OF DIVING DISORDERS

Definitive treatment of DCI begins with early symptom recognition, followed by recompression with hyperbaric oxygen. Supplemental oxygen is considered effective first aid in relieving the signs and symptoms of decompression illness and should be administered as soon as possible. Divers are often dehydrated, either because of incidental causes, immersion, or DCI itself, which can cause a capillary leak. Administration of isotonic glucose-free intravenous fluid is recommended in most cases. Oral rehydration fluids may also be helpful, provided they can be safely administered (i.e., if the diver is conscious). The definitive treatment of DCI is recompression and oxygen administration in a hyperbaric chamber.

The Divers Alert Network (DAN) can be contacted by telephone at (919) 684-2948, ext. 222, or by accessing the website www.diversalertnetwork.org. DAN maintains a 24-hour emergency consultation and evacuation service at (919) 684-8111 or (919) 684-4326. (Collect calls are accepted.) DAN will provide assistance with management of the injured diver, help in deciding if recompression is needed, the location of the closest appropriate recompression facility, and assistance in arranging patient transport.

Bibliography

Bennett PB, Elliott DH. The Physiology and Medicine of Diving, 4th Edition. Saunders, London. 1993.

Moon RE. Treatment of Decompression Illness. In: Diving Medicine, 4th Edition. Bove AA, ed. Saunders, London: 2004. pp. 195–223.

Sheffield PJ, Vann RD. Flying after Recreational Diving Workshop Proceedings. Durham, NC, Divers Alert Network. 2004 ISBN: 0-9673066-4-7.

Thalmann ED. DAN Dive and Travel Medical Guide. Rev. Ed. 2003. Divers Alert Network, Durham, NC.

–DAN NORD

>>Food Poisoning from Marine Toxins

Seafood poisoning occurs after eating contaminated fish or shellfish containing a toxin made by dinoflagellates. These small marine organisms are found throughout the oceans and especially in and near coral reefs. The toxins accumulate in shellfish or are passed up the food chain as smaller fish are eaten by larger fish. Seafood poisonings are divided into those associated with fish and with shellfish.

Symptoms of seafood poisoning vary with the toxin ingested and may be gastrointestinal, neurologic, or allergic. Marine toxins are tasteless, odorless, and not affected by cooking or any food preparation. The risk of seafood poisoning is increasing as we add more seafood in our diet; as the number of toxic algal blooms increase in frequency, intensity, and geographic distribution; and as more people travel to coastal areas and tropical islands.

CIGUATERA FISH POISONING

Description

Ciguatera is a term of Spanish origin that originated in the Caribbean basin to describe the poisoning caused by ingesting a marine snail that the early Spanish settlers called cigua. The term is now used to describe intoxication with a toxin made by a dinoflagellate that can be found in some fish. Large fish become contaminated when they eat reef fish that feed on these small organisms.

Occurrence

Ciguatera is the most commonly reported marine seafood toxin poisoning. About 50,000 to 100,000 people per year who live in or visit tropical and subtropical regions develop ciguatera poisoning. Affected areas lie between and extend slightly beyond the Tropics of Cancer and Capricorn and include the Caribbean Islands, Florida, French Polynesia, American Samoa, Micronesia, Hawaii, and Australia. The following fish have been reported as sources of ciguatera poisoning:

Amberjack	Barracuda	Grouper
Kahala	Parrotfish	Sea Bass
Snapper	Surgeon fish	Ulua

Clinical Presentation

Common symptoms include nausea, vomiting, diarrhea, cramps, excessive sweating, headache, and muscle aches. Sensations of burning or "pins and needles," weakness, itching, and dizziness can occur. Some people experience temperature reversals (hot surfaces feel cold and cold surfaces feel hot), unusual tastes, nightmares, or hallucinations. Rare deaths occur due to hypotension and cardiovascular collapse. Symptoms often occur within 3 hours, but can occur up to a day or more after eating contaminated fish. Neurologic symptoms may begin several days later and continue for months. People who have had a previous ciguatera poisoning develop more severe symptoms with additional exposures.

The diagnosis is based on the clinical signs and symptoms and a history of eating fish known to have ciguatoxin. Laboratory tests have been developed to test for ciguatoxin in fish.

Prevention

Since no country routinely tests for ciguatoxin in locally caught fish, travelers need to be aware of where the problem occurs and which locally caught fish have been associated with the toxin. Ciguatoxins do not affect the taste or smell of the fish, and they are not destroyed by cooking, smoking, or freezing or through any food preparation. Larger fish (>6 lbs) are more likely to have ciguatoxin. Thus, avoiding consumption of very large reef fish is protective, as well as not eating parts of the fish where the toxin is concentrated: the liver, intestines, head, and roe.

Treatment

Treatment of ciguatera poisoning is generally supportive and tailored to symptoms. Arrhythmias, hypotension, and acute neurologic syndromes require emergency treatment.

SCOMBROID

Description

Scombroid poisoning results from eating fish that naturally contain high histidine levels and have not been handled or refrigerated properly. When fish are mishandled, contaminating bacteria are able to chemically convert the histidine to histamine, which may cause what is often referred to a "fish allergy." The poisoning gets its name from the fish most commonly associated with this condition, the family Scombridae. Yellowfin tuna, mackerel, skipjack, and bonito belong to this group. Some nonscombrid fish (e.g., herring, bluefish, sardine, anchovy, amberjack, black marlin, and mahi-mahi) can also cause scombroid poisoning

Occurrence

Scombroid fish poisoning is common and occurs worldwide in the tropics and temperate regions.

Clinical Presentation

A person with scromboid poisoning has flushing of the face and upper body, severe headache, palpitations, abdominal cramping, and diarrhea. Severe itching and partial paralysis may also occur. Symptoms occur within 2 minutes to 2 hours of eating the spoiled fish. This is typically a benign condition and ends in a few hours. The diagnosis is made by the onset of signs and symptoms soon after eating a fish.

Prevention

Fish contaminated with histamine may taste extra sharp, though many of these fish will not have an abnormal odor or taste. Handling fish properly and immediately refrigerating fish after catching will prevent illness. Cooking the fish does not prevent scombroid poisoning.

Treatment

Symptomatic treatment, including the use of antihistamines, can reduce the symptoms.

SHELLFISH POISONING

Description

Shellfish poisonings occur after eating mollusks or crustaceans, such as oysters, clams, cockles, scallops, mussels, crabs, and lobsters, that contain a toxin. These poisonings are rare and are named after the unique symptom the toxins produce: paralytic, neurotoxic, diarrheic, or amnesic. Several small marine plants called dinoflagellates or diatoms produce the toxins responsible for these poisonings. Shellfish either eat or filter these marine animals and concentrate the toxin in their bodies. Symptoms occur when shellfish containing these toxins are ingested.

Occurrence

Contaminated shellfish are usually found along the coast of countries with temperate and tropical marine waters and typically with or shortly after algal blooms ("red tides"), which are favored by warm weather.

Clinical Presentation

Eating shellfish with marine toxins produces a variety of symptoms in a few minutes to several hours. In paralytic shellfish poisoning, symptoms appear 10 to 120 minutes after eating the contaminated shellfish and are usually mild. They begin with a tingling or numbness of the face, arms, and legs, followed by headache, dizziness, nausea, and loss of muscle coordination. In cases of severe poisoning, paralysis and respiratory failure occur, and death may follow in 2–25 hours.

Symptoms of neurotoxic shellfish poisoning occur within a few minutes to a few hours but do not last long. Symptoms include numbness, tingling in the mouth, arms and legs, loss of coordination, stomach upset, and severe muscle aches. Neurotoxic shellfish poisoning is not known to have ever caused any fatalities, and patients normally recover in 2–3 days.

Onset of diarrheic shellfish poisoning usually occurs 30 minutes to 3 hours after eating and includes symptoms such as nausea, vomiting and diarrhea, which resolve within 2–3 days. This disease is not generally life threatening, and patients recover with no long-term sequelae.

Symptoms of amnesic shellfish poisoning occur within 24 hours of eating contaminated shellfish and include nausea, vomiting and diarrhea, headache, disorientation, and possible permanent short-term memory loss. In severe poisoning, seizures, paralysis and death may occur. Persons found to be most susceptible are the elderly and those with kidney problems.

Prevention

Avoidance of eating mollusks locally harvested from areas known to be experiencing red tides is the only method of prevention.

Since these diseases can occur throughout the world, travelers should be aware of local conditions before eating shellfish abroad. Marine shellfish toxins **cannot** be destroyed by cooking or freezing.

Treatment

Treatment for all shellfish poisons is supportive and tailored to symptoms.

Bibliography

CDC. Ciguatera fish poisoning—Texas, 1997. Morbid Mortal Wkly Rep MMWR. 1998;47:692–4.

CDC [homepage on the Internet]. Atlanta: Division of Bacterial and Mycotic Diseases; [updated 2004 Feb 17; cited 2004 Oct 18]. Marine toxins; [about 6 screens]. Available at URL: http://www.cdc.gov/ncidod/dbmd/diseaseinfo/marinetoxins_g.htm.

Hui YH, Kitts D, Stanfield PS, editors. Seafood and environmental toxins. Foodborne disease handbook: Volume 4. 2nd ed. New York: Marcel Dekker; 2001.

U.S. Food & Drug Administration, Center for Food Safety & Applied Nutrition. Foodborne Pathogenic Microorganisms and Natural

Toxins Handbook. Ciguatera. http://vm.cfsan.fda.gov/~mow/chap36.html.

U.S. Food and Drug Administration [homepage on the Internet]. College Park, MD: Center for Food Safety and Applied Nutrition; [updated 2003 Jan 7; cited 2004 Oct 18]. Foodborne pathogenic microorganisms and natural toxins handbook. Ciguatera; [about 3 screens]. Available from: http://vm.cfsan.fda.gov/~mow/chap36.html.

−ALDEN HENDERSON

>>Natural Disasters and Environmental Hazards

NATURAL DISASTERS

Travelers should be aware of the potential for natural phenomena such as hurricanes, tornados, or earthquakes. Natural disasters can contribute to the transmission of some diseases, especially since water supplies and sewage systems may be disrupted. However, transmission cannot take place unless the causative agent is in the environment. Although typhoid can be endemic in developing countries, natural disasters have seldom led to epidemic levels of disease. However, floods have been known to prompt outbreaks of leptospirosis in areas where the organism is found in water sources. (See Chapter 4, *Prevention of Specific Infectious Diseases: Leptospirosis,* for information on how to minimize the risk of infection.)

When water and sewage systems have been disrupted, safe water and food supplies are of great importance in preventing enteric disease transmission. If contamination is suspected, water should be boiled and appropriately disinfected. (See *Risks From Food and Water.*) Travelers who are injured during a natural disaster should have a medical evaluation to determine what additional care may be required for wounds potentially contaminated with feces, soil, or saliva or for wounds that have been exposed to water that may contain parasites or bacteria. Tetanus booster status should always be kept current.

Travelers also should be aware of the risks for injury before, during, and after a natural disaster. In floods, people should avoid driving through swiftly moving water. Travelers should exercise caution during clean-up, particularly when encountering downed power lines, water-affected electrical outlets, interrupted gas lines, and stray or frightened animals. During natural disasters, technological malfunctions may release hazardous materials (e.g., release of toxic chemicals from a point source displaced by strong winds, seismic motion, or rapidly moving water). When arriving at a destination, travelers should be familiar with local risks for seismic, flood-related, landslide-related, and other hazards, as well as evacuation routes and shelters in areas of high risk.

Natural disasters often lead to wide-ranging air pollution in large cities. Uncontrolled forest fires have caused widespread pollution over vast expanses of the world. Natural or manmade disasters resulting in massive structural collapse or dust clouds can cause the release of chemical or biologic contaminants (e.g., asbestos or arthrospores leading to coccidioidomycosis). Health risks associated with these environmental occurrences have not been fully studied. Travelers with chronic pulmonary disease may be more susceptible to adverse effects from these exposures. Breathing and swallowing dust when traveling on unpaved roads or in arid areas can be followed by nausea and malaise. The harmful effects of air pollution are difficult to avoid when visiting some cities; limiting strenuous activity and not smoking can help. Any risk to healthy short-term travelers to such areas is probably small; however, avoidance of dust clouds and areas of heavy dust or haze may be wise. In some very dusty settings, travelers may find it useful to cover the nose and mouth with a handkerchief or disposable surgical mask to reduce the inhalation of larger particles.

ENVIRONMENTAL HAZARDS

Water
Rivers and lakes may be contaminated with organic or inorganic chemical compounds (e.g., heavy metals or other toxins) that can be harmful both to fish and to people who eat the fish or who swim or bathe in the water. Rivers, lakes, and the ocean contaminated with pathogens from human and animal waste may also cause disease in swimmers. Such hazards may not be immediately apparent in a body of water.

Radiation
Travelers should be aware of regions that are known to have been contaminated with radioactive materials, such as the area surrounding the

Chernobyl nuclear power station. In April 1986, this region in Ukraine, about 100 kilometers (62 miles) northwest of Kiev, Ukraine, and 310 km (193 miles) southeast of Minsk, Belarus, had the largest short-term release of radioactive materials into the atmosphere ever recorded. This radiologic contamination primarily affected three republics: Ukraine, Belarus, and Russia. The highest radioactive ground contamination occurred within 30 km (19 miles) of Chernobyl. The level of contamination in any given area is decreasing with time, but it will be many years before levels of radioactivity in some parts of these countries return to those before the event.

Short-term international travelers (those who plan to stay in such regions less than a few months) should not be concerned about residing in areas that are not controlled (marked with signs or fenced). However, long-term travelers are advised that, in some uncontrolled areas, they could receive a radiation dose from the radioactive ground contamination in excess of the international radiologic health standards recommended for the public. Travelers should investigate local conditions before choosing a long-term residence. (For example, ground contamination that exceeds 5 curies per square kilometer [>5 Ci/km^2] of cesium-137 could result in a radiation dose greater than the recommended standards.) Staff of the U.S. embassy should be able to assist in this investigation.

Officials in affected areas attempt to monitor all foodstuffs sold in the public markets for levels of radioactivity. Radioactive concentration limits have been established for various classes of food (e.g., milk, meat, and vegetables). These limits are comparable with standards used by many western nations, including the European Union. Foods with contamination levels in excess of these limits are not allowed to be sold in the markets. Private farmers in affected regions regularly make foods available for sale outside the official market system. These foods are not monitored for radioactivity, and travelers should not eat them. Likewise, travelers are advised not to eat any wild berries, wild mushrooms, or wild game from these regions and to drink only bottled water.

Young children, unborn babies, and nursing infants are potentially at greater risk from exposure to radiation than adults. Pregnant or nursing mothers are advised to acquire food from reliable, well-monitored sources when visiting affected regions.

Travelers should also exercise caution when they encounter objects or equipment that seem to be discarded, misplaced, or abandoned. Lost radioactive sources are still a persisting issue, particularly in countries lacking effective radiation control programs. Such misplaced objects may or may not bear the radioactive symbol. If a questionable object is encountered, appropriate authorities should be notified.

Bibliography

Eisenbud M, Gessel, T. Environmental radioactivity from natural, industrial, and military sources. 4th ed. San Diego, CA: Academic Press; 1997.

Noji EK, editor. The public health consequences of disasters. New York: Oxford University Press; 1996.

Pan American Health Organization. Natural disasters: protecting the public's health [monograph on the Internet]. Washington, DC: PAHO; 2000 [cited 2004 Oct 21]. Available from: http://www.paho.org/English/Ped/SP575/SP575_prelim.pdf.

U.S. Food and Drug Administration. Accidental radioactive contamination of human food and animal feeds: recommendations for state and local agencies [monograph on the Internet]. Rockville, MD: U.S. Food and Drug Administration; 1998 [cited 2004 Oct 21]. Available from: http://www.fda.gov/cdrh/dmqrp/84.html.

Young S, Balluz L, Malilay J. Natural and technologic hazardous material releases during and after natural disasters: a review. Sci Total Environ. 2004;322:3-20.

–JOSEPHINE MALILAY, DAHNA BATTS-OSBORNE, CHARLES W. MILLER, AND ARMIN ANSARI

>>Injuries

Injuries are among the leading causes of death and disability in the world, and they are the leading cause of preventable deaths in travelers. An estimated 5 million people lost their lives from injuries in 2000, for an overall mortality rate of 83.7 per 100,000. More than 90% of these injury deaths occur in lower and middle-income countries. Worldwide, among persons ages 15–44, injuries account for 6 of the 15 leading causes of death.

Injuries can be divided into unintentional and intentional. Examples of the former include road traffic accidents, falls, fires, poisoning, and drowning; examples of the latter are interpersonal and self-inflicted violence. The traditional viewpoint that injuries occur as "accidents" has been challenged over the last decades, as it has been increasingly appreciated that injuries constitute an important public health problem that demands greater research efforts. Risks can be defined, data are being collected, and, more importantly, prevention measures have been implemented that in many cases have had a dramatic effect on the incidence of injuries. Data, however, are lacking in many countries where reporting of injuries is poor. WHO has recently published a document prepared by an international group of scientists who reviewed this subject in depth (see bibliography). Travelers need to understand the increased risk of certain injuries, particularly in developing countries, and have greater awareness of the measures that can be taken to prevent them.

MOTOR VEHICLE AND PEDESTRIAN ACCIDENTS

Worldwide, an estimated 1.2 million people are killed in motor vehicle accidents each year, and as many as 50 million more sustain significant injuries. Within 20 years these figures will increase by an estimated 65%. Road traffic injuries are the leading cause of injury-related deaths worldwide. According to WHO, countries with the highest rates of road traffic injury mortality are Cyprus, India, Kuwait, Qatar, and the United Arab Emirates. Countries in Asia account for more than half of all road traffic deaths in the world. In Thailand, motor vehicle accidents are considered one of the top three public health problems.

Small studies have suggested that traffic accidents are common in foreign tourists for a number of reasons: lack of familiarity with the roads, driving on the opposite side of the road than in one's home country, poor road surfaces without shoulders, unprotected curves and cliffs, and poor visibility due to lack of adequate lighting, both on the road and on the vehicle. Accidents tend to occur more frequently at dusk, whether dawn or evening, in poor weather conditions, at crossroads, while speeding, and while passing other drivers. In many developing areas of the world, building safe highways and an adequate transportation infrastructure has lagged behind other aspects of modernization. As well, a major factor is the mixed vehicle and pedestrian roadways commonly seen in developing countries. The increased lateral mobility associated with the presence of cars, trucks, rickshaws, bicycles, motorbikes, public buses and pedestrians sharing one lane promotes vehicular accidents.

Other variables contribute not only to increased accidents but also to increased injuries such as lack of use of safety measures. For example, a study in Kenya found that only 26% of persons injured in crashes were wearing seat belts. In developing countries more than half of adult motorized two-wheeler drivers do not wear helmets properly (if at all), and child passengers rarely wear helmets. For the traveler, this translates into lack of availability of helmets, but even when helmets are available, into discomfort in acting differently from the local population. The rapid increase in the number of motorcycles (about 10% every year) in Vietnam has contributed to traffic accidents. Almost half of the motorcycle drivers there are unlicensed, and an estimated 75% do not follow any road laws, which are difficult to enforce. A study from Bermuda reported that tourists sustain a much higher rate of motorbike injuries than the local population, with the highest rate in persons age 50–59 (126.7 per 1,000). Loss of vehicular control, unfamiliar equipment, and inexperience with motorized two-wheelers contributed to accidents and injuries, even when traveling at speeds <30 mph. In addition, age ≥65 has been suggested as an independent risk factor for motor vehicle injuries, especially if the driver has a chronic illness or a hearing impairment.

By far the most important risk factor for road traffic injuries is the presence of alcohol in the blood of a driver or a pedestrian who is injured. Studies show that 20%–70% of fatally injured drivers have blood alcohol levels higher than legal limits. As well, travelers may have a more carefree attitude while away from home that predisposes to driving under the influence of alcohol. An alcohol-impaired driver has a 17 times greater risk of being involved in a fatal crash.

OTHER UNINTENTIONAL INJURIES

Falls and burns are important causes of injuries in travelers. Falls from stairs, jumping or climbing accidents, and falls from trees (most frequently coconut and mango) are reported. Burns may occur with vehicular accidents but are more likely due to careless use of small kerosene stoves and candles. When visiting or living in rural destinations, particularly in developing countries, injuries from burns, animals, and older farming equipment used without protection may occur.

Travel by local commercial air carriers in many countries carries a far greater risk than appreciated. Pilots may not be as well trained and mechanical maintenance may not be regulated as well as it is in the United States. A survey of crashes of commercial jets at airports showed that rates in Latin America and Africa were 7 times that in North America. Travel on unscheduled flights and in small aircraft has the highest risk.

Poisoning in travelers can occur in several settings. Persons traveling with children should carry antimalarial medication in child-proof containers; similarly, when planning for housing in developing areas, risks such as exposed wires and lead paint should be considered.

Prevention

Injuries account for a substantial proportion of evacuations of tourists from developing countries. Travelers should consider purchasing special health and evacuation insurance if their destinations include countries where there may not be access to good medical care. In many countries, victims of injuries never reach a hospital, and there is no coordinated ambulance service. CDC recommends that long-term travelers or those who will be using public transportation, bicycles, and motorbikes prepare by taking first-aid courses, bringing first-aid equipment, a communications device, and equipment that will add visibility to themselves and/or their vehicles (e.g., reflecting vest or highly visible, brightly colored clothing and accessories, and portable vehicle lights [high-mounted brake lights are best]). In addition, travelers planning to bicycle should carry their own light-colored helmet. Helmets have significantly reduced the number of injuries and deaths wherever laws have been implemented (e.g., Italy and Malaysia). Protective clothing should be worn when riding on motorbikes. When renting vehicles, travelers should choose those with seat belts and should test the vehicle to be sure that brakes and lights are functional. Bringing child seats is advisable, as they can reduce infant deaths in car crashes by 71% and toddler deaths by 54%. Children <12 years of age should ride in the back seat. Careful consideration to safe public transportation within country destinations requires planning ahead and avoidance of trips using local unscheduled small aircraft, riding in the back of open trucks, and traveling at night.

Recommendations for avoiding other injuries include staying on one of the lower floors of high-rise hotels, choosing lodging that has smoke detectors and a sprinkler system, and checking to see where the fire exits are on one's floor. Overall, the use of common sense and avoiding alcohol excess, which contributes to risky behaviors, can prevent many injuries in travelers.

INTENTIONAL INJURIES

Violence and collective violence (conflicts among nations and groups, terrorism, torture and rape as a consequence of war, kidnappings, and refugee movements resulting in bloodshed) are leading worldwide public health problems and are growing concerns of travelers. The 20th century was one of the most violent periods in history. Of the hundreds of millions who lost their lives because of violence, more than half were civilians. In 2000, about 1.6 million persons lost their lives to violence, and only $\frac{1}{5}$ were casualties of armed conflicts. Rates of violent deaths in low to middle-income countries are more than 3 times those in higher-income countries, although there are great variations within countries, depending on regional demographic differences.

Risk factors that travelers should remain alert to and that should alert travelers to reconsider a particular itinerary are destinations where the government is unstable, even for short periods of time; where recent coups have taken place; where there is marked social inequality; where there have been rapid demographic changes, or where the government is under control by a single group that identifies itself by a particular ethnic background or religious fundamentalism. These same regions usually lack emergency response systems should there be violence.

Homicide and suicide risk may be different for the traveler than at home. Unfamiliarity with a destination, not being vigilant to one's surroundings, and attention-seeking behaviors may increase risk of assault. For longer-term travelers (e.g., missionaries and volunteers), social isolation and substance abuse, particularly in the face of living in areas of poverty and rigid gender roles, may increase the risk of depression and suicide.

Prevention

Education about and greater awareness of regions of the world where political and civil unrest is present are important for all travelers. Remaining vigilant and aware of one's surroundings at all times is essential. The U.S. State Department maintains a website that features a section on Travel and Living Abroad (www.state.gov/travel), which covers issues such as warnings, emergencies, crisis awareness and preparedness, consular information, and special services. The following commercial site also contains useful travel safety advice for international travelers: www.kevincoffee.com/safety_tips_index.htm. Organizations sending people to remote areas of the world or areas of unrest should strongly consider screening measures to try to avoid premature returns because of risk-taking behaviors, substance abuse, or suicide attempts. For travelers, the use of common sense is most important, with moderation in alcohol consumption and avoidance of illegal substances.

SUMMARY

The increasing acceptance of injuries and violence as major public health problems has lead to the development of preventive strategies, particularly for travelers who find themselves in new environments and who may be more likely to be unaware of risks or complacent in exotic surroundings. Despite greater understanding and increased research efforts in this field, much is still unknown in many countries about the extent of injury-related morbidity and mortality. Travel health advisors need to bring greater awareness to other health-care providers and to the public about these risks and especially about preventive measures that have been shown to be effective and simple to implement. The creation of an International Society for Violence and Injury Prevention has been proposed (www.who.int/violence_injury_prevention/isvip/en).

Bibliography

Barss P, Smith G, Baker S, et al. Injury prevention: an international perspective. New York: Oxford University Press; 1998.

Carey MJ, Aitken ME. Motorbike injuries in Bermuda: a risk for tourists. Ann Emerg Med. 1996;28:424–9.

Hargarten SW, Baker TD, Guptill K. Overseas fatalities of United States citizen travelers: an analysis of deaths related to international travel. Ann Emerg Med. 1991;20:622–6.

Hargarten S, Bouc G. Emergency air medical transport of U.S. citizen tourists: 1988 to 1990. Air Med J. 1993;12:398–402.

Krug EG, Dahlberg LL, Mercy JA, et al. World report on violence and health [monograph on the Internet]. Geneva, Switzerland: World Health Organization; 2002 [cited 2004 Oct 18]. Available from: www.who.int/violence_injury_prevention/violence/world_report/en.

Krug EG, Sharma GK, Lozano R. The global burden of injuries. Am J Public Health. 2000;90:523–6.

McInnes RJ, Williamson LM, Morrison A. Unintentional injury during foreign travel: a review. J Travel Med. 2002;9:297–307.

Peden M, McGee K, Sharma G. The injury chart book: a graphical overview of the global burden of injuries. Geneva, Switzerland: World Health Organization; 2002.

Peden M, Scurfield R, Sleet D, et al. World report on road traffic injury prevention [monograph on the Internet]. Geneva, Switzerland: World Health Organization; 2004 [cited 2004 Oct 18]. Available from: www.who.int/world-health-day/2004/infomaterials/world_report/en.

Petridou E, Dessypris N, Skalkidou A, et al. Are traffic injuries disproportionally more common among tourists in Greece? Struggling with incomplete data. Accid Anal Prev. 1999;31:611–5.

–PHYLLIS KOZARSKY AND PAUL ARGUIN

>>Animal-Associated Hazards

Animals in general tend to avoid human beings, but they can attack if they perceive threat, are protecting their young or territory, or are injured or ill. Although attacks by wild animals are more dramatic, attacks by domestic animals are by far more common. Animals cause injury through bites, kicks, blunt trauma, or the use of horns or claws.

Further damage can occur if injuries become secondarily infected, and may result in serious systemic disease. As a general rule, travelers should never try to pet, handle, or feed unfamiliar animals, domestic or wild, particularly in areas of endemic rabies. Young children should be closely supervised while around wild or domestic animals not known to have been properly vaccinated against rabies. All bite wounds should receive prompt attention and cleansing to reduce the risk of infection. (See Rabies section for more information.) CDC also recommends that travelers receive a tetanus booster before departure, if they have not had one within the last 5 to 10 years, in the event of a puncture wound or bite.

Macaques, a type of monkey, pose an additional threat as potential sources of herpes B virus. Herpes B virus is related to the herpes simplex viruses, which cause oral and genital ulcers. Herpes B infection is rare in humans, and all documented cases have resulted from occupational exposures. No case of herpes B infection has been documented in travelers or others exposed to monkeys in the wild. However, travelers to areas where free-ranging macaques exist should be aware of the potential risk. An infected monkey may appear completely healthy, and herpes B infection rates may be high in some populations. Documented routes of infection include animal bites and scratches, exposure to infected tissue or body fluids, cage scratches, and human-to-human spread. Some exposures resulting in human infection were considered trivial at the time they occurred. Disease may start as an influenza-like illness within 1 month after exposure. Neurologic symptoms develop as the virus infects the central nervous system and may lead to ascending paralysis and respiratory failure. If the disease is untreated, the death rate in humans from herpes B infection reaches 80%. Recent guidelines have been published for the prevention of herpes B infection after exposure and for the treatment of established infection. Travelers should never attempt to feed, pet, or otherwise handle any monkeys.

Poisonous snakes are hazards in many locations, although deaths from snakebites are relatively rare. Snakebites occur in areas where dense human populations coexist with dense snake populations (e.g., Southeast Asia, sub-Saharan Africa, and Tropical America). The Australian brown snake; Russell's viper and cobras in southern Asia; carpet vipers in the Middle East; and coral snakes and rattlesnakes in the Americas are particularly dangerous. Most snakebites are the direct result of startling, handling, or harassing snakes. Because snakes tend to be active at night and in warm weather, as a precaution, travelers should wear boots and long pants when walking outdoors at night in areas possibly inhabited by venomous snakes. Attempts to kill snakes are dangerous. The venom of a small or immature snake can be even more concentrated than that of larger ones; therefore, all snakes should be left alone. Fewer than half of all snakebite wounds actually contain venom, but travelers should be advised to seek immediate medical attention any time a bite wound breaks the skin. Immobilization of the affected limb and application of a pressure bandage that does not restrict blood flow are recommended first-aid measures while the victim is moved as quickly as possible to a medical facility. Incision of the bite site and tourniquets that impair blood flow to the affected limb are not recommended. Specific therapy for snakebites is controversial and should be left to the judgment of local emergency medical personnel.

The bites and stings of some arthropods may cause unpleasant reactions. Travelers should be advised to seek medical attention if an insect bite or sting causes redness, swelling, bruising, or persistent pain. Those who have a history of severe allergic reactions to insect bites or stings should also consider carrying an epinephrine autoinjector (EpiPen) in case of recurrence. Many insects can transmit communicable diseases, even without the traveler's being aware of the bite. This is particularly true when camping or staying in rustic accommodations. Travelers to many parts of the world should be advised to use insect repellents containing DEET, protective clothing, and mosquito netting. (See *Protection Against Mosquitoes and Other Arthropods*.) Stings from scorpions can be painful but, with a few exceptions, are seldom dangerous. Stings in infants and children have the highest morbidity and mortality. In general, exposure to scorpion envenomations can be avoided by sleeping under mosquito nets and by shaking clothing and shoes before putting them on.

Bibliography

CDC. Dog-bite-related fatalities—United States, 1995-1996. Morbid Mortal Wkly Rep MMWR. 1997;46:463–7.

CDC. Nonfatal dog bite-related injuries treated in hospital emergency departments—United States, 2001. Morbid Mortal Wkly Rep MMWR. 2003;52:605–10.

Cohen JI, Davenport DS, Sterwart JA, et al; B Virus Working Group. Recommendations for prevention of and therapy for exposure to B virus (Cercopithecine Herpesvirus 1). Clin Infect Dis. 2002;35:1191–203.

Gold BS, Dart RC, Barish RA. Bites of venomous snakes. N Engl J Med. 2002;347:347–56.

Huff JL, Barry PA. B-virus (Cercopithecine herpesvirus 1) infection in humans and macaques: potential for zoonotic disease. Emerg Infect Dis. 2003;9:246–50.

–DEBORAH NICOLLS AND PAUL ARGUIN

CHAPTER 7

Conveyance and Transportation Issues

>>Air Travel

For most healthy persons, air travel may be more cumbersome than in the past but should not pose any specific health risks. However, for travelers with underlying medical problems, conditions in an aircraft can increase the risk of a number of health-related problems. At cruising altitude (approximately 11,500 m, or 37,000 feet), the aircraft cabin pressure is equivalent to the atmospheric pressure at approximately 1,500–2,500 m (5,000–8,000 ft) above sea level. Therefore, within the pressurized cabin, the inspired oxygen pressure is lower than the oxygen pressure at sea level. Most healthy travelers will not notice these changes. However, passengers with cardiopulmonary diseases (especially those who normally require supplemental oxygen), cerebrovascular disease, anemia, and sickle cell disease may suffer from signs or symptoms related to exacerbations of their underlying conditions.

People with chronic illnesses, particularly those whose condition may be unstable, should have a pre-travel examination by a physician to ensure they are fit for travel. Those who require supplemental in-flight oxygen should notify the airline as far in advance as possible, at least 48 hours before departure. Not all airlines provide in-flight supplemental oxygen. Furthermore, some airlines offer oxygen only on certain types of aircraft, or they may limit the number of oxygen-requiring passengers per flight or per day. Travelers should also be aware that they are responsible for arranging their own oxygen supply while on the ground, both at departure and on arrival. Passengers should make arrangements with their oxygen supplier as soon as possible to have a representative meet them at the airport. The National Home Oxygen Patients Association (www.homeoxygen.org) provides a brochure, *Airline Travel with Oxygen,* to assist patients who require supplement oxygen during travel. They also provide a list of specific requirements and prices for individual airlines. The brochure and list are available through the website.

Air in the middle ear and sinuses expands and contracts during ascent and descent to equalize with the cabin air pressure. People with ear, nose, and sinus infections or severe congestion should avoid flying because the obstruction of air flow may cause pain and injury. If flying cannot be postponed or avoided, decongestants and anti-inflammatory agents may help reduce air flow obstruction and discomfort. Abdominal gases also expand during flight, causing abdominal bloating and discomfort. Travelers who are particularly sensitive to these changes should avoid carbonated beverages and foods that can increase gas production. Furthermore, because of the potential damage that may result from gas expansion, patients who have had recent surgery, particularly intra-abdominal or intraocular procedures, should consult with their physicians before arranging air travel.

Aircraft cabin air is typically very dry, usually 10%–20% humidity. It is easy, therefore, to become dehydrated, and small children are especially susceptible. Passengers should try to limit consumption of alcoholic and caffeinated beverages, which can worsen dehydration. Instead, they should drink plenty of water before departure and during the flight. Travelers with underlying reactive airway disease (e.g., asthma) may also notice increased reaction to the dry cabin air. Steroid-dependent asthmatics should consult their physicians about the potential need to increase steroid dosing during travel. Inhalers should be readily available in carry-on baggage to be used in the event of an exacerbation. Finally, some travelers may notice irritation due to dryness of the skin, eyes, and airway passages. Moisturizers, saline eye drops (or rewetting drops for contact lenses), and saline nasal spray can alleviate these symptoms.

Immobility coupled with long flights increases the risk of venous stasis and the formation of blood clots (deep vein thrombosis or DVT) in the legs. Although most people with DVT have mild or no symptoms, severe pulmonary emboli have been reported in passengers up to several days after travel. People at increased risk for DVT include those who have had DVT in the past, have undergone recent surgery (especially abdominal or orthopedic surgery), are pregnant, have a malignancy, or have genetic blood-clotting abnormalities. People with such conditions should consult with a physician before traveling. However, travelers should be aware that DVT can occur in people without known risk factors. Measures to combat stasis include ensuring adequate hydration, wearing compression stockings and loose-fitting clothing, periodically walking through the cabin, and stretching. Occasionally, people who are at higher risk are advised to use an anticoagulant medication, such as aspirin or low molecular-weight heparins.

For the most part, the quality of air in the cabin should not pose a hazard for travelers. Commercial aircraft are equipped with environmental control systems that monitor and control pressurization, air flow, air filtration, and temperature. Older model airplanes provide 100% fresh air in the cabin, while newer models, in an effort to conserve fuel, provide up to 50% recycled air in the cabin. The recycled air passes through filters, typically high-efficiency particulate air (HEPA) filters, similar to those used in hospital respiratory isolation rooms. Moreover, the air in the cabin is recirculated 20–30 times per hour (approximately one cycle every 3 minutes). The recycled air has not been found to adversely affect air quality in the cabin.

IN-FLIGHT DISEASE TRANSMISSION

Concern has been increasing about the possible spread of communicable diseases during air travel. Infections of particular concern include tuberculosis, *Neisseria meningitidis*, measles, influenza, and SARS.

Tuberculosis

Only one investigation has documented transmission of *Mycobacterium tuberculosis* (TB) from a symptomatic passenger to six other passengers who were seated in the same section of a commercial aircraft during a long flight ($\geq$8 hours). These six passengers were identified by conversion to a positive tuberculin skin test; none had evidence of active tuberculosis. The HEPA filters used in newer commercial aircraft (described above) are able to filter out TB bacteria from the recycled air and are used in hospital respiratory isolation rooms to prevent the spread of TB within the hospital setting. Furthermore, the number of air exchanges per hour in airplanes exceeds the number recommended for hospital isolation rooms. The risk of TB transmission on commercial aircraft, therefore, remains low. People known to have infectious TB should travel by private transportation, rather than a commercial carrier, if travel is required. See CDC web site for more information (http://www.cdc.gov/travel/tb_risk.htm).

Neisseria meningitidis

Meningococcal disease has been documented in travelers, particularly those traveling for the Hajj; however, transmission due to exposure while aboard an aircraft has not been documented. Guidelines for the management of airline passengers who have been exposed to meningococcal disease are available at http://www.cdc.gov/travel/menin-guidelines.htm.

Measles

Measles is a highly contagious viral disease. Most cases diagnosed in the United States are imported from countries where measles is still endemic (see *Measles* section). Furthermore, a person infected with measles is contagious from the first onset of vague symptoms (up to 4 days before rash) to approximately 4 days after the development of rash; therefore, the potential for disease transmission during air travel is a concern. Despite this risk, very few cases of measles have been documented as a direct result of in-flight exposure. Travelers should ensure they are immunized if they have not had the disease.

Influenza

Influenza is highly contagious, particularly among people in enclosed spaces. Transmission of infection has been documented aboard an aircraft, with most risk being associated with proximity to source. (See *Influenza* section and http://www.cdc.gov/flu for more information.) Since December 2003, a new strain of avian influenza virus has been shown to cause infection in humans, with limited human-to-human spread. Because influenza viruses are very adept at changing, there is concern that this strain could eventually become a threat and thus affect air travel. See the CDC Avian Flu website for more general information and guidelines (http://www.cdc.gov/flu/avian/index.htm).

SARS

SARS was first identified in Southern China in November 2002 and recognized as a global threat by March 2003. It is caused by a new coronavirus, the SARS-associated coronavirus (http://www.cdc.gov/ncidod/sars/factsheetcc.htm). Despite the clear role of international travel in the spread of SARS during the 2003 outbreak, only one case of in-flight transmission has been confirmed. The CDC SARS web site (http://www.cdc.gov/ncidod/sars/index.htm) has up-to-date information regarding the management of travel-related risk and guidelines for flight crews.

From investigations of disease outbreaks associated with air travel, two main risk factors for the spread of communicable diseases have been identified: flight duration (≥ 8 hours, including ground time) and seating proximity to the source. There is also increased risk of spread when the aircraft ventilation system is off. (In general, the environmental systems are on when the engines are on or when an auxiliary unit is used, such as when the aircraft is on the ground at the gate.) To reduce the spread of disease, standard respiratory and hand hygiene practices should always be encouraged. People with febrile illnesses or other possible communicable diseases should postpone air travel. Furthermore, airline regulations require that passengers be removed from an aircraft within 30 minutes of shutting off the ventilation system.

DISINSECTION

To reduce the international spread of mosquitoes and other vectors, a number of countries require disinsection of all in-bound flights. WHO and the International Civil Aviation Organization (ICAO) specify two approaches for aircraft disinsection: either spray the aircraft cabin with an aerosolized insecticide (usually 2% phenothrin) while passengers are on board, or treat the aircraft's interior surfaces with a residual insecticide while the aircraft is empty. Some countries use a third method, in which aircraft are sprayed with an aerosolized insecticide while passengers are not on board. Although disinsection, when done appropriately, was declared safe by the WHO in 1995, there is still much debate about the safety of the agents and methods used for disinsection. Although passengers and crew members have reported reactions to both the aerosols and residual insecticides, including rashes, respiratory irritation, burning eyes, and tingling and numbness of the lips and fingertips, there are no data to support a cause-and-effect relationship. Guidelines for disinsection are being updated for the revised International Health Regulations. While only a few countries require disinsection for all in-bound flights, many countries reserve the right to increase the use of disinsection in the setting of increased threat of vector or disease spread. An updated list of countries that require disinsection and the types of methods used are available at the U.S. Department of Transportation website: (http://ostpxweb.dot.gov/policy/Safety%20Energy%20Env/disinsection.htm).

Useful Links

International Travel and Health. Travel by Air. International Travel and Health. WHO. Available at: http://www.who.int/ith

Aerospace Medical Association. Useful Tips for Airline Travel. Available at http ://www.asma.org/Publication/Tips_For_Travelers2001.pdf

Transportation Security Administration (TSA) website: http://www.tsa.gov/public/interapp/editorial/editorial_1568.xml

Bibliography

Aerospace Medical Association, Medical Guidelines Task Force. Medical Guidelines for Airline Travel, 2nd edition. Aviation, Space, and Environ Med. 2003;74(5): section II: A1-A20. Also available at http://www.asma.org/Publication/medguid.pdf (accessed 9/14/04)

Amornkul P, Takahashi H, Bogard A, Nakata M, Harpaz R, Effler PV. Low risk of measles transmission after exposure on an international airline flight. J Infect Diseases. 2004;189:81–5.

Ferrari E, Chevallier T, Chapelier A, Baudouy M. Travel as a risk factor for venous thromboembolic disease: a case-control study. Chest 1999;115:440–4.

Kenyon TA, Valway SE, Ihle WW, Onorato IM, Castro KG. Transmission of multidrug-resistant *Mycobacterium tuberculosis* during a long airplane flight. N Engl J Med. 1996;334:933–8.

Moser MR, Bender TR, Margolis HS, Noble GR, Kendal AP, Ritter DG. An outbreak of influenza aboard a commercial airliner. Am.J Epidemiol. 1979;10:1–6.

National Academies. Subcommittee on Aviation. Hearing on the Aircraft Cabin Environment. June 5, 2003. available at: http://www.house.gov/transportation/aviation/06-05-03/06-05-03memo.html (accessed 9/14/04)

Wilder-Smith A, Tai Goh K, Paton N. Experience of Severe Acute Respiratory Syndrome in Singapore: importation of cases, and defense strategies at the airport. J Travel Med. 2003;10:25962.

World Health Organization. (1998). Tuberculosis and Air Travel: Guidelines for Prevention and Control. Available at: http://www.who.int/gtb/publications/aircraft/index.html (Accessed 10/5/04)

World Health Organization (2003). Consensus document on the epidemiology of severe acute respiratory syndrome (SARS) — 17 October 2003. Available at http://www.who.int/csr/sars/en/WHO consensus.pdf. (Accessed 10/6/04)

–PHYLLIS KOZARSKY AND DEBORAH NICOLLS

>>Cruise Ship Travel

BACKGROUND

In 2003, over 8 million passengers embarked from North American ports for cruise travel. Popular destinations for cruises from the United States include the Caribbean, Mexico, Central and South America, Canada, Alaska, and Florida. Worldwide, 10 million passengers travel on cruise ships annually, and more than 70 million cruise ship bed-days are available. The Caribbean and the Mediterranean rank as the most popular destinations for cruises, but cruise itineraries include all continents and areas not easily accessible by other means of travel. Given the broad appeal and relative high value of cruise ship travel, the cruise industry has had overall passenger occupancies at full capacity in recent years. While the industry average for the duration of a cruise is about 7 days, cruise voyages can last from several hours (e.g., gambling cruises) to several months (e.g., around-the-world and semester-at-sea cruises).

Cruise ships and all ocean-sailing vessels engaged in international commerce show flags of registry, which are required for operation in international waters. Ships are most often registered in the United Kingdom, Liberia, Panama, Norway, the Netherlands, the Bahamas, and the United States. Flag registry states provide comprehensive maritime expertise and administrative services; require annual safety inspections before issuance of a passenger vessel certificate; and monitor vessel compliance with international and flag state standards. International Health Regulations stipulate health and sanitation requirements for international conveyances. In the United States, the U.S. Coast Guard enforces maritime safety requirements and CDC has regulatory responsibilities for sanitation and public health on cruise ships.

Today's typical large cruise ship can be considered a gathering place for the global community, where opportunities for interpersonal interactions and sharing common activities and food and beverages are plentiful. The diversity of passengers and crew members on a typical large cruise ship also means diverse background in health and immunization status, medical and public health tendencies and behavior, and potential for disease exposure. Moreover, the cruise ships' rapid movement from one port city to another, where there may be differences in sanitation standards and infectious disease exposure risks, can result in frequent and recurrent introduction of communicable diseases by embarking passengers and crew members. This movement may result in disease spread to other passengers and crew members in a ship's relatively closed and crowded environment, as well as dissemination of those diseases to the home communities of disembarking passengers and crew members.

CDC VESSEL SANITATION PROGRAM (VSP)

In 1975, in response to several large gastrointestinal disease outbreaks on cruise ships, CDC established VSP, a joint cooperative program with the cruise industry to establish and maintain a high level of sanitation and hygiene on cruise ships. VSP encourages the cruise industry to establish and maintain a comprehensive sanitation program and conducts biannual unannounced sanitation inspections on each cruise ship arriving in the United States with an international itinerary and 13 or more passengers. VSP is also actively engaged in the design and construction of new ships as well as retrofitting older ones to enhance facilities and provisions that promote shipboard sanitation and environmental control.

Official shipboard sanitation inspections are conducted in ports in the United States and its territories and cover environmental health and control measures, including 1) water supply, storage, distribution, disinfection, and protection; 2) food-handling practices, including storage, preparation, and service; 3) product temperature control; 4) potential contamination of food, water, and ice; 5) personal hygiene and sanitation practices followed by crew members; 6) general cleanliness, facility repair, and vector control; and 7) training programs in environmental and public health practices. A score of 86 or higher out of 100 at the time of inspection indicates an acceptable level of sanitation. In general, the higher the score, the higher the level of sanitation. VSP could recommend or require that a cruise ship not sail if sanitation deficiencies could pose a public health threat. VSP sanitation scores and reports for specific ships are available at http://www.cdc.gov/nceh/vsp.

CRUISE SHIP MEDICAL FACILITIES

In 2000, the American College of Emergency Physicians (ACEP) Cruise Ship and Maritime Medicine Section published *ACEP Health Care Guidelines on Cruise Ship Medical Facilities*, a consensus report on facilities and staffing needs that are considered appropriate aboard cruise ships within the recognized limitations of the sea environment. These recommendations, found at http://www.acep.org/1,593,0.html, include communicable disease control measures such as isolation rooms, medications for infectious diseases, and emergency and mass casualty preparedness. Large cruise lines that operate in the United States are generally well equipped and staffed. However, cruise travelers should note that these guidelines for large cruise lines may not be followed by smaller ships or those run by independent operators where there may be no medical provisions on board. Cruise ship travelers who have chronic diseases, who require more comprehensive facilities or who may require medical treatment should consult with their health-care providers.

TRANSMISSION OF ILLNESS ON CRUISE SHIPS

Communicable disease occurrences on board cruise ships reflect similar events on shore and may be magnified by increased interpersonal interaction. However, heightened disease surveillance efforts by cruise lines and awareness among cruise ship travelers have yielded the detection of illnesses of potential public health significance that might have otherwise gone unnoticed. Clusters of various communicable diseases—including measles, rubella, varicella, meningococcal meningitis, hepatitis A, Legionnaire's disease, and respiratory and gastrointestinal illnesses—among cruise ship travelers have been reported and investigated. In recent years, influenza and norovirus outbreaks have posed particularly difficult public health challenges for the cruise industry. Information on these and other diseases can be found at http://www.cdc.gov/travel.

The extent of communicable disease control programs and expertise within the cruise industry is highly variable, ranging from less than optimal to a level of sophistication that exceeds CDC recommendations. Cruise ship travelers who suspect that they have become ill with a communicable disease exposure during their cruise travel should contact VSP (for gastrointestinal illness) or one of the CDC Quarantine Stations (other illnesses).

OTHER ILLNESS OR INJURY CONSIDERATIONS FOR CRUISE SHIP TRAVEL

Because of temperature and weather variations, environmental exposure to pollutants and contaminants, changes in diet and physical activities, and generally increased level of stress being away from the comforts of home, the cruise ship traveler may be subject to exacerbation of existing chronic health conditions. A prospective cruise ship traveler with health conditions that might increase his or her potential for injury or illness should consult his or her health-care provider before embarking on a cruise. Special cruises are now available for travelers who have certain medical conditions, including those on dialysis.

PREVENTIVE HEALTH FOR CRUISE SHIP TRAVELERS

Because of multiple ports visited and the resultant exposures, cruise ship travelers often are uncertain what prevention behaviors and immunizations are appropriate for their itineraries. Among cruise ship passengers and crew members, risk of exposure to infectious diseases is difficult to quantify because of the broad spectrum of cruise ship experiences and limited data. In general, prospective cruise ship travelers should 1) ensure that their routinely recommended age- and medical condition-specific immunizations are up to date, particularly influenza vaccine if indicated; 2) follow the prevention and immunization recommendations that apply to each country on the itinerary; 3) pay particular attention to hand hygiene, either with soap and water or by using an alcohol-based hand sanitizer; and 4) consult a travel health specialist who may tailor prevention guidelines and immunizations according to the health status of the cruise ship traveler, duration of travel, countries to be visited, and shore-side activities.

Useful Link

Cruise Line International Association. Cited in http://www.cruising.org. Accessed on October 26, 2004.

Bibliography

American College of Emergency Physicians. Health care guidelines for cruise ship medical facilities. Ann Emerg Med. 1998;31:535.

CDC. Vessel Sanitation Program Operations Manual. [monograph on the Internet]. Atlanta, GA: CDC;2000 [cited 2004 Oct 26]. Available from: http://www.cdc.gov/nceh/vsp/manual/VSP%20Operations%20Manual%202000.pdf.

Koo D, Maloney K, Tauxe R. Epidemiology of diarrheal disease outbreaks on cruise ships, 1986 through 1993. JAMA 1996;275:545–7.

Minooee A, Rickman LS. Infectious diseases on cruise ships. Clin
Infect Dis 1999;29:737–44.

Peake DE, Gray CL, Ludwig, Hill CD. Descriptive epidemiology of
injury and illness among cruise ship passengers. Ann Emerg Med
1999;33:67–72.

–DAVID KIM

>>Death Overseas

IMPORTATION OR EXPORTATION OF HUMAN REMAINS

Federal quarantine regulations (42 CFR 71) govern the importation of
persons, animals, or things that may be infected with a communicable
disease. These regulations place explicit restrictions on the importation of
the uncremated remains of humans who are known or suspected to have
died from one of the following communicable diseases: cholera, diphtheria, infectious tuberculosis, plague, smallpox, yellow fever, viral hemorrhagic fevers (Lassa, Marburg, Ebola, Congo-Crimean, or others not yet
isolated or named) or severe acute respiratory syndrome (SARS). If the
death was suspected to be the result of one of these diseases, permission
to import the remains should be obtained from CDC, Division of Global
Migration and Quarantine (CDC/DGMQ). Granting this permission is
contingent on an assurance that the remains will be handled according to
specified standards, which include a requirement that the remains be
placed in a hermetically sealed casket. In addition, the remains must be
interred in a below-ground grave by a facility licensed to perform these
services in the United States and in accordance with local burial standards. The remains are cleared for entry into the United States by the
CDC Quarantine Officer assigned to the port of arrival, upon review of a
copy of the signed permission from CDC/DGMQ and the death certificate, which has been translated in English and which states the cause of
death. Copies of both documents should therefore accompany the
remains during shipment. The local mortician handling the remains following their importation will be subject to the regulations of the state and
local health authorities for interstate and intrastate shipment and is

requested to submit a letter to CDC/DGMQ certifying the appropriate disposition of the remains according to the terms of the permission.

Federal regulations also provide CDC with the authority to restrict the importation of the remains of persons who died of other communicable diseases. While such restrictions are not generally employed, CDC reserves the right to do so on a case-by-case basis when necessary to prevent the spread of disease. There are no federal restrictions on the importation of cremated human remains or the remains of persons who have died of noncommunicable diseases.

The U.S. Consulate will generally assist family members in making arrangements with local authorities for preparation and transportation of the remains. The authority and responsibilities of a U.S. Consular Officer relating to the return of remains of a deceased U.S. citizen abroad are based on established U.S. laws, treaties, and international practice. Local law and protocols of the foreign country may affect the options available to the family of the deceased.

The United States has no requirements for the exportation of human remains; however, travelers should be advised that the requirements of the country of destination must be met. Travelers should also be advised that information regarding these requirements may be obtained from the appropriate foreign embassy or consulate.

Additional, detailed information on death overseas is available through the U.S. Department of State website at http://travel.state.gov/family/issues_death.html. Information on the return of the remains of a deceased U.S. citizen can also be obtained by calling the Office of American Citizens Services, Department of State, at 202-647-5226. Information on procedures for obtaining permission for importation of the remains of persons who died of communicable disease may be obtained by contacting CDC/DGMQ at 404-498-1600.

Bibliography

CDC. Interim guidance for autopsy and safe handling of human remains of monkeypox patients [monograph on the Internet]. Atlanta, GA: CDC; 2003 [cited 2004 Oct 21]. Available from: http://www.cdc.gov/ncidod/monkeypox/pdf/autopsy.pdf.

U.S. Department of Health and Human Services. Title 42, Part 71. Foreign quarantine [monograph on the Internet]. Washington, DC: Government Printing Office; 2003 [cited 2004 Oct 25]. Available from: http://www.access.gpo.gov/nara/cfr/waisidx_03/42cfr71_03.html.

—RAM KOPPAKA

>>Animal Importation and Reentry

Travelers should be advised that animals, including pets, which are transported internationally should be free of communicable diseases. CDC has jurisdiction over and places restrictions on the importation of dogs, cats, turtles, monkeys, other animals, and animal products capable of causing human disease (see http://www.cdc.gov/ncidod/dq/faq_animal_importation.htm). Pets taken out of the United States are subject upon return to the same regulations as those entering for the first time. The U.S. Department of Agriculture and the U.S. Fish and Wildlife Service also have jurisdiction over animals and should be consulted for additional information.

DOGS

Dogs >3 months of age presented for importation from countries where rabies is known to occur (see Prevention of Specific Infectious Diseases: Rabies, Table 4–14) must be accompanied by a valid rabies vaccination certificate that includes the following information:

- The breed, sex, age, color, markings, and other identifying information.
- A vaccination date at least 30 days before importation (see following).
- The vaccination expiration date. If not shown, the date of vaccination must be within 12 months of date of importation.
- The signature of a licensed veterinarian.

A dog not accompanied by the previously described certificate may be admitted providing the importer completes a confinement agreement. Such a dog must be kept in confinement during transit to the United States, be vaccinated within 4 days of arrival at the destination, and remain in confinement for at least 30 days after the date of vaccination. These requirements apply equally to service animals such as Seeing Eye dogs. A copy of the confinement agreement (CDC 75.37) can be found on the CDC website at http://www.cdc.gov/ncidod/dq/pdf/cdc 7537-05-24-04.pdf.

A dog <3 months of age may be admitted provided the importer completes a confinement agreement (Table 7–1). Such a dog must be kept in confinement during transit and at the U.S. destination until it is vaccinated at 3 months of age and for at least 30 days after vaccination. Routine rabies vaccination of dogs is recommended in the United States and required by most state and local health authorities.

CATS

Although proof of rabies vaccination is not required for importation of cats, routine rabies vaccination of cats is recommended in the United States and required by most state and local health authorities.

RESTRICTED ANIMALS, ANIMAL PRODUCTS AND VECTORS

Certain live animals, hosts, or vectors of human disease, including insects, biological materials, tissues, and other unprocessed animal products may require a CDC permit for importation or transfer within the United States.

Monkeys and Other Nonhuman Primates

Nonhuman primates can transmit a variety of serious diseases to humans. Live monkeys and other nonhuman primates may be imported into the United States only by importers registered with CDC and only for scientific, educational, or exhibition purposes. Monkeys and other nonhuman primates may not be imported for use as pets. Nonhuman primates transported from the United States to other countries may only return to the United States via a registered importer for the approved indications listed above.

Turtles

Turtles can transmit salmonellosis to humans, and because small turtles are often kept as pets, restrictions apply to their importation. An individual may import no more than six live turtles with a carapace (shell) length of <4 inches. Viable turtle eggs may be imported into the

TABLE 7-1. REQUIREMENTS FOR ENTRY OF PET DOGS INTO THE UNITED STATES

SITUATION	REQUIREMENTS FOR ENTRY
Dog is of any age and from a country reporting no rabies (see Table 4–14). The dog has been in the rabies-free country since birth or for the past 6 months.	No rabies vaccination requirement. If the dog appears to be ill upon arrival, examination by a veterinarian may be required. A local veterinarian should be consulted after arrival at final destination in U.S. to ensure local requirements are met.
Dog is >3 months old and is arriving from a country **not** free of rabies.	If the dog appears to be ill upon arrival, examination by a veterinarian may be required. Owner must present a certificate upon arrival showing that the dog was vaccinated against rabies at least 30 days prior to entry into the United States. The certificate must be current (unexpired), signed by a licensed veterinarian and in English or accompanied by a translation. A local veterinarian should be consulted after arrival at final destination in U.S. to ensure local requirements are met.
Dog is >3 months old and is arriving from a country not free of rabies, but no rabies vaccination certificate is presented.	The dog will be released if it appears to be well and after the owner agrees on form CDC 75.37 (Notice to Owners and Importers of Dogs) to confine the dog immediately upon arrival at the final destination and to have it vaccinated against rabies within 4 days. Confinement may be at a place of the owner's choosing, including the home. The dog must then be confined for an additional 30 days following vaccination. Confinement is defined as restriction of the animal to a building or other enclosure, in isolation from other animals and people except for contact necessary for its care. If the dog is allowed out of the enclosure, the owner must muzzle the dog and use a leash. If the dog appears to be ill upon arrival, examination by a veterinarian may be required. A local veterinarian should be consulted after arrival at final destination in U.S. to ensure local requirements are met.
Dog is <3 months old and is arriving from a country not free of rabies.	A vaccination certificate presented for a puppy <3 months old cannot be accepted. The dog will be released if it appears to be well and after the owner agrees on form CDC 75.37 to confine the dog until it is 3 months old, then have it vaccinated and confined for 30 additional days. Confinement is defined as restriction of the animal to a building or other enclosure, in isolation from other animals and people except for contact necessary for its care. If the dog is allowed out of the enclosure, the owner must muzzle the dog and use a leash. A local veterinarian should be consulted after arrival at final destination in the U.S. to ensure local requirements are met.

TABLE 7-1. REQUIREMENTS FOR ENTRY OF PET DOGS INTO THE UNITED STATES-CONT'D

SITUATION	REQUIREMENTS FOR ENTRY
Dog is >3 months old and is arriving from a country not free of rabies. A rabies vaccination certificate is presented showing vaccination <30 days before arrival in the U.S.	The dog will be released if it appears to be well and after the owner agrees on form CDC 75.37 to confine the dog for the balance of the 30 days since vaccination. Confinement is defined as restriction of the animal to a building or other enclosure, in isolation from other animals and people except for contact necessary for its care. If the dog is allowed out of the enclosure, the owner must muzzle the dog and use a leash. A local veterinarian should be consulted after arrival at final destination in the U.S. to ensure local requirements are met.
Dog of any age arriving in Hawaii or Guam from any location worldwide, including the mainland U.S.	Quarantine requirements apply. For further information: In Hawaii: http://www.hawaiiag.org/hdoa/ai_aqs_info.htm or call 808-483-7151 In Guam: http://ns.gov.gu/pets.html or call 671-735-7222

United States if the importation is not for commercial purposes. CDC has no restrictions on the importation of live turtles with a carapace length >4 inches.

African Rodents and Civets

To reduce the risk of introducing monkeypox and the SARS coronavirus, live African rodents and civets and unprocessed African rodent and civet products may not be imported into the United States. CDC may issue permission for an importation of these animals and unprocessed animal products when the importation is for a bona-fide noncommercial scientific or educational purpose. Rodent and civet products that have been processed to render them noninfectious may be imported without permission.

Bats and Other Vectors

Any animal, including snails and insects, known or suspected of being infected with an organism capable of causing disease in humans may require a permit issued by CDC. All live bats require an import permit from the CDC and the U.S. Department of Interior, Fish and Wildlife Services. The applications for a CDC import permit for these animals can be found at http://www.cdc.gov/od/ohs/biosfty/imprtper.htm.

MEASURES AT PORTS OF ENTRY

CDC regulations provide for the examination of admissible animals presented for importation into the United States. Animals with evidence of disease that might be transmissible to humans may be subject to additional disease control measures. For additional information regarding importation of these animals, travelers should be advised to contact CDC, Attention: National Center for Infectious Diseases, Division of Global Migration and Quarantine, Mailstop E03, Atlanta, Georgia 30333 (1-404-498-1670).

Travelers planning to import horses, ruminants, swine, poultry, birds, and dogs used for handling livestock should be advised to contact the U.S. Department of Agriculture Animal Plant Health Inspection Service (1-301-734-8364) or at http://www.aphis.usda.gov/ regarding additional requirements.

Travelers planning to import fish, reptiles, spiders, wild birds, rabbits, bears, wild members of the cat family, or other wild or endangered animals should be advised to contact the U.S. Department of the Interior, Fish and Wildlife Service (1-703-358-1949) or at http://permits.fws.gov/ImportExport/ImportExport.shtml.

Travelers planning to take a companion animal to a foreign country should be advised to meet the entry requirements of the country of destination. To obtain this information, travelers should write or call the country's embassy in Washington, D.C., or the nearest consulate.

Bibliography

CDC. Compendium of animal rabies prevention and control, 2004: National Association of State Public Health Veterinarians, Inc. (NASPHV). MMWR Morbid Mortal Wkly Rep 2004;53(No. RR-9):1–6.

CDC. Human rabies prevention — United States, 1999: recommendations of the Advisory Committee on Immunization Practices (ACIP). MMWR Morbid Mortal Wkly Rep 1999;48(No. RR-1):1–21.

DeMarcus TA, Tipple MA, Ostrowski SR. US policy for disease control among imported nonhuman primates. J Infect Dis. 1999; 179 Suppl 1:S281–2.

Foreign Quarantine Regulations. 42 CFR 71. Available at URL: http://www.access.gpo.gov/nara/cfr/waisidx_03/42cfr71_03.html

Stam F, Romkens TE, Hekker TA, Smulders YM. Turtle-associated human salmonellosis. Clin Infect Dis. 2003;37(11):167–9.

–PAUL ARGUIN

CHAPTER 8

International Travel with Infants and Young Children

>>Traveling Safely with Infants and Children

INTRODUCTION

The number of children who travel or live outside their home countries has increased dramatically. An estimated 1.9 million children travel overseas each year. Health issues related to pediatric international travel are complex, reflecting varied activities, exposures, and age-specific health risks. While some travel health concerns are similar for children and adults, international pediatric travelers have unique problems because of variable immunity and different age-based behavior; for example, a newly mobile toddler will have different health risks than a sexually active adolescent. Furthermore, many travel-related vaccinations and preventive medications used for adults are not licensed or recommended for pediatric use.

Pediatric travelers have also been impacted by trends in the travel industry. The adventure travel industry is growing rapidly, and a large number of programs are now available for young children, adolescents, and their families. Adventure travelers have diverse geographic and environmental exposures. They participate in unconventional activities, ranging from visiting remote villages in developing countries to mountain climbing and rafting. These trips frequently involve more health hazards than traditional tourism or business travel. Travel opportunities for children with chronic medical conditions have also increased, leading to additional health challenges related to host susceptibility.

Although data about the incidence of pediatric illnesses associated with international travel are limited, studies of pediatric travelers have reported serious morbidity and mortality. The most common reported health problems are diarrheal illnesses, malaria, and motor vehicle- and water-related accidents. Children who are visiting family and relatives living in developing countries are at high risk for a variety of travel-related health problems, including malaria, intestinal parasites, and tuberculosis. In addition, travelers visiting friends and relatives are less likely to seek pre-travel preventive care.

Clinicians should obtain a complete assessment of travel-related activities and provide preventive counseling and interventions tailored to specific risks. Adults traveling with young children should be counseled to monitor the children carefully for signs of illness. Irritability may be a response to changes in time zone and environment but may also indicate illness in young children. Excessive or persistent irritability, fevers, or signs of dehydration should be evaluated promptly. Children with chronic diseases or immunocompromising conditions require travel preparations and treatment tailored to their specific underlying condition.

DIARRHEA AND DEHYDRATION

Diarrhea and associated gastrointestinal illness are among the most common travel-related problems affecting children. Young children and infants are at high risk for diarrhea and other food- and waterborne illnesses because of limited pre-existing immunity and behavioral factors such as frequent hand-to-mouth contact. Infants and children with diarrhea can become dehydrated more quickly than adults.

Prevention
Causes of travelers' diarrhea in children are similar to those in adults. (See *Travelers' Diarrhea.*) For young infants, breastfeeding is the best way to prevent foodborne and waterborne illness. Travelers should use only purified water for drinking, preparing ice cubes, brushing teeth, and mixing infant formula and foods. Scrupulous attention should be paid to handwashing and cleaning pacifiers, teething rings, and toys that fall to the floor or are handled by others. When proper handwashing facilities are not available, an alcohol-based hand sanitizer can be used as a disinfecting agent. However, alcohol does not remove organic material; visibly soiled hands should be washed with soap and water before application.

Travelers should ensure that dairy products are pasteurized. Fresh fruits and vegetables must be adequately cooked or washed well and peeled without recontamination. Bringing finger foods or snacks (self-prepared or from home) will reduce the temptation to try potentially risky foods between meals. Meats and fish should be well cooked and eaten just after they have been prepared. Travelers should avoid food from street vendors.

Management of Diarrhea in Infants and Young Children
Adults traveling with children should be counseled about the signs and symptoms of dehydration and the proper use of World Health Organiza-

tion oral rehydration solutions (ORS). Immediate medical attention is required for an infant or young child with diarrhea who has signs of moderate to severe dehydration (Table 8–1), bloody diarrhea, fever >38.5° C (>101.5° F), or persistent vomiting. ORS should be provided to the infant by bottle or spoon while medical attention is being obtained.

Assessment and Treatment of Dehydration

The greatest risk to the infant with diarrhea and vomiting is dehydration. Fever or increased ambient temperature increases fluid losses and speeds dehydration. Parents should be advised that dehydration is best prevented and treated by use of ORS, in addition to the infant's usual food (Table 4–19). Rice and other cereal-based ORS, in which complex carbohydrates are substituted for glucose, are also available and may be more acceptable to young children. Adults traveling with children should be counseled that sports drinks, which are designed to replace water and electrolytes lost through sweat, do not contain the same proportions of electrolytes as the solution recommended by WHO for rehydration during diarrheal illness.

ORS packets are available at stores or pharmacies in almost all developing countries. [See information below regarding ORS availability in the United States.] ORS is prepared by adding one packet to boiled or treated water. Travelers should be advised to check packet instructions carefully to ensure that the salts are added to the correct volume of water. ORS solution should be consumed or discarded within 12 hours if held at room temperature or 24 hours if kept refrigerated. A dehydrated child will drink ORS avidly; travelers should be advised to give it to the child as long as the dehydration persists. An infant or child who vomits the ORS will usually keep it down if it is offered by spoon in frequent small sips.

Children weighing <10 kilograms who have mild to moderate dehydration should be administered 60–120 mL ORS for each diarrheal stool or vomiting episode. Children who weigh ≥10 kg should receive 120–240 mL ORS for each diarrheal stool or vomiting episode. Severe dehydration is a medical emergency that usually requires administration of fluids by IV or intraosseous routes.

Dietary Modification

Breastfed infants should continue nursing on demand. Formula-fed infants should continue their usual formula during rehydration. They

TABLE 8-1. ASSESSMENT OF DEHYDRATION LEVELS IN INFANTS.

SIGNS	SEVERITY		
	MILD	MODERATE	SEVERE
General condition	Thirsty, restless, agitated	Thirsty, restless, irritable	Withdrawn, somnolent, or comatose; rapid deep breathing
Pulse	Normal	Rapid, weak	Rapid, weak
Anterior fontanelle	Normal	Sunken	Very sunken
Eyes	Normal	Sunken	Very sunken
Tears	Present	Absent	Absent
Mucous membranes	Slightly dry	Dry	Dry
Skin turgor	Normal	Decreased	Decreased with tenting
Urine	Normal	Reduced, concentrated	None for several hours
Weight loss	4%–5%	6%–9%	$\geq$10%

should receive a volume that is sufficient to satisfy energy and nutrient requirements. Lactose-free or lactose-reduced formulas are usually unnecessary. Diluting formula may slow resolution of diarrhea and is not recommended. Older infants and children receiving semi-solid or solid foods should continue to receive their usual diet during the illness. Recommended foods include starches, cereals, yogurt, fruits, and vegetables. Foods that are high in simple sugars, such as soft drinks, undiluted apple juice, gelatins, and presweetened cereals, can exacerbate diarrhea by osmotic effects and should be avoided. In addition, foods high in fat may not be tolerated because of their tendency to delay gastric emptying. The practice of withholding food for $\geq$24 hours is inappropriate. Early feeding can decrease changes in intestinal permeability caused by infection, reduce illness duration and improve nutritional outcome. Highly specific diets (e.g., the BRAT [bananas, rice, applesauce, and toast] diet) have been commonly recommended;

however, similar to juice-centered and clear fluid diets, such severely restrictive diets used for prolonged periods of time can result in malnutrition and should be avoided.

ORS packets are available in the United States from Jianas Brothers Packaging Company, 2533 Southwest Boulevard, Kansas City, Missouri 64108, USA (1-816-421-2880). In addition, Cera Products, 8265 I Patuxent Range Road, Jessup, Maryland 20794, USA (1-301-490-4941 or 1-888-Ceralyte; www.ceralyte.com), markets a rice cereal- rather than a glucose-based product, Ceralyte, in several different flavors. ORS packets may also be available at stores that sell outdoor recreation and camping supplies.

Other Measures
Parents should be particularly careful to wash hands well after diaper changes in infants with diarrhea to avoid spreading infection to themselves and other family members.

The use of antimotility agents (e.g., loperamide, lomotil) in children <2 years of age is not recommended. Because overdoses of these types of drugs can be fatal, they should be used with extreme caution in children. Side effects of these drugs in adults include opiate-induced ileus, drowsiness, and nausea. Lomotil has been associated with fatal overdoses and other severe complications, including coma and respiratory depression.

Antibiotics
Few data are available regarding empiric administration of antibiotics for travelers' diarrhea in children. Furthermore, the antimicrobial options for empiric treatment in children are limited. Trimethoprim-sulfamethoxazole (TMP/SMX) was previously used for empiric treatment of travelers' diarrhea in children; however, its effectiveness has been reduced by widespread drug resistance and it is no longer routinely recommended. Fluoroquinolones, which are frequently used for empiric treatment in adults, are not approved for children <18 years of age because of the potential for cartilage injury, although some travel medicine experts report safely using very short-term (1-3 days) ciprofloxacin for TD treatment for some older children. Tetracyclines can cause teeth staining if used in children <8 years of age.

In some studies, azithromycin has been found to be as effective as fluoro-quinolones in treating travelers' diarrhea in adults. In practice, some clinicians prescribe azithromycin either as a single dose or at 10 mg/kg for 3–5 days for empiric treatment. Flavored oral suspension of azithromycin is available. The suspension does not require refrigeration; however, it should be used within 10 days of mixing. The unreconstituted form of azithromycin has a longer expiration period. In certain circumstances, the unreconstituted form can be provided with clear instructions for preparation and may be useful for children traveling for <10 days.

MALARIA

Malaria is one of the most serious, life-threatening diseases affecting pediatric international travelers. In the United States, 5,794 cases of malaria in US civilians were reported to CDC from 1992 through 2000. Of these cases, 976 (17%) occurred in children <18 years of age. Among children with malaria, 343 (35%) were 1 month to 5 years old, 215 (22%) were 6–9 years old, 226 (23%) were 10–14 years old, and 192 (20%) were 15–17 years old. The largest percentage of cases occurred in persons who were visiting family and friends.

Children with malaria can rapidly develop a high level of parasitemia. They are at increased risk of severe complications of malaria, including shock, seizures, coma, and death. Initial symptoms of malaria in children may mimic may other common causes of pediatric febrile illness and therefore may result in delayed diagnosis and treatment. Clinicians should counsel adults traveling in malarious areas with children to be aware of the signs and symptoms of malaria and to seek prompt medical attention if they develop.

Detailed information about malaria risk and chemoprophylaxis, as well as precautions for avoiding mosquito bites, is presented in Chapter 4. Medications used in infants and young children are the same as those recommended for adults except that doxycycline should not be given to children <8 years of age. Aatovaquone/proguanil (Malarone) should not be used for prophylaxis in children weighing <11 kg (24 lbs) because of lack of data on safety and efficacy. Pediatric doses for malaria chemoprophylaxis are provided in Tables 4–9 and 4–10. Pediatric doses of medications used for self-treatment are included in Table 4–11. Pyrimethamine-sulfamethoxazole should not be used.

Because overdose of antimalarial drugs can be fatal, medication should be stored in childproof containers and kept out of the reach of infants and children. Mefloquine and chloroquine phosphate are manufactured in the United States in tablet form. Atovaquone/proguanil is available in pediatric tablet form. Pediatric doses should be calculated carefully according to body weight. Before departure, pharmacists can be asked to pulverize tablets and prepare gelatin capsules with calculated pediatric doses. Chloroquine, mefloquine, and atovaquone/proguanil have a bitter taste. Mixing the powder in food or drink can facilitate the administration of antimalarial drugs to infants and children. Additionally, any compounding pharmacy can alter the flavoring of malaria medication tablets so that they are more willingly ingested by children. A list of compounding pharmacies is available at http://www.iacprx.org/referral_service/index.html. Physicians should calculate the dose and volume to be administered based on body weight because the concentration of chloroquine base varies in different suspensions.

INSECT AND OTHER ARTHROPOD PRECAUTIONS

Personal protection against mosquitoes, ticks, and biting flies is an important part of prevention against malaria, yellow fever, and other diseases for which no other prophylaxis is available, such as dengue fever. While outdoors, children should wear as much protective clothing (long sleeves and long pants) as they can tolerate. They should sleep in rooms with air conditioning or screened windows or under bed nets. Mosquito netting should be used over infant carriers. Clothing and mosquito nets can be treated with the repellent permethrin, which is derived from chrysanthemum flowers. However, permethrin should not be applied to the skin. DEET-containing insect repellents should be applied to exposed areas of skin. Repellent should not be applied to skin under clothing. To avoid accidental ingestion, it should not be applied to children's faces or hands. It can be used sparingly around the ears. Children should not be allowed to apply their own repellent. DEET should not be used on children <2 months of age.

There had been some controversy regarding the recommended concentration of DEET for pediatric use. In 1998, the Environmental Protection Agency conducted an extensive review of DEET safety. The agency concluded that there is no evidence that DEET is toxic to infants and/or children. Additional evaluations have not demonstrated a link between seizures and topical use.

The concentration of DEET affects the duration of protection. Higher concentrations provide longer protection; however, the duration of protection reaches a plateau at approximately 30%–50%. In a laboratory study, a product with 23.8% DEET provided an average of 5 hours of protection (range 3–6 hours) and a product with 6.65% DEET provided an average of 2 hours of protection (range 1.5–2.8 hours). Duration of protection may be affected by the environmental temperature, sweating, wind conditions, and mosquito density. Thus, DEET formulations as high as 50% are recommended for both adults and children >2 months of age.

Other products have been evaluated for repellent activity. However, they have not been as well studied as DEET and may not be safe for use in children. Products containing 7.5% of IR3535, a repellent that has recently become available in the United States, provided approximately 23 minutes of protection. Most botanical products provide relatively limited or no protection.

Products that contain repellents and sunscreen are generally not recommended because of the need to reapply sunscreen more frequently than repellent. Mosquito coils should be used with extreme caution in the presence of children to avoid burns and inadvertent ingestion.

INFECTION AND INFESTATION FROM SOIL CONTACT

Children are more likely than adults to have contact with soil or sand and therefore may be exposed to infectious stages of parasites present in soil, including ascariasis, hookworm, cutaneous larva migrans, trichuriasis, and strongyloidiasis. Children and infants should wear protective footwear and play on a sheet or towel rather than directly on the ground. Clothing should not be dried on the ground. Clothing or diapers dried in the open air should be ironed before use to prevent infestation with fly larvae (myiasis).

ANIMAL BITES AND RABIES

Worldwide, rabies is more common in children than adults. In addition to the potential for increased contact with animals, children are also more likely to be bitten on the head or neck, leading to more severe injuries. They are also less likely to report a bite. Children and their families should be counseled to avoid all stray or unfamiliar animals and to inform parents of any contact or bites. Animal exposure abroad is not limited to rural areas, since stray dogs are common in many urban areas. Children may approach or be unable to avoid animals. Mammal-associated injuries should be washed thoroughly with water and soap (and povidone iodine if available), and the child should be evaluated promptly for the need for rabies postexposure prophylaxis and other measures. (See *Rabies* section for details.)

AIR TRAVEL

Injuries and deaths can occur in children held on adult laps during turbulence and nonfatal crashes. The American Academy of Pediatrics recommends that children should be placed in a rear-facing Federal Aviation Authority (FAA)-approved child-safety seat until they are at least 1 year old and weigh at least 20 pounds. Children >1 year old and 20–40 pounds in body weight should use a forward-facing FAA-approved child safety seat, while children weighing >40 pounds can be secured in the aircraft seat belt. Air travel is safe for healthy newborns and infants; however, children with chronic heart or lung problems or with upper or lower respiratory symptoms at the time of travel may be at risk for hypoxia during flight, and a physician should be consulted before travel.

Ear pain can be very troublesome for infants and children during descent. Equalization of pressure in the middle ear can be facilitated by swallowing or chewing; infants should nurse or suck on a bottle. Older children can try chewing gum. Antihistamines and decongestants have not been shown to have benefit. There is no evidence that air travel exacerbates the symptoms or complications associated with otitis media.

Travel to different time zones, "jet lag," and schedule disruptions can disturb sleep patterns in infants and children, as well as adults. Attempts to adjust sleep schedules 2–3 days before departure may be helpful. After arrival, children should be encouraged to be active outside or in brightly lit areas during daylight hours to promote adjustment. Sedative medications may cause oversedation or paradoxical agitation, and melatonin may have effects on sexual development in infants and children. In general, these medications should be avoided in infants and children. Diphenhydramine can be useful for some children but, similar to any medication for sedation, should be administered as a test dose before travel to determine the effect on the individual child.

MOTION SICKNESS

Motion sickness can present as ataxia, dizziness, and nausea in children. Other symptoms include pallor and cold sweats. For symptomatic treatment of children, dimenhydrinate, 1–1.5 mg/kg per dose or diphenhydramine, 0.5–1 mg/kg per dose, up to 25 mg, can be given 1 hour before travel and every 6 hours during the trip. Because some children have paradoxical agitation with these medicines, a test dose should be given at home before departure. Scopalamine causes potentially dangerous adverse effects in children and should not be used; prochloperazine and metoclopramide are minimally effective in children.

ACCIDENTS

Vehicle-Related

Vehicle-related accidents are the leading cause of death in children who travel. While traveling in automobiles and other vehicles, children weighing <40 pounds should be restrained in age-appropriate car seats or booster seats. These seats often must be carried from home, since availability of well-maintained and approved seats may be limited abroad. In general, children are safest traveling in the rear seat; they should never travel in the bed of a pick-up truck. Families should be counseled that many developing countries have cars without rear seatbelts.

Drowning and Water-Related Illness and Injuries

Drowning is the second leading cause of death in young travelers; close supervision is essential. Appropriate water safety devices such as life vests may not be available abroad, and families should consider bringing these from home. A variety of diarrheal and parasitic illnesses can be transmitted by swallowing even small amounts of fecally contaminated water, and other infections, such as schistosomiasis, result from skin contact with contaminated water. Thus, while in schistosomiasis-endemic areas, children should not swim in fresh, unchlorinated water and should be carefully supervised while being washed in a bathtub. Protective footwear is important to avoid injury in many marine environments.

Other Injuries

Conditions at hotels and other lodging may not be as safe as those in the United States and should be carefully inspected for exposed wiring, pest poisons, paint chips, or inadequate stairway or balcony railings (See *Injuries* section in Chapter 6).

ALTITUDE

Children and infants are more susceptible to acute mountain sickness and the more serious complications of high-altitude cerebral edema and high-altitude pulmonary edema. Young children may present with unexplained fussiness and change in sleep and activity patterns; older children may complain of headache or shortness of breath. Acetazolamide (Diamox) is not approved for use for this indication in children, but it is generally safe for use in children when used for other indications. It is contraindicated in children who are allergic to sulfa medications.

SUN EXPOSURE

Sun exposure and particularly sunburn before age 15 are strongly associated with melanoma and other forms of skin cancer. Exposure to UV light is highest near the equator, at high altitudes, during midday (10 a.m. to 4 p.m.), and where light is reflected off water or snow. Sunscreens (or sun blocks), either physical (titanium or zinc oxides) or chemical, at least SPF 15 and providing protection from both UVA and UVB, should be applied every 2 hours, especially after sweating and water exposure. If both sunscreen and insect repellent are applied separately or as a combined product, the efficacy of the sunscreen is diminished by one third, and covering attire should be worn or time in the sun decreased accordingly. Hats and sunglasses also reduce sun injury to skin and eyes. Babies <6 months of age require extra protection from the sun because of their thinner and more sensitive skin; severe sunburn for this age group is considered a medical emergency. Babies should be kept in the shade and wear clothing that covers the entire body; a minimal amount of sunscreen can be applied to small exposed areas, including the infant's face and hands. However, in general, sunscreens are generally recommended for use in children >6 months of age.

OTHER GENERAL CONSIDERATIONS

Changes in schedule, activities, and environment can be stressful for children. Including them in planning for the trip and bringing along familiar toys or other objects can decrease these stresses. For children with chronic illnesses, decisions regarding timing and itinerary should be made in consultation with a health-care provider(s).

As for any traveler, insurance coverage for illnesses and accidents while abroad should be verified before departure. Consideration should be given to purchasing special travel insurance for airlifting or air ambulance to an area with adequate medical care. In case family members become separated, each infant or child should carry identifying information and contact numbers in their own clothing or pockets. **Because of concerns about illegal transport of children across international borders, if only one parent is traveling with the child he or she may need to carry relevant custody papers or a notarized permission letter from the other parent.** See section on *Seeking Health Care Abroad,* regarding U.S. embassy contact information in case of illness or medical emergency abroad.

PEDIATRIC TRAVEL HEALTH KIT

In addition to the kit recommended for all travelers (Chapter 2), parents should carry safe water and snacks; waterless, alcohol-based hand sanitizer; child-safe hand wipes; ORS packets; diaper rash ointment; and a water- and insect-proof ground sheet for play outside. In addition, many countries may not provide medications and child-care products of the same type and quality as are available at home. As a precaution, travelers with children should consider bringing additional items they might need, such as baby formula and medications specific to the child.

Useful Links

American Academy of Pediatrics. http://www.aap.org

Office of Travel and Tourism. www.tinet.ita.doc.gov

Bibliography

Adachi J, Ericsson C, Jiang Z, et al. Azithromycin found to be comparable to levofloxacin for the treatment of US travelers with acute diarrhea acquired in Mexico. Clin Infect Dis 2003;37:1165–1171.

American Academy of Pediatrics. Restraint use on aircraft. Pediatrics 2001;5:1218–22.

American Academy of Pediatrics. Summer safety tips. http://www.aap.org/advocacy/releases/summertips.htm (accessed May 26, 2004).

Bell JW, Veltri JC, Page BC. Human exposures to N,N-diethyl-m-toluamide insect repellents reported to the American Association of Poison Control Centers 1993-1997. Int J Toxicol 2002;21:341–352.

Boyce J, Pittet D. Guideline for hand hygiene in health-care settings. MMWR Morb Mortal Wkly Rep. 2002;51:1–44.

King C, Glass R, Bresee J, et al. Managing acute gastroenteritis among children. Oral rehydration, maintenance, and nutritional therapy. MMWR Morb Mortal Wkly Rep 2003;52:1–16.

Moraga F, Osorio J, Vargas M. Acute mountain sickness in tourists with children at Lake Chungara (4400 m) in northern Chile. Wilderness Environ Med. 2002;1:31–35.

Pitzinger B, Steffen R, Tschopp A. Incidence and clinical features of travelers' diarrhea in infants and children. Pediatr Infect Dis J. 1991;10:719–723.

Sadé J, Amos A, Fuchs C. Barotrauma vis-à-vis the "chronic otitis media syndrome": two conditions with middle ear gas deficiency. Is secretory otitis media a contraindication to air travel? Ann Otol Rhinol Laryngol 2003;112:230–235.

Weiss M, Frost J. May children with otitis media with effusion safely fly? Clin Pediatr 1987;11:567–568.

—NICHOLAS WEINBERG, MICHELLE WEINBERG, AND SUSAN MALONEY

>>Vaccine Recommendations for Infants and Children

For all children, decisions regarding vaccinations should be made in cooperation with a health-care provider who will review the traveler's medical history and itinerary. Each traveler should be up to date with their routine childhood vaccinations because many of the diseases prevented by these vaccines are rare or nonexistent in the United States but are still common in other parts of the world. The recommended childhood and adolescent immunization schedule is depicted in Table 8–2. Table 8–3 depicts the catch-up schedule for children and adolescents who start their vaccination schedule late or who are >1 month behind. This table also describes the recommended minimal intervals between doses for children who need to be vaccinated on an accelerated schedule, which is sometimes required for international travel. Proof of yellow fever vaccination is required for entry into certain countries (see *Yellow Fever Vaccine Requirements and Information on Malaria Risk and Prophylaxis, by Country*). Recommendations for other vaccines and immunobiologics depend on the traveler's medical history and itinerary and do not alter the schedule for recommended childhood immunizations.

MODIFYING THE IMMUNIZATION SCHEDULE FOR INADEQUATELY IMMUNIZED INFANTS AND YOUNGER CHILDREN BEFORE INTERNATIONAL TRAVEL

Factors influencing recommendations for the age at which a vaccine is administered include the age-specific risks of the disease and its complications, the ability of people of a given age to respond to the vaccine, and the potential interference with the immune response by passively transferred maternal antibody. Vaccines are recommended for the youngest age group at risk for developing the disease whose members are known to develop an adequate antibody response to vaccination.

The routine immunization recommendations and schedules for infants and children in the United States do not provide specific guidelines for infants and young children who will travel internationally before the age when specific vaccines and toxoids are routinely recommended. When

TABLE 8-2. RECOMMENDED CHILDHOOD AND ADOLESCENT IMMUNIZATION SCHEDULE – UNITED STATES, 2005.

Recommended Childhood and Adolescent Immunization Schedule UNITED STATES • 2005

Vaccine ▼ / Age ▶	Birth	1 month	2 months	4 months	6 months	12 months	15 months	18 months	24 months	4–6 years	11–12 years	13–18 years
Hepatitis B[1]	HepB #1	HepB #2			HepB #3						HepB Series	
Diphtheria, Tetanus, Pertussis[2]			DTaP	DTaP	DTaP		DTaP			DTaP	Td	Td
Haemophilus influenzae type b[3]			Hib	Hib	Hib	Hib						
Inactivated Poliovirus			IPV	IPV		IPV				IPV		
Measles, Mumps, Rubella[4]						MMR #1				MMR #2	MMR #2	MMR #2
Varicella[5]						Varicella					Varicella	
Pneumococcal[6]			PCV	PCV	PCV	PCV			PCV	PPV		
Influenza[7]					Influenza (Yearly)					Influenza (Yearly)		
Hepatitis A[8]										Hepatitis A Series		

Vaccines below red line are for selected populations

This schedule indicates the recommended ages for routine administration of currently licensed childhood vaccines, as of December 1, 2004, for children through age 18 years. Any dose not given at the recommended age should be given at any subsequent visit when indicated and feasible.

 Indicates age groups that warrant special effort to administer those vaccines not previously given. Additional vaccines may be licensed and recommended during the year. Licensed combination vaccines may be used whenever any components of the combination are indicated and the vaccine's other components are not contraindicated. Providers should consult the manufacturers' package inserts for detailed recommendations. Clinically significant adverse events that follow immunization should be reported to the Vaccine Adverse Event Reporting System (VAERS). Guidance about how to obtain and complete a VAERS form can be found on the Internet: www.vaers.org or by calling 800-822-7967.

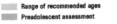 Range of recommended ages   Only if mother HBsAg(−)

Preadolescent assessment   Catch-up immunization

DEPARTMENT OF HEALTH AND HUMAN SERVICES
CENTERS FOR DISEASE CONTROL AND PREVENTION

The Childhood and Adolescent Immunization Schedule is approved by:
Advisory Committee on Immunization Practices www.cdc.gov/nip/acip
American Academy of Pediatrics www.aap.org
American Academy of Family Physicians www.aafp.org

Footnotes
Recommended Childhood and Adolescent Immunization Schedule
UNITED STATES • 2005

1. Hepatitis B (HepB) vaccine. All infants should receive the first dose of hepatitis B vaccine soon after birth and before hospital discharge; the first dose may also be given by age 2 months if the infant's mother is hepatitis B surface antigen (HBsAg) negative. Only monovalent HepB can be used for the birth dose. Monovalent or combination vaccine containing HepB may be used to complete the series. Four doses of vaccine may be administered when a birth dose is given. The second dose should be given at least 4 weeks after the first dose, except for combination vaccines which cannot be administered before age 6 weeks. The third dose should be given at least 16 weeks after the first dose and at least 8 weeks after the second dose. The last dose in the vaccination series (third or fourth dose) should not be administered before age 24 months.

Infants born to HBsAg-positive mothers should receive HepB and 0.5 mL of Hepatitis B Immune Globulin (HBIG) within 12 hours of birth at separate sites. The second dose is recommended at age 1–2 months. The last dose in the immunization series should not be administered before age 24 months. These infants should be tested for HBsAg and antibody to HBsAg (anti-HBs) at age 9–15 months.

Infants born to mothers whose HBsAg status is unknown should receive the first dose of the HepB series within 12 hours of birth. Maternal blood should be drawn as soon as possible to determine the mother's HBsAg status; if the HBsAg test is positive, the infant should receive HBIG as soon as possible (no later than age 1 week). The second dose is recommended at age 1–2 months. The last dose in the immunization series should not be administered before age 24 weeks.

2. Diphtheria and tetanus toxoids and acellular pertussis (DTaP) vaccine. The fourth dose of DTaP may be administered as early as age 12 months, provided 6 months have elapsed since the third dose and the child is unlikely to return at age 15–18 months. The final dose in the series should be given at age ≥4 years. **Tetanus and diphtheria toxoids (Td)** is recommended at age 11–12 years if at least 5 years have elapsed since the last dose of tetanus and diphtheria toxoid-containing vaccine. Subsequent routine Td boosters are recommended every 10 years.

3. Haemophilus influenzae type b (Hib) conjugate vaccine. Three Hib conjugate vaccines are licensed for infant use. If PRP-OMP (PedvaxHIB or ComVax [Merck]) is administered at ages 2 and 4 months, a dose at age 6 months is not required. DTaP/Hib combination products should not be used for primary immunization in infants at ages 2, 4 or 6 months but can be used as boosters following any Hib vaccine. The final dose in the series should be given at age ≥12 months.

4. Measles, mumps, and rubella vaccine (MMR). The second dose of MMR is recommended routinely at age 4–6 years but may be administered during any visit, provided at least 4 weeks have elapsed since the first dose and both doses are administered beginning at or after age 12 months. Those who have not previously received the second dose should complete the schedule by the visit at age 11–12 years.

5. Varicella vaccine. Varicella vaccine is recommended at any visit at or after age 12 months for susceptible children (i.e., those who lack a reliable history of chickenpox). Susceptible persons aged ≥13 years should receive 2 doses, given at least 4 weeks apart.

6. Pneumococcal vaccine. The heptavalent **pneumococcal conjugate vaccine (PCV)** is recommended for all children aged 2–23 months. It is also recommended for certain children aged 24–59 months. The final dose in the series should be given at age ≥12 months. **Pneumococcal polysaccharide vaccine (PPV)** is recommended in addition to PCV for certain high-risk groups. See *MMWR* 2000;49(RR-9):1-35.

7. Influenza vaccine. Influenza vaccine is recommended annually for children aged ≥6 months with certain risk factors (including but not limited to asthma, cardiac disease, sickle cell disease, HIV, and diabetes), healthcare workers, and other persons (including household members) in close contact with persons in groups at high risk (see *MMWR* 2004;53(RR-6):1-40) and can be administered to all others wishing to obtain immunity. In addition, healthy children aged 6–23 months and close contacts of healthy children aged 0–23 months are recommended to receive influenza vaccine, because children in this age group are at substantially increased risk for influenza-related hospitalizations. For healthy persons aged 5–49 years, the intranasally administered live, attenuated influenza vaccine (LAIV) is an acceptable alternative to the intramuscular trivalent inactivated influenza vaccine (TIV). See *MMWR* 2004;53(RR-6):1-40. Children receiving TIV should be administered a dosage appropriate for their age (0.25 mL if 6–35 months or 0.5 mL if ≥3 years). Children aged ≤8 years who are receiving influenza vaccine for the first time should receive 2 doses (separated by at least 4 weeks for TIV and at least 6 weeks for LAIV).

8. Hepatitis A vaccine. Hepatitis A vaccine is recommended for children and adolescents in selected states and regions and for certain high-risk groups; consult your local public health authority. Children and adolescents in these states, regions, and high-risk groups who have not been immunized against hepatitis A can begin the hepatitis A immunization series during any visit. The 2 doses in the series should be administered at least 6 months apart. See *MMWR* 1999;48(RR-12):1-37.

TABLE 8-3. RECOMMENDED CHILDHOOD AND ADOLESCENT IMMUNIZATION SCHEDULE – UNITED STATES, 2005. FOR CHILDREN AND ADOLESCENTS WHO START LATE OR WHO ARE >1 MONTH BEHIND

Recommended Immunization Schedule
for Children and Adolescents Who Start Late or Who Are More Than 1 Month Behind
UNITED STATES • 2005

The tables below give catch-up schedules and minimum intervals between doses for children who have delayed immunizations. There is no need to restart a vaccine series regardless of the time that has elapsed between doses. Use the chart appropriate for the child's age.

CATCH-UP SCHEDULE FOR CHILDREN AGED 4 MONTHS THROUGH 6 YEARS

Vaccine	Minimum Age for Dose 1	Minimum Interval Between Doses			
		Dose 1 to Dose 2	Dose 2 to Dose 3	Dose 3 to Dose 4	Dose 4 to Dose 5
Diphtheria, Tetanus, Pertussis	6 wks	4 weeks	4 weeks	6 months	6 months[1]
Inactivated Poliovirus	6 wks	4 weeks	4 weeks	4 weeks[2]	
Hepatitis B[3]	Birth	4 weeks	8 weeks (and 16 weeks after first dose)		
Measles, Mumps, Rubella	12 mo	4 weeks[4]			
Varicella	12 mo				
Haemophilus influenzae type b[5]	6 wks	4 weeks if first dose given at age <12 months / 8 weeks (as final dose) if first dose given at age 12-14 months / No further doses needed if first dose given at age ≥15 months	4 weeks[6] if current age <12 months / 8 weeks (as final dose)[6] if current age ≥12 months and second dose given at age <15 months / No further doses needed if previous dose given at age ≥15 mo	8 weeks (as final dose) This dose only necessary for children aged 12 months–5 years who received 3 doses before age 12 months	
Pneumococcal[7]	6 wks	4 weeks if first dose given at age <12 months and current age <24 months / 8 weeks (as final dose) if first dose given at age ≥12 months or current age 24–59 months / No further doses needed for healthy children if first dose given at age ≥24 months	4 weeks if current age <12 months / 8 weeks (as final dose) if current age ≥12 months / No further doses needed for healthy children if previous dose given at age ≥24 months	8 weeks (as final dose) This dose only necessary for children aged 12 months–5 years who received 3 doses before age 12 months	

CATCH-UP SCHEDULE FOR CHILDREN AGED 7 YEARS THROUGH 18 YEARS

Vaccine	Minimum Interval Between Doses		
	Dose 1 to Dose 2	Dose 2 to Dose 3	Dose 3 to Booster Dose
Tetanus, Diphtheria	4 weeks	6 months	6 months[8] if first dose given at age <12 months and current age <11 years / 5 years[8] if first dose given at age ≥12 months and third dose given at age <7 years and current age ≥11 years / 10 years[8] if third dose given at age ≥7 years
Inactivated Poliovirus[9]	4 weeks	4 weeks	IPV[2,9]
Hepatitis B	4 weeks	8 weeks (and 16 weeks after first dose)	
Measles, Mumps, Rubella	4 weeks		
Varicella[10]	4 weeks		

Footnotes
Children and Adolescents Catch-up Schedules   UNITED STATES • 2005

1. **DTaP.** The fifth dose is not necessary if the fourth dose was given after the fourth birthday.
2. **IPV.** For children who received an all-IPV or all-oral poliovirus (OPV) series, a fourth dose is not necessary if third dose was given at age ≥4 years. If both OPV and IPV were given as part of a series, a total of 4 doses should be given, regardless of the child's current age.
3. **HepB.** All children and adolescents who have not been immunized against hepatitis B should begin the HepB immunization series during any visit. Providers should make special efforts to immunize children who were born in, or whose parents were born in, areas of the world where hepatitis B virus infection is moderately or highly endemic.
4. **MMR.** The second dose of MMR is recommended routinely at age 4–6 years but may be given earlier if desired.
5. **Hib.** Vaccine is not generally recommended for children aged ≥5 years.
6. **Hib.** If current age <12 months and the first 2 doses were PRP-OMP (PedvaxHIB or ComVax [Merck]), the third (and final) dose should be given at age 12–15 months and at least 8 weeks after the second dose.
7. **PCV.** Vaccine is not generally recommended for children aged ≥5 years.
8. **Td.** For children aged 7–10 years, the interval between the third and booster dose is determined by the age when the first dose was given. For adolescents aged 11–18 years, the interval is determined by the age when the third dose was given.
9. **IPV.** Vaccine is not generally recommended for persons aged ≥18 years.
10. **Varicella.** Give 2-dose series to all susceptible adolescents aged ≥13 years.

Report adverse reactions to vaccines through the federal Vaccine Adverse Event Reporting System. For information on reporting reactions following immunization, please visit www.vaers.org or call the 24-hour national toll-free information line 800-822-7967. Report suspected cases of vaccine-preventable diseases to your state or local health department.

For additional information about vaccines, including precautions and contraindications for immunization and vaccine shortages, please visit the National Immunization Program Web site at www.cdc.gov/nip or call the National Immunization Information Hotline at 800-232-2522 (English) or 800-232-0233 (Spanish).

deciding when to travel with a young infant or child, parents should be advised that the earliest opportunity to receive routine immunizations recommended in the United States (except for the dose of hepatitis B vaccine administered at birth) is at 6 weeks if an accelerated schedule is followed. Parents should also be aware of the youngest age at which vaccinations can be administered for diseases endemic at their destination. The following section provides additional guidance for active and passive immunization of such infants and children. Additional information about all the diseases and vaccines mentioned below can be found in Chapter 4 *(Prevention of Specific Infectious Diseases)*.

ROUTINE INFANT AND CHILDHOOD VACCINATIONS

Hepatitis B Vaccine

Hepatitis B virus is a cause of acute and chronic hepatitis, cirrhosis, and hepatocellular carcinoma. There are 200 to 300 million chronic carriers worldwide. Infants and children who have not previously been vaccinated and who are traveling to areas with intermediate and high hepatitis B virus (HBV) endemicity are at risk if they are directly exposed to blood from the local population. Circumstances in which HBV transmission could occur in children include receipt of blood transfusions not screened for HBV surface antigen (HBsAg), exposure to unsterilized medical or dental equipment, or continuous close contact with local residents who have open skin lesions (impetigo, scabies, or scratched insect bites).

Hepatitis B vaccine is recommended for all infants, with the first dose administered soon after birth and before hospital discharge. Infants and children who will travel should receive the three doses of HBV vaccine before traveling. The interval between doses one and two should be 1–2 months. Between doses two and three, the interval should be a minimum of 2 months; the interval between doses one and three should be at least 4 months. The third dose should not be given before the infant is 6 months of age. Adolescents not previously vaccinated with hepatitis B vaccine should be vaccinated at 11–12 years of age. For adolescents, the usual schedule is two doses separated by at least 4 weeks, followed by a third dose 4–6 months after the second dose.

Diphtheria and Tetanus Toxoid and Pertussis Vaccine

Diphtheria, tetanus, and pertussis each occur worldwide and are endemic in countries with low immunization levels. Infants and children leaving the United States should be immunized before traveling. Optimum protection against diphtheria, tetanus, and pertussis in the first year of life is achieved with at least three but preferably four doses of diphtheria and tetanus toxoids and acellular pertussis vaccine (DTaP), the first administered when the infant is 6–8 weeks of age and the next two at 4- to 8-week intervals. A fourth dose of DTaP should be administered 6–12 months after the third dose when the infant is 15–18 months of age. A fifth (booster) dose is recommended when the child is 4–6 years of age. The fifth dose is not necessary if the fourth dose in the primary series was given after the child's fourth birthday.

Two doses of DTaP received at intervals at least 4 weeks apart can provide some protection; however, a single dose offers little protective benefit. Parents should be informed that infants and children who have not received at least three doses of DTaP might not be fully protected against pertussis. For infants and children <7 years of age, if an accelerated schedule is required to complete the series before travel, the schedule may be started as soon as the infant is 6 weeks of age, with the second and third doses given 4 weeks after each preceding dose. The fourth dose should not be given before the infant is 12 months of age and should be separated from the third dose by at least 6 months. The fifth (booster) dose should not be given before the child is 4 years of age.

Haemophilus influenzae Type b Conjugate Vaccine

Haemophilus influenzae type b (Hib) is an endemic disease worldwide that can cause fatal cases of meningitis, epiglottitis, and other invasive diseases. Infants and children should have optimal protection before traveling. Routine Hib vaccination beginning at 2 months of age is recommended for all U.S. children. The first dose may be given when an infant is as young as 6 weeks of age. Hib vaccine should never be given to an infant <6 weeks of age. A primary series consists of two or three doses (depending on the type of vaccine used) separated by 4–8 weeks. A booster dose is recommended when the infant is 12–15 months of age.

If Hib vaccination is started when the infant or child is ≥7 months of age, fewer doses may be required. If different brands of vaccine are administered, a total of three doses of Hib conjugate vaccine completes the primary series. After completion of the primary infant vaccination series, any of the licensed Hib conjugate vaccines may be used for the booster dose when the infant is 12–15 months of age.

If previously unvaccinated, infants <15 months of age should receive at least two vaccine doses before travel. An interval as short as 4 weeks between these two doses is acceptable. Unvaccinated infants and children 15–59 months of age should receive a single dose of Hib vaccine. Children >59 months of age do not need to be vaccinated unless a specific condition exists such as functional or anatomic asplenia, immunodeficiency, immunosuppression, or HIV infection.

Polio Vaccine

While polio has been eradicated in the United States, poliovirus continues to circulate in parts of Africa and Asia. In the United States, all infants and children should receive four doses of inactivated poliovirus vaccine (IPV) at 2, 4, and 6–18 months and 4–6 years of age. If accelerated protection is needed, the minimum interval between doses is 4 weeks, although the preferred interval between the second and third doses is 2 months. Infants and children who had initiated the poliovirus vaccination series with one or more doses of oral poliovirus vaccine (OPV) should receive IPV to complete the series.

Measles, Mumps, and Rubella Vaccine

Measles is an endemic disease in countries where measles immunization levels are low, and the risk for contracting measles in many countries is greater than in the United States. Infants and children should be as well protected as possible against measles and should complete the immunization series before traveling. While the risk for serious disease in infants from either mumps or rubella is low, these diseases do circulate in many parts of the world and vaccination is recommended.

In addition to the measles, mumps, and rubella vaccine (MMR), monovalent measles, monovalent mumps, monovalent rubella, and combinations of the components are available. However, the Advisory Committee on Immunization Practices (ACIP) recommends that MMR be administered when any of the individual components is indicated.

According to the recommended childhood immunization schedule (Table 8–2), a child should receive MMR at age 12 months and again at age 4–6 years. For children who are ≥12 months of age, the second dose of MMR may be given 28 days after the first dose.

Infants 6–11 months of age should receive a dose of MMR before departure. However, MMR given before age 12 months should not be counted as part of the series. Children who receive MMR before age 12 months will need two more doses of MMR, the first of which should be administered at age 12 months.

If MMR is unavailable, monovalent vaccines may be used. However, a child receiving monovalent vaccines will still need two doses of MMR beginning at age 12 months.

Varicella Vaccine

Varicella (chickenpox) is an endemic disease throughout the world. The varicella vaccine is recommended for all children ≥12 months of age.

A single dose of varicella vaccine is also recommended for all susceptible children by their 13th birthday. Efforts should be made to ensure varicella immunity by this age, because varicella disease can be more severe among older children and adults. Children >13 years of age need to receive two doses of varicella vaccine at least 4 weeks apart to optimize protection.

Vaccination is not necessary for children with a reliable history of chickenpox. When a prior history of chickenpox is unclear, the vaccine may be given.

Pneumococcal Vaccine

Streptococcus pneumoniae causes substantial morbidity and mortality throughout the world each year. The vaccine is available in two forms: the pneumococcal conjugate vaccine (PCV7) and the pneumococcal polysaccharide vaccine (PPV23).

All infants should be vaccinated with PCV7. Infant vaccination provides the earliest protection, and infants <23 months of age have the highest incidence of pneumococcal disease. The primary series for PCV7 includes three doses given at 2, 4, and 6 months of age with a fourth (booster) dose at 12–15 months of age (see Table 4–13). Children ≥24 months of age at high risk for the development of pneumococcal disease (with sickle cell disease, asplenia, HIV, chronic illness, or immunocompromising conditions) should receive a dose of PPV23 at least 2 months following their last dose of PCV7. If the child is ≤10 years of age, one revaccination with PPV23 should be considered 3–5 years after the first dose of PPV 23.

Unvaccinated children 7–11 months of age should receive two doses at least 4 weeks apart and a booster dose at age 12–15 months. Unvaccinated children 12–23 months of age should receive two doses at least 8 weeks apart. Previously unvaccinated healthy children 24–59 months of age should receive a single dose of PCV7. However, previously unvaccinated children 24–59 months of age at high risk for pneumococcal disease should receive two doses separated by at least 8 weeks. Children 24–59 months of age who are at increased risk for pneumococcal disease (as previously described) and who were previously vaccinated with PPV23 should receive two doses of PCV7 separated by at least 8 weeks. The PCV7 vaccine is not routinely recommended for children >59 months (5 years) of age.

Influenza Vaccine

Influenza vaccine can be used to reduce risk of influenza infection in transmission season (November-February in the Northern Hemisphere, April-September in the Southern Hemisphere, and throughout the year in the tropics). The vaccine is prepared in two forms: an intramuscular trivalent inactivated vaccine (TIV) and a live, attenuated, intranasal vaccine (LAIV).

All children 6–23 months of age should receive TIV annually. In addition, all children with risk factors for influenza (including but not limited to asthma, cardiac disease, sickle cell disease, HIV, and diabetes) should also receive TIV annually. In addition, all children who have close contact with healthy children <24 months of age or with persons at high risk should be vaccinated annually. For healthy children ≥5 years of age, LAIV is an acceptable alternative to TIV. (LAIV can be given to healthy persons 5–49 years of age).

Children receiving TIV should be administered an age-appropriate dose (0.25 mL for those 6–35 months of age and 0.5 mL for those ≥36 months of age). Children ≤8 years of age who are receiving influenza vaccine for the first time should receive two doses (separated by at least

4 weeks for TIV and at least 6 weeks for LAIV). Children ≥9 years of age should receive one injection of the 0.5-mL dose.

Hepatitis A Vaccine or Immune Globulin for Hepatitis A

Hepatitis A virus (HAV) is endemic in most parts of the world, and infants and children traveling to these areas are at increased risk for acquiring HAV infection. Although HAV is often not severe in infants and children <5 years of age, those infected efficiently transmit infection to other infants and children and to adults.

Children ≥2 years of age who will be traveling to areas where there is a high risk of HAV infection should be immunized. The HAV vaccine series consists of two doses at least 6 months apart. The first dose should be administered 4 weeks before travel to allow time for an adequate immune response to develop. The second dose is necessary for long-term protection.

The vaccine is not approved for children <2 years of age. Children <2 years of age and children who will be traveling less than 4 weeks after receipt of the first dose should be administered immune globulin (IG) (See Chapter 4, *Hepatitis A* section). The vaccine and IG can be administered at the same time at different anatomic sites.

IG interferes with the response to live injected vaccines (e.g., measles, mumps, rubella, and varicella vaccines). Administration of live vaccines should be delayed for at least 3 months after administration of IG. Moreover, IG should not be administered for 2 weeks after measles-, mumps-, and rubella-containing vaccines and for 3 weeks after vaccination with varicella vaccine. If IG is given during this time, the child should be revaccinated with the live vaccine at least 3 months after administration of IG. When travel plans do not allow adequate time for administration of live vaccines and IG before travel, the severity of the diseases and epidemiology of the diseases at destination points will help determine the most appropriate course of preparation.

OTHER VACCINES AND IMMUNE GLOBULIN

Yellow Fever Vaccine

Yellow fever, a disease transmitted by mosquitoes, is endemic in certain areas of Africa and South America (Maps 4–12 and 4–13). Proof of yellow fever vaccination is required for entry into some countries (see *Yellow Fever Vaccine Requirements and Information on Malaria Risk and Prophylaxis, by Country*).

Infants are at high risk for developing encephalitis from yellow fever vaccine, a live virus vaccine. Vaccination of infants should be considered on an individual basis. Although the incidence of these adverse events has not been clearly defined, 14 of 18 reported cases of post-vaccination encephalitis were in infants <4 months old. One fatal case confirmed by viral isolation was in a 3-year-old child.

Travelers with infants <9 months of age should be strongly advised against traveling to areas within the yellow fever-endemic zone. The ACIP recommends that yellow fever vaccine never be given to infants <6 months of age. Infants 6-8 months of age should be vaccinated only if they must travel to areas of ongoing epidemic yellow fever and a high level of protection against mosquito bites is not possible. Infants and children >9 months of age can be vaccinated if they travel to countries within the yellow fever-endemic zone. Physicians considering vaccinating infants <9 months of age should contact the Division of Vector-Borne Infectious Diseases (970-221-6400) or the Division of Global Migration and Quarantine (404-498-1600) at CDC for advice.

Typhoid Vaccine
Typhoid fever is an acute, life-threatening febrile illness caused by the bacterium *Salmonella enterica* Typhi.

Two typhoid vaccines are available: a Vi capsular polysaccharide vaccine (ViCPS) administered intramuscularly and an oral, live, attenuated vaccine (Ty21a). Both vaccines induce a protective response in 50%–80% of recipients. The ViCPS vaccine can be administered to children ≥2 years of age, with a booster dose 2 years later if continued protection is needed. The Ty21a vaccine, which consists of a series of four capsules ingested every other day, can be administered to children ≥6 years of age. All the capsules should be taken at least 1 week before potential exposure. A booster series for Ty21a can be taken every 5 years.

Because neither vaccine is fully protective, preventing contamination of food and beverages remains extremely important.

Meningococcal Vaccine

Meningitis primarily affects children and adolescents, with high morbidity and mortality rates. Epidemics are recurrent in sub-Saharan Africa during the dry season (December through June), and CDC recommends travelers be vaccinated before traveling to this region during the dry season. Meningococcal vaccination is a requirement to enter Saudi Arabia when traveling to Mecca during the annual Hajj.

Two meningococcal vaccines are licensed for use in the United States; both are quadrivalent A, C, Y, and W-135 vaccines. The serogroup A polysaccharide in the vaccine induces an antibody response in some children as young as 3 months. Thus, vaccinating infants traveling to high-risk areas can provide some degree of protection. For children vaccinated at <4 years of age, revaccination in 2–3 years should be considered if they remain at high risk for infection. For children vaccinated at ≥4 years of age, revaccination should be considered in 3–5 years if they remain at high risk.

Japanese Encephalitis Vaccine

Primarily night-biting mosquitoes in rural areas of Asia and the Pacific Rim transmit Japanese encephalitis (JE). In temperate climates, their numbers are greatest from June through September; they are inactive during the winter. Most reported cases occur in children. Although most infections are asymptomatic, the mortality rate can be as high as 30%, and neurologic sequelae are reported in 50% of survivors. Serious neurologic sequelae occur more frequently in the very young. The risk to short-term travelers and those who confine their travel to urban centers is very low. Expatriates and travelers living for prolonged periods in rural areas where JE is endemic or epidemic are at greatest risk. Travelers with extensive unprotected outdoor, evening, and nighttime exposure in rural areas, such as might be experienced while bicycling, camping, or engaging in certain occupational activities, might be at high risk even if their trip is brief. The decision to vaccinate a child should take into consideration the itinerary, expected activities, and level of JE activity in the country.

JE vaccine is administered as a series of three injections on days 0, 7, and 30. A booster dose is administered at least 24 months later. Children 1–2 years of age receive 0.5 mL of vaccine per dose; those

≥3 years of age receive 1.0 mL of vaccine per dose. No data are available on vaccine efficacy for infants <1 year of age.

JE vaccine is associated with local reactions and mild systemic side effects (fever, headache, myalgias, and malaise). Serious allergic reactions, including anaphylaxis, have occurred up to 1 week after immunization. Children receiving the vaccine series should be observed for 30 minutes after immunization. Moreover, the series should be completed at least 10 days before departure, and during that time, vaccine recipients should be remain in areas with access to medical care.

Rabies Vaccine

Rabies is an acute, fatal encephalomyelitis usually transmitted by the bite of an infected mammal. Rabies occurs throughout the world and is endemic in most countries. As with other vaccines, the decision to vaccinate will depend on the itinerary and expected activities during international travel. Children should always be instructed to avoid contact with unfamiliar animals because those animals could be infected with rabies.

Three rabies vaccines are licensed for use in the United States. Each may be administered to infants and children. All the rabies vaccines, when used in a preexposure regimen, are given as a series of injections on days 0, 7, and 21 or 28 days. Even if a child has completed the preexposure prophylaxis, any mammal bite warrants immediate medical evaluation to determine the need for postexposure immunization.

Bibliography

Centers for Disease Control and Prevention. Preventing pneumococcal disease among infants and young children: recommendations of the Advisory Committee on Immunization Practices (ACIP). MMWR Morbid Mortal Wkly Rep 2000;49(No. RR-9):1–35.

Centers for Disease Control and Prevention. Prevention and control of meningococcal disease and Meningococcal disease and college students: recommendations of the Advisory Committee on Immunization Practices (ACIP). MMWR Morbid Mortal Wkly Rep 2000;49(No. RR-7):1–22.

Centers for Disease Control and Prevention. Prevention and control of influenza: recommendations of the Advisory Committee on Immunization Practices (ACIP). MMWR Morbid Mortal Wkly Rep 2004;53(No. RR-6):1–40.

Epidemiology and prevention of vaccine-preventable diseases. Seventh edition. Eds. William Atkinson, Charles Wolfe. Washington: Public Health Foundation; 2003.

Mackell SM. Vaccinations for the pediatric traveler. Clin Infect Dis 2003;37:1508–16.

—DREW POSEY

>>Breastfeeding and Travel

DECIDING ABOUT TRAVEL AND BREASTFEEDING

Travel need not be a reason to stop breastfeeding. A mother traveling with a nursing infant may find breastfeeding makes travel easier than it would be if traveling with a bottle-fed infant. A mother traveling without her nursing infant or child may take steps to preserve breastfeeding and maintain her milk supply while separated. The major factors for a mother traveling without her nursing infant or child to consider are the amount of time she has to prepare for her trip, her flexibility of time while traveling, her options for storing expressed milk while traveling, the duration of her travel, and her destination. Mothers planning travel away from a nursing infant may access information from her pediatrician or from an International Board Certified Lactation Consultant (IBCLC) at http://gotwww.net/ilca/, or from the international organization at www.iblce.org/international%20registry.htm.

PREPARATION FOR TRAVEL WHILE BREASTFEEDING

Breastfeeding mothers may wish to find local breastfeeding support before beginning travel and keep pertinent contact information handy throughout the trip. La Leche League International has breastfeeding experts in many countries (www.lalecheleague.org).

A mother traveling with a nursing infant <6 months old need not plan on supplementing breastfeeding because of international travel.

Breastfed infants do not require water supplementation, even in extreme heat environments, if the mother is adequately hydrated. A breastfeeding mother traveling without her nursing infant or child may wish to build a supply of milk to be fed to the infant or child during her absence by expressing milk and storing it for later use by another caregiver.

Depending on her destination, a mother may need to plan for milk expression without a reliable electrical power source. Expressing milk without an electrical power source is less reliable for maintaining milk supply over a long period of time than expressing milk with a hospital-grade electric breast pump. Intermittent milk expression can be successful with battery and manual breast pumps, as well as manual expression.

The destination for travel can impact decisions for milk storage. Once milk is cooled, a cold chain needs to be maintained until milk is consumed. Refrigerated milk can subsequently be frozen; however, once frozen milk is fully thawed, it should be used within 1 hour. Guidance on human milk storage is found in Table 8–4.

Most nursing mothers may be immunized routinely, based on recommendations for the specific travel itinerary. Breastfeeding is not a contraindication to the administration of vaccines, including live-virus vaccines (see Table 8–5); however, there is a theoretical risk to the infant with the use of the yellow fever vaccine in breastfeeding mothers (See Chapter 4, *Yellow Fever* section). Breastfed infants should be vaccinated according to routine recommended schedules (see *Vaccine Recommendations for Infants and Children*).

Breastfeeding mothers should take the usual adult dose of the antimalarial drug appropriate for the itinerary. Nursing mothers with infants weighing <11 kg (approximately 24 pounds) should not take atovaquone/proguanil (Malarone) for prophylaxis. Data are limited on the use of doxycycline during breastfeeding; however, most experts consider its short-term use compatible with breastfeeding. Primaquine is contraindicated during lactation unless both the mother and breastfed infant have normal G6PD levels. It is critical to note that breastfed infants require their own antimalarial medication if traveling to an endemic area. Mother's milk does not provide malaria protection, even when the mother is taking an adequate medication and dose for herself.

TABLE 8-4. HUMAN MILK STORAGE FOR HEALTHY INFANTS[1]

LOCATION	TEMPERATURE	DURATION	COMMENTS
Countertop, table	Room temperature (up to 77° F or 25° C)	6–8 hours	Containers should be covered and kept as cool as possible; covering the container with a cool towel may keep milk cooler.
Insulated cooler bag	5–39° F or −15–4° C	24 hours	Keep ice packs in contact with milk containers at all times, limit opening cooler bag.
Refrigerator	39° F or 4° C	5 days	Store milk in the back of the main body of the refrigerator.
Freezer			
Compartment of refrigerator	5° F or −15° C	2 weeks	Store milk toward the back of the freezer, where tempera-
Refrigerator/freezer with separate doors	0° F or −18° C	3–6 months	ture is most constant. Milk stored for longer durations in the ranges listed is safe, but
Chest or upright manual-defrost deep freezer	−4° F or −20° C	6–12 months	some of the lipids in the milk undergo degradation, resulting in lower quality.

[1]Academy of Breastfeeding Medicine Clinical Protocol Number #8: Human Milk Storage Information for Home Use for Healthy Full-Term Infants, Academy of Breastfeeding Medicine, Princeton Junction, NJ, 2004.

TRAVELING WITH A BREASTFED INFANT

Infants are particularly susceptible to painful pressure due to eustachian tube collapse as a result of pressure changes during air travel. Breastfeeding during ascent and descent often relieves this discomfort.

No special precautions are necessary for airport security screenings while breastfeeding. Breast milk does not need to be declared at US Customs when returning to the United States. Electric breast pumps are considered personal items during air travel and may be carried on and stowed underneath the passenger seat, similar to a laptop computer, purse, or diaper bag.

TABLE 8-5. VACCINATION OF BREASTFEEDING MOTHERS

VACCINE/ IMMUNOBIOLOGIC	PRECAUTIONS FOR BREASTFEEDING
Immune globulins, pooled or hyperimmune	None
Diphtheria-Tetanus	None
Hepatitis A	Data on safety in breastfeeding are not available; it is unlikely that vaccination would cause untoward effects in breastfed infants. Consider immune globulin rather than vaccine.
Hepatitis B	None
Influenza	Vaccination with inactivated influenza vaccine is encouraged when feasible for children aged 6–23 months and their close contacts and caregivers.
Japanese encephalitis	Data on safety in breastfeeding are not available; vaccine should not be routinely administered.
Measles	None
Meningococcal meningitis	None
Mumps	None
Pneumococcal	Data on safety in breastfeeding are not available; it is unlikely that vaccination would cause untoward effects in breastfed infants.
Polio, inactivated	None
Rabies	Data on safety in breastfeeding are not available; however, this vaccine is commonly given to breastfeeding mothers without any observed untoward effects in breastfed infants.
Rubella	None
Tuberculosis (BCG)	Data on safety in breastfeeding are not available.
Typhoid (ViCPS)	Specific information concerning use during breastfeeding is not available. However, the vaccine may be used when risk of exposure to typhoid fever is high.

TABLE 8-5. VACCINATION OF BREASTFEEDING MOTHERS-cont'd

VACCINE/ IMMUNOBIOLOGIC	PRECAUTIONS FOR BREASTFEEDING
Typhoid (Ty21a)	Specific information concerning use during breastfeeding is not available. However, the vaccine may be used when risk of exposure to typhoid fever is high.
Varicella	None
Yellow fever	Vaccination of nursing mothers should be avoided because of the theoretical risk for transmission of 17D virus to the breastfed infant. When travel to high-risk yellow fever-endemic areas cannot be avoided or postponed, nursing mothers can be vaccinated.
Vaccinia (Smallpox)	**Women who are breastfeeding should not be given this vaccine. If there is a smallpox outbreak, recommendations on who should get vaccinated may change.**

Breastfed infants are protected from travelers' diarrhea, and thus it is often recommended that a nursing mother try, if reasonable, to continue to breastfeed until returning home. A nursing mother with travelers' diarrhea should increase her own fluid intake and frequency of breastfeeding; she should not stop breastfeeding because of travelers' diarrhea. The use of oral rehydration salts (ORS) is fully compatible with breastfeeding.

In addition to the usual contents of the travel health kit (see Chapter 2), breastfeeding mothers may wish to include an antifungal cream, which can be used to treat periareolar yeast.

Bibliography

American Academy of Pediatrics. The transfer of drugs and other chemicals into human milk. Pediatrics 2001;108(3):776–789.

CDC. Protection against viral hepatitis: Recommendations of the Immunization Practices Advisory Committee (ACIP).MMWR Morbid Mortal Wkly Rep 1990;39(RR-2);1–26.

CDC. Recommendations of the Advisory Committee on Immunization Practices (ACIP) and the American Academy of Family Physicians (AAFP) MMWR Morbid Mortal Wkly Rep 2002;51(RR-2):1-36.

Lawrence RA. Breastfeeding: A guide for the medical profession. 4th ed. Mosby: New York, 1994.

Marmet C. Technique for Manual Expression of Breastmilk. http://www.lactationinstitute.org/MANUALEX.html

Nikem VC, Hofmeyr GJ. Secretion of the antidiarrhoeal agent loperamide oxide in breastmilk. Eur J Clin Pharmacol 1992;42(6): 695–696.

Popkin BM, Adair L, Akin JS, Black R, Briscoe J, Fledger W. Breastfeeding and diarrheal morbidity. Pediatrics 1990;86(6):874–882.

Sachdev HPS, Krishna J, Puri RK, Satyanarayana L, Kumar S. Water supplementation in exclusively breastfed infants during summer in the tropics. Lancet 1991;337(8747):929–933.

–KATHERINE SHEALY

>>International Adoptions

GENERAL INFORMATION

Approximately 20,000 infants and children are adopted from abroad each year by citizens of the United States. Infants and children from Asia, Central and South America, and Eastern Europe account for >90% of international adoptions. To complete an international adoption and bring an infant or a child to the United States, prospective parents must fulfill the requirements set by the Bureau of Citizenship and Immigration Services (BCIS) http://uscis.gov/graphics/index.htm (formerly the Immigration and Naturalization Service [INS]), the foreign country where the infant or child resides, and sometimes the state of residence of the adoptive parent(s). The adoption of a foreign-born orphan does not automatically guarantee the child's eligibility to immigrate to the United States. The adoptive parent needs to be aware of U.S. immigration law and legal regulatory procedures. An orphan cannot legally immigrate to the United States without BCIS processing.

An infant or child cannot be brought to the United States without an immigrant visa, issuance of which is based on a BCIS-approved petition (BCIS Form I-600A: Application for Advance Processing of Orphan Petition, which can be found at: http://uscis.gov/graphics/formsfee/ forms/i-600a.htm). Detailed information about the procedures and requirements for international adoptions is available on the BCIS website at http://www.bcis.gov/graphics/services/index2.htm. When the Orphan Petition has been approved by the BCIS, the adoptive parent(s) can apply for an immigrant visa (IR-3) at the appropriate U.S. consular office abroad. In addition to the approved Orphan Petition, the consular officer will also require specific documentation, including a medical examination of the adoptee.

Adoptive parents who travel overseas to pick up their child should obtain pre-travel advice. They should be aware that unexpected complications in the adoption process may prolong their stay and should plan accordingly, especially if malaria prophylaxis or other important medication is needed. In addition, they need to take precautions regarding proper rest, food, water, and insect exposure to protect their own health, so that they can care for the child. Recently, an outbreak of measles was identified among children being adopted from China and their family members. Therefore, all traveling family members should be sure that they are up to date on recommended vaccinations, including MMR, prior to travel.

OVERSEAS MEDICAL EXAMINATIONS

All immigrants, including infants and children adopted overseas by U.S. citizens, and refugees coming to the United States must have a medical examination overseas by a designated physician. The medical examination focuses primarily on detecting certain serious contagious diseases that may be the basis for visa ineligibility; prospective adoptive parents should be advised not to rely on this medical examination to detect all possible disabilities and illnesses. If an infant or a child is found to have an illness or disability that may make the child ineligible for a visa, a visa may still be issued after the illness has been adequately treated or after a waiver of the visa eligibility has been approved by the BCIS. If the physician notes that the infant or child has a serious disease or disability, the prospective parent(s) will be notified and asked if they wish to proceed with the infant's or child's immigration.

The medical examination consists of a brief physical examination and a medical history. A chest radiograph examination for tuberculosis and blood tests for syphilis and HIV are required for immigrants ≥15 years of age. Applicants <15 years of age are tested only if there is reason to suspect any of these diseases.

A new subsection of the U.S. Immigration and Nationality Act requires that any person seeking an immigrant visa for permanent residency must show proof of having received the vaccines recommended by the Advisory Committee on Immunization Practices (ACIP) before immigration. While this new subsection now applies to all immigrant infants and children entering the United States, internationally adopted children <11 years of age have been exempted from the overseas immunization requirements. Adoptive parents are required to sign a waiver indicating their intention to comply with the immunization requirements within 30 days after the infant's or child's arrival in the United States.

Additional information about the medical examination and the vaccination exemption form for internationally adopted children are available on the Department of State website at http://www.travel.state.gov/adopt.html.

FOLLOW-UP MEDICAL EXAMINATION AFTER ARRIVAL IN THE UNITED STATES

The varied geographic origins of internationally adopted infants and children, their unknown backgrounds before adoption (including parental history and living circumstances), and the inadequacy of health care in many developing countries make appropriate medical evaluation of internationally adopted children a complex and important task. An internationally adopted infant or child should be examined within 2 weeks of his or her arrival in the United States, but an adoptee who has an acute illness or a chronic condition needs immediate attention. All adopted infants and children should have a complete physical examination, a review of any available medical records, and age-appropriate screening tests, including evaluation for possible anemia, vision and hearing impairments, and assessment of growth and development. Children >18 months of age should also have a dental evaluation.

Screening for Infectious Diseases

Infectious diseases, among the most common medical diagnoses, have been found in up to 60% of internationally adopted children, depending on their country of origin; many of these infections can be asymptomatic. Screening for these diseases is important for the health of the adopted infant or child as well as that of their adoptive family. The American Academy of Pediatrics recommends that all internationally adopted children be screened with the following: hepatitis B serology; HIV serology, syphilis serology, Mantoux intradermal skin test for tuberculosis, stool examination for ova and parasites, and complete blood count with red blood cell indices. Other screening tests may be recommended based on country of origin, risk factors, symptoms, or clinical findings. Laboratory reports from the country of origin should not be considered reliable.

Viral Hepatitis

Routine serologic screening for hepatitis A infection is not indicated. Many adopted children acquire hepatitis A virus infection early in life and are immune thereafter. However, for adopted children who will be residing in an area of the United States where routine hepatitis A vaccination is recommended, it may be cost effective to screen these children for previous immunity before initiating the vaccination series.

All internationally adopted children should be screened for hepatitis B infection, including hepatitis B surface antigen (HBsAg), hepatitis B surface antibody (anti-HBs) and hepatitis B core antibody (anti-HBc). If a child is hepatitis B surface antigen (HBsAg) positive, all unvaccinated household contacts should receive the full vaccine series. Children who test positive for HBsAg should receive a medical evaluation for chronic hepatitis B infection. Children who do not have serologic evidence of previous infection should receive the full vaccine series.

Screening for hepatitis C should be considered for all infants and children adopted from Asia, Eastern Europe, or Africa. Hepatitis C testing for children adopted from other areas should be considered if the records indicate potential risk factors such as receipt of blood products or maternal drug use. Testing for hepatitis D, which is available at CDC, should be considered for children from the Mediterranean area, Africa, Eastern Europe, and Latin America who have chronic infection with hepatitis B virus.

HIV

Risk of HIV depends on country of origin and individual risk factors. However, because of the rapidly changing global epidemiology of HIV and often unknown backgrounds, screening for antibodies to HIV should be considered for all internationally adopted children. If test results are available from the adopted child's country of origin, repeat testing should be performed to confirm the overseas results. Antibodies in a child <18 months of age may reflect maternal infection without transmission to the infant, and infection in the infant should be confirmed with an assay for HIV DNA by polymerase chain reaction. Two negative tests obtained 1 month apart are required for the child to be considered uninfected.

Syphilis

Regardless of overseas testing results and/or history of treatment, internationally adopted children should be tested for syphilis by nontreponemal and treponemal serologic tests upon arrival. Children who have positive tests should receive further evaluation for treatment.

Tuberculosis

Mantoux tuberculin skin testing (TST) is recommended for international adoptees because their rates of TB infection are several times higher than those of U.S.-born children. The definition of a positive TST for children born in regions of the world with high TB prevalence is ≥10 mm of induration. If the TST is positive, a chest radiograph must be performed to evaluate for active TB disease. If evidence of TB disease is found, efforts to isolate an organism for sensitivity testing are very important because of the high proportions of drug resistance in many other countries, including countries in Eastern Europe, the former Soviet Union, and Asia.

Receipt of BCG vaccine is not a contraindication for TST. After BCG immunization, however, distinguishing between a positive TST result caused by *M. tuberculosis* infection and that caused by BCG can be difficult. However, infection with *M. tuberculosis* should be strongly suspected in any asymptomatic child with a positive TST result, regardless of history of BCG immunization. Circumstances that increase the likelihood that a positive TST is due to TB infection include contact with a person with active TB, immigration from a country with high TB prevalence, or a long interval since the last BCG immunization. Because BCG does not prevent infection with TB and because of the high risk for exposure in most countries where BCG is given, the AAP recommends that children with a positive TST be given 9 months of isoniazid therapy.

Parasites and Intestinal Pathogens

Up to 35% of internationally adopted children have ova or parasites identified on stool examinations. Internationally adopted children should have a complete blood count with a peripheral eosinophil count, which may be an indicator of parasitic disease infection. Regardless of the eosinophil count, all internationally adopted children should be screened initially with three separate stool samples, collected on 3 separate days, analyzed for ova and parasites. If enteric symptoms develop in the future, these tests should be repeated, even if it has been several years after arrival in the United States. For *Giardia intestinalis* and *Cryptosporium parvum* infection, stool examination for antigen by enzyme immunoassay may be more sensitive than microscopic exam. Giardiasis is particularly prevalent in internationally adopted children from Eastern Europe. *Strongyloides stercoralis* serologic testing, available at CDC on request through the state public health laboratory, should be considered for children who have a high eosinophil count.

Children from schistosomiasis-endemic areas should have serologic tests for schistosomiasis performed at CDC. These tests may be requested through the state public health laboratory.

Children with diarrhea should also be evaluated for bacterial organisms, including *Escherichia coli* species, *Salmonella* species, *Shigella* species, and *Campylobacter* species.

Ectoparasites

Internationally adopted children should be carefully examined for scabies and lice, so that they can be appropriately treated and to prevent infestation of family members and contacts.

Evaluation for Other Medical Problems
Lead
Potentially dangerous levels of lead have been reported in internationally adopted children, particularly those from China, Cambodia, Russia, and other countries in Eastern Europe. Lead exposure in other countries can result from a variety of sources, including leaded gasoline exhaust, ceramic ware, and traditional medicines. All children from these areas of the world and any others in whom lead toxicity is suspected should be screened, with follow-up and treatment based on standard guidelines. Information about lead poisoning is available at www.cdc.gov/nceh/lead/lead.htm or by calling 1-800-232-6789.

G6PD Deficiency
This enzyme deficiency is relatively common in persons from Asia, the Mediterranean area, and Africa. Screening for this deficiency in children from these areas should be considered before drugs are prescribed that can cause hemolysis in persons who have G6PD deficiency.

Vaccination
Internationally adopted children <11 years of age are not required to have vaccinations before arrival in the United States as long as the adoptive family signs a waiver stating that they will have the child vaccinated within 30 days of arrival in the United States.

Internationally adopted infants and children frequently are underimmunized and should receive necessary immunizations according to recommended schedules in the United States (see Table 8–2). In a retrospective review of records of 504 children, 65% had no written records of overseas vaccination. Among the 178 children with documented overseas vaccination, 167 (94%) had valid records and some vaccine doses that were acceptable and up to date under the U.S. schedule.

In assessing the immunization status of an internationally adopted child, only written documentation should be accepted as proof of receipt of immunization. In general, written records are deemed valid if the vaccine type, date of administration, number of doses, intervals between doses, and age of the patient at the time of administration are comparable with the current U.S. schedule. Although some vaccines with inadequate potency have been produced in other countries, most vaccines used worldwide are produced with adequate quality control standards and are reliable. However, immunization records for some internationally adopted children, particularly those from orphanages, may not reflect protection because of inaccurate or unreliable records, lack of vaccine potency, poor nutritional status, or other problems. For any child, if there is any question as to whether the immunizations were administered or were immunogenic, the best course is to repeat them. Vaccination is generally safe and avoids the need to obtain and interpret serologic tests.

In an older infant or child who is thought to have been vaccinated appropriately, judicious use of serologic testing can be helpful in determining which immunizations may be needed and can decrease the number of injections required. Verification of protection from MMR vaccine requires testing for antibodies to each virus. Serology is of limited availability or difficult to interpret for *Haemophilus influenzae* type b (Hib) and poliovirus. Vaccination for these as well as varicella and pneumococcal disease, which are not administered in most countries, should be administered to internationally adopted children based on age and medical history.

Data indicate increased risk of local adverse reactions after the fourth and fifth doses of DTP or DtaP. In some circumstances, judicious use of serologic testing of antibody levels to assess immunity may be helpful in decreasing the possibility of vaccine side effects. For children whose records indicate that they have received >3 doses, options include initial serologic testing or administration of a single booster dose of DTaP, followed by serologic testing after 1 month. If a severe local reaction occurs after revaccination, serologic testing for specific IgG antibody to tetanus and diphtheria toxins can be measured before additional doses are administered. No established serologic correlates exist for protection against pertussis, but protective concentrations of antibody to both diphtheria and tetanus toxin can serve to validate the vaccination record.

In the United States, multiple outbreaks of measles have been reported in children who were recently adopted from China and in their U.S. contacts. Measles outbreaks among children in Chinese orphanages were also reported. In 2002 and 2004, adoptions from the affected orphanages were temporarily suspended while Chinese authorities implemented measures to control and prevent further transmission of measles among adopted children. Prospective parents who are traveling internationally to adopt children, as well as their household contacts, should ensure that they have a history of natural disease or have been vaccinated against measles according to guidelines of the Advisory Committee on Immunization Practices. All persons born after 1957 should receive two doses of measles-containing vaccine.

Bibliography

American Academy of Pediatrics. Medical evaluation of internationally adopted children for infectious diseases. In: Pickering LK, editor. Red book: 2003 report of the Committee on Infectious Diseases. 26th ed. Elk Grove Village, IL: American Academy of Pediatrics; 2003. p. 173–180.

Atkinson WL, Pickering LK, Schwartz B, et al. General recommendation on immunizations. Recommendations of the Advisory Committee on Immunization Practices (ACIP) and the American Academy of Family Physicians (AAFP). Morbid Mortal Wkly Rep MMWR. 2002;51(RR-2):1–35.

CDC. Measles outbreak among internationally adopted children arriving in the United States, February - March 2001. Morbid Mortal Wkly Rep MMWR. 2002;51:1115–6.

CDC. Multistate investigation of measles among adoptees from China — April 9, 2004. Morbid Mortal Wkly Rep MMWR. 2004;53:309–10.

CDC. Update: measles among children adopted from China. Morbid Mortal Wkly Rep MMWR. 2004;53:459.

Schulte JM, Maloney S, Aronson J, et al. Evaluating acceptability and completeness of overseas immunization records of internationally adopted children. Pediatrics. 2002;109:e22.

–MICHELLE WEINBERG AND SUSAN MALONEY

CHAPTER 9

Advising Travelers with Specific Needs

>>The Immunocompromised Traveler

RISK ASSESSMENT IN THE IMMUNOCOMPROMISED TRAVELER

The main risk for the immunocompromised traveler is a complication or exacerbation of the underlying disease. In addition, endemic infectious diseases that may be acquired at the destination(s) may cause disease of increased severity in that traveler. Each proposed preventive intervention must be examined from two perspectives: 1) safety in the context of the underlying immunocompromise and ongoing medication; and 2) the possibility of decreased effectiveness of the intervention in that context. Before proceeding, the medical provider should ensure a complete understanding by the traveler of the wisdom of the proposed itinerary, based on his/her medical needs and the traveler's individual tolerance for the risks of the proposed interventions and of the travel itself.

SPECIFIC IMMUNOCOMPROMISING CONDITIONS

The degree to which a person is immunocompromised should be determined by a health-care provider. For practical purposes, immunocompromised travelers can be categorized into one of four groups, each with a general approach for that patient.

Severe Immunocompromise (non-HIV)

Persons considered as having severe immunosuppression include those with active leukemia or lymphoma, generalized malignancy, aplastic anemia, solid organ transplant, bone marrow transplant within 2 years of transplantation, or transplants of longer duration still on immunosuppressive drugs or with graft-versus-host disease, congenital immunodeficiency, and current or recent radiation therapy. For solid organ transplants, much higher risk of infection occurs within the first year of transplant, so particularly high-risk travel might be postponed until beyond that time.

Medications that cause severe immunosuppression include high-dose corticosteroids, alkylating agents (e.g., cyclophosphamide), antimetabolites (e.g., methotrexate in any dose, azathioprine, 6-mercaptopurine), transplant-related immunosuppressive drugs (e.g., cyclosporine, tacrolimus, sirolimus, and mycophenolate mofetil), mitoxantrone (used in multiple sclerosis), and most cancer chemotherapeutic agents (not tamoxifen). The immunosuppressive effects of steroid treatment vary, but most clinicians consider a dose of ≥20 mg/day of prednisone or equivalent administered for ≥2 weeks as causing severe immunocompromise. Tumor necrosis factor (TNF)-blocking agents such as etanercept and infliximab are known to activate latent mycobacterial infection, but the degree of overall susceptibility to other microorganisms is unclear. Although the benefits of live viral and bacterial vaccines in persons receiving TNF-blocking agents need to be carefully weighed against potential risk, most practicing clinicians would be reluctant to use such vaccines in this situation.

Severe Immunocompromise Due to Symptomatic HIV/AIDS

Consultation with the HIV-infected traveler cannot be performed without knowledge of a current CD4 lymphocyte count. HIV-infected persons with CD4 counts <200, history of an AIDS-defining illness, or clinical manifestations of symptomatic HIV are considered to have severe immunosuppression. (See also the section on AIDS in Chapter 4.)

Asymptomatic HIV Infection

Asymptomatic HIV-infected persons with CD4 counts from 200 to 500 are considered to have limited immune deficits. Antiretroviral drug-induced increased CD4 counts and not nadir counts should be used in categorizing HIV-infected persons. The exact time at which reconstituted lymphocytes are fully functional is not well defined. To achieve maximal vaccine response with minimal risk, if possible, a wait of 3 months post-reconstitution before immunization is advised by many clinicians.

Chronic Diseases with Limited Immune Deficits

These chronic diseases include asplenia, chronic renal disease, chronic hepatic disease (cirrhosis and alcoholism), diabetes, and nutritional deficiencies. Patients taking ribavirin and interferon for hepatitis C infection are at risk for neutropenia, although no clinically apparent increase in opportunistic infections has been described. No information on possible decreased vaccine efficacy or increased adverse events with live viral antigens is available for this group.

PERSONS CONSIDERED TO HAVE NO IMMUNOLOGIC COMPROMISE

For the purpose of pretravel preparation, travelers with the following conditions are not considered to be immunocompromised and should be prepared as any other traveler, although the nature of previous or underlying disease needs to be kept in mind:

1) Corticosteroid therapy under the following circumstances: short-term (i.e., <2 weeks); ≤20 mg per day of prednisone or equivalent; long-term, alternate-day treatment with short-acting preparations; maintenance physiologic doses (replacement therapy); steroid inhalers; topical steroids (skin, ears, or eyes); intra-articular, bursal, or tendon injection of steroids; or if >1 month has passed since high-dose steroids (>20 mg/day prednisone equivalent for >2 weeks) have been used.

2) HIV patients with >500 CD4 lymphocytes.

3) >3 months since chemotherapy for leukemia/lymphoma or cancer and the malignancy is in remission. Although some clinicians suggest waiting only >1 month since a last dose of immunosuppressive medications that are not being used for the chemotherapy of cancer, data are inconclusive. This recommendation may primarily refer to corticosteroids, but it remains unknown exactly how long is safest.

4) Bone marrow transplant >2 years post-transplant, not on immunosuppressive drugs and without graft-versus-host disease.

5) Definitive data do not exist with respect to autoimmune diseases in the absence of any overlay of immunosuppressive drugs (e.g., lupus, inflammatory bowel disease, rheumatoid arthritis, or multiple sclerosis). The ACIP advice for the normal use of live-virus vaccines in multiple sclerosis (MS) patients who are not undergoing a current exacerbation of disease is reinforced by the National MS Society (www.nationalmssociety.org/Sourcebook-vaccinations.asp), a source well respected by MS patients and their physicians. In the past, many practicing neurologists have strongly advised their patients against the use of live-virus vaccines at any time. If possible, MS patients should not receive any vaccine for 6 weeks after the onset of a disease exacerbation. Immunomodulatory agents such as interferons and glatiramer acetate commonly used in MS patients are not thought to impact vaccine response or safety, but definitive data are lacking. In these special circumstances, travel health advisors

should confer with the traveler's other physicians in developing an appropriate plan.

VACCINE ADMINISTRATION

Travelers with symptomatic HIV or severe non-HIV immunocompromise: 1) cannot be given live-virus or bacterial vaccines; 2) may require additional vaccines when compared with the healthy traveler; and 3) may have decreased protection from some or all vaccines administered. Use of vaccines for different categories of immunocompromised adults is shown in Table 9–1. Overall destination and risk behavior considerations for travel-related vaccines are the same as for other travelers, although the consequences of not administering an indicated vaccine may be more severe. Sufficiently high risk for acquiring infections should prompt discussion of trip deferral or consideration of an alternate destination.

Vaccine Considerations for Certain Hosts

1) Transient increases in HIV viral load, which return quickly to baseline, have been observed after administration of several different vaccines to HIV-infected persons. The clinical significance of these increases is not known but they do not preclude the use of any vaccine.

2) Patients receiving any vaccines while receiving immunosuppressive therapy or in the 2 weeks before starting therapy because of imminent travel are not considered to have received valid vaccine doses. They should be revaccinated >3 months after therapy is discontinued with all vaccines that are still indicated at that time.

3) Complete revaccination with standard childhood vaccines should begin 12 months after bone marrow transplantation. However, MMR vaccine should be administered at 24 months of age if the recipient is presumed to be immunocompetent. Influenza vaccine should be administered at 6 months of age and annually thereafter.

4) Persons with chronic lymphocytic leukemia have poor humoral immunity even early in the disease course and rarely respond to vaccines.

5) Household contacts of severely immunocompromised patients may be given live-virus vaccines such as yellow fever, MMR, or varicella vaccine but should not be given live intranasal influenza vaccine.

TABLE 9-1. VACCINATION OF IMMUNOCOMPROMISED ADULTS

	ASYMPTOMATIC HIV	SYMPTOMATIC HIV INFECTION/AIDS	SEVERELY IMMUNOCOMPROMISED (NON-HIV RELATED)	POST-SOLID ORGAN TRANSPLANT / CHRONIC IMMUNOSUPPRESSIVE THERAPY	ASPLENIA	RENAL FAILURE	CHRONIC HEPATIC DISEASE, CIRRHOSIS, DIABETES
Live Vaccines							
Bacille Calmette-Guérin	X	X	X	X	U	U	U
Influenza (LAIV)	X	X	X	X	U	X	X
MMR (MR/M/R)[1]	R	W	X	X	U	U	U
Typhoid, Ty21a	X	X	X	X	U	U	U
Varicella (Adults)[2]	U	X	X	X	U	U	U
Yellow Fever[3]	W	X	X	X	U	U	U
Killed (Inactivated) Vaccines							
Haemophilus influenzae (Hib)	C[4]	C[4]	R	R	R	U	U

Key: R = Recommended for all in this patient category.
      U = Use as indicated for normal hosts.
      C = Consider.
      W = Warning.
      X = Contraindicated

[1]MMR vaccination should be considered for all symptomatic HIV-infected persons with CD4 counts >200/mL without evidence of measles immunity. Immune globulin may be administered for short-term protection of those facing high risk of measles in whom MMR vaccine is contraindicated.
[2]Varicella vaccine should not be administered to persons who have cellular immunodeficiencies, but persons with impaired humoral immunity (including congenital or acquired hypo- or dysglobulinemia) may be vaccinated. Immunocompromised hosts should receive two doses of vaccine spaced at 3-month intervals.
[3]Yellow fever vaccine. See detailed text below.
[4]Decision based on consideration of the individual patient's risk of Hib disease and the effectiveness of the vaccine for that person. In some settings, the incidence of Hib disease may be higher among HIV-infected adults than non-HIV-infected adults, and the disease can be severe in these patients.

TABLE 9-1. VACCINATION OF IMMUNOCOMPROMISED ADULTS-CONT'D

	ASYMPTOMATIC HIV	SYMPTOMATIC HIV INFECTION/AIDS	SEVERELY IMMUNOCOMPROMISED (NON-HIV RELATED)	POST-SOLID ORGAN TRANSPLANT / CHRONIC IMMUNOSUPPRESSIVE THERAPY	ASPLENIA	RENAL FAILURE	CHRONIC HEPATIC DISEASE, CIRRHOSIS, DIABETES
Killed (Inactivated) Vaccines							
Hepatitis A	U[5]	U[5]	U	U	U[5]	U[5]	U[5]
Hepatitis B	U[5]	U[5]	U	U	U	R[6]	U
Influenza (inactivated)	R	R	R	R	R	R	R
Japanese encephalitis	U	U	U	U	U	U	U
Meningococcal	U	U	U	U	R	U	U
Pneumococcal polysaccharide	R	R	R	R	R	R	R
Polio (IPV)	U	U	U	U	U	U	U
Rabies	U	U	U	U	U	U	U
Td	R	R	R	R	R	R	R
Typhoid, Vi	U	U	U	U	U	U	U

[5]Routinely indicated for all men who have sex with men, persons with multiple sexual partners, patients with chronic hepatitis, and injection drug users
[6]Use special double-dose vaccine formulation. Test for anti-Hbs response after vaccination and revaccinate if initial response is absent.

Considerations for Certain Vaccines
Yellow Fever Vaccine
Severely immunosuppressed travelers should be strongly discouraged from travel to destinations that present true risk of yellow fever. If travel to a yellow fever-endemic zone (see *Yellow Fever* section) by

such individuals is unavoidable and the vaccine is not given, travelers should be instructed carefully in methods to avoid mosquito bites and should be provided a vaccination waiver letter. Travelers should be warned that vaccination waiver documents may not be accepted by some countries and that if this waiver is rejected, the option of deportation might be preferable to yellow fever vaccination at the destination. Patients with limited immune deficits or asymptomatic HIV should be offered the choice of vaccination and monitored closely for possible adverse effects. As vaccine response may be sub-optimal, such vaccinees are candidates for serologic testing 1 month post-vaccination. (Contact a state health department or the CDC Division of Vector-Borne Diseases [970] 221-6400.) Diligent insect precautions are similarly recommended in this situation. Despite the theoretical risk for neuroinvasion and encephalitis due to vaccine, clinical or epidemiologic studies to evaluate the risk of yellow fever vaccination among severely compromised recipients have not been reported. If international travel requirements and not true exposure risk are the only reasons to vaccinate an asymptomatic HIV-infected person or person with a limited immune deficit, a waiver letter should be given.

Hib Vaccine

This vaccine is recommended or should be considered for many categories of compromised host. Normally only one dose is recommended for persons >5 years of age. This dose may be insufficient to induce immunity in immunosuppressed persons, but the data are insufficient to recommend more than one dose.

Pneumococcal Polysaccharide Vaccine

This vaccine is recommended for many categories of compromised host, followed by a single booster at 5 years of age. Data are insufficient on the use of pneumococcal conjugate vaccine to recommend its use in compromised older children and adults.

Influenza Vaccine

Influenza is a year-round infection in the tropics, and in the Southern Hemisphere the influenza season is April through September. Immuno-compromised patients should be protected according to influenza risk at the destination; they should not be given live intranasal influenza vaccine. (See *Influenza* section.)

PREVENTION AND SELF-TREATMENT OF INFECTIONS

Travelers with symptomatic HIV or severe non-HIV immuno-compromise are at risk for increased severity of some diseases.

Enteric infections

The risk for foodborne and waterborne infections among immuno-suppressed persons is magnified during travel to developing countries. Many enteric infections, such as those caused by *Salmonella, Campylobacter,* and *Cryptosporidium,* can be very severe or become chronic in immunocompromised persons.

Foods and beverages, specifically raw fruits and vegetables, raw or undercooked seafood or meat, tap water, ice made with tap water, unpasteurized milk and dairy products, and items purchased from street vendors, may be contaminated. Immunocompromised travelers need to be extraordinarily diligent in adhering to the food and water precautions recommended for all travelers. (See *Risks from Food and Drink* section.) Waterborne infections might result from swallowing water during recreational activities. To reduce the risk for cryptosporidiosis and giardiasis, patients should avoid swallowing water during swimming and should not swim in water that might be contaminated (e.g., with sewage or animal waste). Attention to hand hygiene, including frequent and thorough hand washing, is the best prevention against gastroenteritis and is especially important on cruise ships. Since diarrhea is a frequent complication of highly active antiretroviral therapy for HIV, such patients should receive counseling regarding the symptoms of enteric infections.

Antimicrobial prophylaxis for travelers' diarrhea is not recommended routinely for immunocompromised persons traveling to developing countries because of the potential for adverse effects. Nonetheless, many studies (none involving an immunocompromised population) have reported that prophylaxis can reduce the risk for travelers' diarrhea. In circumstances in which the risk for infection is high, the period of travel brief, and the patient severely immunocompromised, the health-care provider and patient may opt for antibiotic prophylaxis with a quinolone antibiotic once a day (e.g., 500 mg ciprofloxacin).

Loperamide can be used to treat mild diarrhea. As for immuno-competent travelers, antimicrobial agents (e.g., fluoroquinolones or azithromycin (see *Travelers' Diarrhea* section) should be provided to travelers before their departure, to be taken for self-treatment if diarrhea occurs. Severely immunocompromised travelers should have a lower threshold than other travelers for initiating self-therapy.

Malaria

Meticulous malaria prevention should always be advised, as for immunocompetent travelers. (See *Malaria* section.) Malaria does not appear to occur more frequently or pose a greater risk for adverse outcomes in immunocompromised travelers (including those with advanced HIV or asplenia), except in travelers who are both HIV infected and pregnant. Both atovaquone and mefloquine have theoretical potential for competition with protease inhibitors for metabolic enzymes (e.g., cytochrome P450) in the liver, but published evidence for clinically significant interaction is lacking. For malaria treatment, the use of quinidine (and by implication quinine) in patients on nelfinavir or ritonavir is contraindicated because of potential cumulative cardiotoxicity. This drug should be used only with close monitoring in those taking amprenivir, delaviridine, or the lopinavir/ritonavir combination.

Reducing Risk for Other Diseases

Travelers should be informed about other region-specific risks and instructed in ways to reduce those risks. Geographically focal infections that pose an increased risk of severe outcome to immunocompromised persons include visceral leishmaniasis (a protozoan infection transmitted by the sandfly) and several inhalationally acquired fungal infections (e.g., *Penicillium marneffei* infection in Southeast Asia and coccidioidomycosis in the Americas). Many developing areas have high rates of tuberculosis and obtaining a baseline tuberculin skin test should be considered. Patients with advanced HIV and transplant recipients are frequently taking either primary or secondary prophylaxis for one or more opportunistic infections (e.g., pneumocystis, mycobacteria, and toxoplasma). Complete adherence to all indicated regimens should be confirmed before travel.

GENERAL PREPARATION: PRACTICAL CONSIDERATIONS

■ Identify specific sources of medical care at the destination before departure and seek medical attention promptly when ill.

- Avoid changes in the medication regimen shortly before travel to ensure that no side effects or complications of a new regimen occur while traveling.
- Verify medical insurance coverage, purchase additional travel insurance if necessary and possible, and understand that many policies will not cover pre-existing conditions.
- Carry an oversupply of medications, along with copies of prescriptions. Medications should be divided between carry-on and checked baggage, as either one can be lost or stolen. Long-stay travelers should ensure the availability of adequate medication at the destination or a reliable source for its importation.
- HIV-positive travelers should be informed that many countries restrict entry of travelers with HIV infection. Antiretroviral drugs found in baggage at customs may lead to exclusion. Many countries require HIV antibody testing for students, workers, and others applying for long-term entry permits. (See http://www.travel.state.gov/law/HIVtestingreqs.html for an unofficial list of requirements.) Travelers should ascertain whether tests conducted in their home countries before travel will be accepted.
- Seek medical assistance early in case of any febrile illness while in a developing country. Asplenic or functionally asplenic patients are predisposed to rapidly overwhelming sepsis with encapsulated bacteria. If competent medical help is not readily available, febrile asplenic patients should carry a broad-spectrum antibiotic such as levofloxacin to initiate self-therapy immediately. Widespread bacterial resistance now precludes most clinicians from recommending oral penicillins as in the past.

Bibliography

Atkinson WL, Pickering LK, Schwartz B, et al. General recommendations on immunization. Recommendations of the Advisory Committee on Immunization Practices (ACIP) and the American Academy of Family Physicians (AAFP). Morbid Mortal Wkly Rep MMWR. 2002;51(RR-2):1–35.

CDC. Recommendations of the Advisory Committee on Immunization Practices (ACIP): use of vaccines and immune globulins for persons with altered immunocompetence. Morbid Mortal Wkly Rep MMWR. 1993;42(RR-4):1–18.

Castelli F, Patroni A. The human immunodeficiency virus-infected traveler. Clin Infect Dis. 2000;31:1403–8.

Kaplan JE, Masur H, Holmes KK. Guidelines for preventing opportunistic infections among HIV-infected persons—2002. Morbid Mortal Wkly Rep MMWR 2002;51(RR-8):1–52.

Ljungman P. Vaccination in the immunocompromised host. In: Plotkin SL, Orenstein WA, editors. Vaccines. 4th ed. Philadelphia: Saunders; 2004. p. 155–68.

Mileno MD. Preparation of immunocompromised travelers. In: Keystone JS, Kozarsky P, Freedman DO, Nothdurft HD, Connor BA, editors. Travel medicine. St. Louis: Mosby; 2004. p. 249–55.

Schreibman T, Bia FJ. Travel immunizations for special risk groups: pregnant and immune compromised. In: Jong EC, Zuckerman JN. Travelers' vaccines. Hamilton, Ontario: BC Decker; 2004. p. 387–408.

–DAVID FREEDMAN

>>Preconceptional Planning, Pregnancy and Travel

FACTORS AFFECTING THE DECISION TO TRAVEL BEFORE AND DURING PREGNANCY

Reproductive-aged women who may be planning both pregnancy and international travel should consider preconceptional immunization, when practical, to prevent disease in the offspring. Since as many as 50% of pregnancies are unplanned, reproductive-aged women should consider maintaining current immunizations during routine check-ups in case of an unplanned pregnancy and a need to travel. Preconceptional immunizations are preferred to vaccination of pregnant women, because they decrease risk to the unborn child. A woman should defer pregnancy for at least 28 days after receiving live vaccines (e.g., MMR, yellow fever), because of theoretical risk of transmission to the fetus. Vaccination of susceptible women during the postpartum period, especially for rubella and varicella, is another opportunity for prevention, and these vaccines should be encouraged and administered (even for breastfeeding mothers) before discharge from the hospital. For women taking malarial prophylactic medications in anticipation of travel, no data link these medications to congenital malformations, so CDC does not recommend that women planning pregnancy need to wait a specific period of time after their use before becoming pregnant.

Pregnant women considering international travel should be advised to evaluate the potential problems associated with international travel as well as the quality of medical care available at the destination and during transit. According to the American College of Obstetrics and Gynecology, the safest time for a pregnant woman to travel is during the second trimester (18–24 weeks), when she usually feels best and is in least danger of spontaneous abortion or premature labor. A woman in the third trimester should be advised to stay within 300 miles of home because of concerns about access to medical care in case of problems such as hypertension, phlebitis, or premature labor. Pregnant women should be advised to consult with their health-care providers before making any travel decisions. Collaboration between travel health experts and obstetricians is helpful in weighing benefits and risks based on destination and recommended preventive and treatment measures. Table 9–2 lists relative contraindications to international travel during pregnancy. In general, pregnant women with serious underlying illnesses should be advised not to travel to developing countries.

PREPARATION FOR TRAVEL DURING PREGNANCY

Once a pregnant woman has decided to travel, a number of issues need to be considered before her departure.

■ An intrauterine pregnancy should be confirmed by a clinician and ectopic pregnancy excluded before beginning any travel.

■ Health insurance should provide coverage while abroad and during pregnancy. In addition, a supplemental travel insurance policy and a prepaid medical evacuation insurance policy should be obtained, although most may not cover pregnancy-related problems.

TABLE 9-2. POTENTIAL CONTRAINDICATIONS TO INTERNATIONAL TRAVEL DURING PREGNANCY

OBSTETRICAL RISK FACTORS	GENERAL MEDICAL RISK FACTORS	TRAVEL TO POTENTIALLY HAZARDOUS DESTINATIONS
• History of miscarriage • Incompetent cervix • History of ectopic pregnancy (ectopic with current pregnancy should be ruled out before travel) • History of premature labor or premature rupture of membranes • History of or existing placental abnormalities • Threatened abortion or vaginal bleeding during current pregnancy • Multiple gestation in current pregnancy • Fetal growth abnormalities • History of toxemia, hypertension, or diabetes with any pregnancy • Primigravida at ≥35 years of age or ≤15 years of age	• History of thromboembolic disease • Pulmonary hypertension • Severe asthma or other chronic lung disease • Valvular heart disease (if NYHA class III or IV heart failure) • Cardiomyopathy • Hypertension • Diabetes • Renal insufficiency • Severe anemia or hemoglobinopathy • Chronic organ system dysfunction requiring frequent medical interventions	• High altitudes • Areas endemic for or with ongoing outbreaks of life-threatening food- or insect-borne infections • Areas where chloroquine-resistant *P. falciparum* malaria is endemic • Areas where live-virus vaccines are required and recommended

- Check medical facilities at her destination. For a woman in the last trimester, medical facilities should be able to manage complications of pregnancy, toxemia, and cesarean sections.
- Determine beforehand whether prenatal care will be required abroad and, if so, who will provide it. The pregnant traveler should also make sure prenatal visits requiring specific timing are not missed.
- Determine, before traveling, whether blood is screened for HIV and hepatitis B at the destination. The pregnant traveler should also be advised to know her blood type, and Rh-negative pregnant women should receive the anti-D immune globulin (a plasma-derived product) prophylactically at about 28 weeks' gestation. The immune globulin dose should be repeated after delivery if the infant is Rh-positive.

General Recommendations for Travel

A pregnant woman should be advised to travel with at least one companion; she should also be advised that, during her pregnancy, her level of comfort may be adversely affected by traveling. Typical problems of pregnant travelers are the same as those experienced by any pregnant woman: fatigue, heartburn, indigestion, constipation, vaginal discharge, leg cramps, increased frequency of urination, and hemorrhoids. Preventive measures including avoidance of gas-producing food or drinks before scheduled flights (entrapped gases can expand at higher altitudes) and periodic movement of the legs (to decrease venous stasis) can be followed by pregnant women during travel. However, pregnant women should continuously use seatbelts while seated, as air turbulence is not predictable and may cause significant trauma.

Signs and symptoms that indicate the need for immediate medical attention are bleeding, passing tissue or clots, abdominal pain or cramps, contractions, ruptured membranes, excessive leg swelling or pain, headaches, or visual problems.

Greatest Risks for Pregnant Travelers

Motor vehicle accidents are a major cause of morbidity and mortality for pregnant women. When available, safety belts should be fastened at the pelvic area. Lap and shoulder restraints are best; in most accidents, the fetus recovers quickly from the safety belt pressure. However, even after seemingly mild blunt trauma, a physician should be consulted.

Hepatitis E (see Chapter 4), which is not vaccine preventable, can be especially dangerous for pregnant women, for whom the case-fatality rate is 17%–33%. Therefore, pregnant women should be advised that the best preventive measures are to avoid potentially contaminated water and food, as with other enteric infections.

Scuba diving at any depth should be avoided in pregnancy because of the risk of decompression syndrome in the fetus.

Specific Recommendations for Pregnancy and Travel
Air Travel during Pregnancy

Commercial air travel poses no special risks to a healthy pregnant woman or her fetus. The American College of Obstetricians and Gynecologists (ACOG) states that women (with healthy, single pregnancies) can fly safely up to 36 weeks' gestation. The lowered cabin pressures (kept at the equivalent of 1,524–2,438 meters [5,000–8,000 feet]) affect fetal oxygenation minimally because of the favorable fetal hemoglobin-oxygen dynamics. If required for some medical indications, supplemental oxygen can be ordered in advance. Severe anemia, sickle-cell disease or trait, or history of thrombophlebitis are relative contraindications to flying. Pregnant women with placental abnormalities or risks for premature labor should avoid air travel. Each airline has policies regarding pregnancy and flying; it is always safest to check with the airline when booking reservations, because some will require medical forms to be completed. Domestic travel is usually permitted until the pregnant traveler is in her 36th week of gestation, and international travel may be permitted until weeks 32–35, depending on the airline. A pregnant woman should be advised always to carry documentation stating her current gestational age and expected date of delivery.

Airport security radiation exposure is minimal for pregnant women and has not been linked to an increase in adverse outcomes for unborn children to date. However, because of early reports of a possible association of radiation exposure during pregnancy and subsequent increased risk of childhood leukemia and cancer, a pregnant passenger may request a hand or wand search rather than being exposed to the radiation of the airport security machines.

An aisle seat at the bulkhead will provide the most space and comfort, but a seat over the wing in the midplane region will give the smoothest ride. A pregnant woman should be advised to walk every half hour during a smooth flight and flex and extend her ankles frequently to prevent phlebitis. The safety belt should always be fastened at the pelvic level. Dehydration can lead to decreased placental blood flow and hemoconcentration, increasing risk of thrombosis. Thus, pregnant women should drink plenty of fluids during flights.

For flight attendants and pilots, working air travel is restricted by most airlines by 20 weeks' gestation.

Travel to High Altitudes during Pregnancy
Acclimatization responses at altitude act to preserve fetal oxygen supply, but all pregnant women should avoid altitudes >3,658 meters (>12,000 feet). In addition, altitudes >2,500 meters (>8,200 feet) should be avoided in late or high-risk pregnancy. Pregnant air travelers with medical problems that may be exacerbated by a hypoxic, high-altitude environment but who must travel by air should be prescribed supplemental oxygen during air travel. All pregnant women who have traveled to high altitude should postpone exercise until acclimatized.

Food- and Waterborne Illness during Pregnancy
Pregnant travelers should be advised to exercise dietary vigilance while traveling because dehydration from travelers' diarrhea can lead to inadequate placental blood flow and increased risk for premature labor. Suspect drinking water should be boiled to avoid long-term use of iodine-containing purification systems. Iodine tablets can probably be used for travel up to several weeks, but congenital goiters have been reported in association with administration of iodine-containing drugs during pregnancy. Pregnant travelers should eat only well-cooked meats and pasteurized dairy products, while avoiding pre-prepared salads; this will help to avoid diarrheal disease as well as infections such as toxoplasmosis and *Listeria*, which can have serious sequelae in pregnancy.

Oral rehydration is the mainstay of therapy for travelers' diarrhea. Bismuth subsalicylate compounds are contraindicated because of the theoretical risks of fetal bleeding from salicylates and teratogenicity from the bismuth. The combination of kaolin and pectin may be used, and loperamide should be used only when necessary. The antibiotic treatment of travelers' diarrhea during pregnancy can be complicated. Azithromycin or an oral third-generation cephalosporin may be the best options for treatment if an antibiotic is needed.

Malaria during Pregnancy

Malaria in pregnancy carries significant morbidity and mortality for both the mother and the fetus. Pregnant women should be advised to avoid travel to malaria-endemic areas if possible. Women who do choose to go to malarious areas can reduce their risk of acquiring malaria by following several preventive approaches, including personal protection to avoid infective mosquito bites and using prophylactic malaria medication as directed. Because no preventive method is 100% effective, they should seek care promptly if symptoms of malaria develop. Pregnant women traveling to malarious areas should 1) remain indoors between dusk and dawn, if mosquitoes are active outdoors during this time; 2) if outdoors at night, wear light-colored clothing, long sleeves, long pants, and shoes and socks; 3) stay in well-constructed housing with air-conditioning and/or screens; 4) use permethrin-impregnated bed nets; and 5) use insect repellents containing DEET as recommended for adults, sparingly, but as needed. (See also *Protection against Mosquitoes and Other Arthropods*.) Pyrethrum-containing house sprays may also be used indoors if insects are a problem. If possible, remaining in cities or areas of cities that are at low (or lower) risk for malaria can help reduce the chances of infection. Pregnant travelers should be under the care of providers knowledgeable in the care of pregnant women in tropical areas.

For pregnant women who travel to areas with chloroquine-sensitive *Plasmodium falciparum* malaria, chloroquine has been used for malaria chemoprophylaxis for decades with no documented increase in birth defects. For pregnant women who travel to areas with chloroquine-resistant *P. falciparum*, mefloquine should be recommended for chemoprophylaxis during the second and third trimesters. For women in their first trimester, most evidence suggests that mefloquine prophylaxis causes no significant increase in spontaneous abortions or congenital malformations if taken during this period. (Also see section *Chemoprophylaxis during Pregnancy*, in the Malaria section, Chapter 4.)

Because there is no evidence that chloroquine and mefloquine are associated with congenital defects when used for prophylaxis, CDC does not recommend that women planning pregnancy need to wait a specific period of time after their use before becoming pregnant. However, if women or their health-care providers wish to decrease the amount of antimalarial drug in the body before conception, Table 9–3 provides information on the half-lives of selected antimalarial drugs. After 2, 4, and 6 half-lives, approximately 25%, 6%, and 2% of the drug remain in the body.

Avoidance of Insects during Pregnancy

Like malaria, other vector-borne illnesses may be more severe in pregnancy, bear potential harm to the fetus, or both. Pregnant travelers should scrupulously avoid insects by wearing clothing that covers most of the body, bed nets, permethrin treatment for clothing and nets, and application of DEET-containing repellents. (See also *Protection against Mosquitoes and Other Arthropods*.) The recommendations for DEET use in pregnant women do not differ from those for nonpregnant adults. Women choosing lower concentrations of DEET must increase the frequency of application if staying outdoors for long periods.

Malaria must be treated as a medical emergency in any pregnant returning traveler. A woman who has traveled to an area that has chloroquine-resistant strains of *P. falciparum* should be treated as if she has illness caused by chloroquine-resistant organisms. Because of the serious nature of malaria, quinine or intravenous quinidine should be initiated and the case should be managed in consultation with an infectious disease or tropical medicine specialist. The management of malaria in a pregnant woman should include frequent blood glucose determinations and careful fluid monitoring: these requirements may necessitate intensive care supervision.

Immunizations

Risk to a developing fetus from vaccination of the mother during pregnancy is primarily theoretical. No evidence exists of risk from vaccinating pregnant women with inactivated virus or bacterial vaccines or toxoids. The benefits of vaccinating pregnant women usually outweigh potential risks when the likelihood of disease exposure is high, when infection would pose a risk to the mother or fetus, and when the vaccine is unlikely to cause harm.

Pregnant women should be advised to avoid live-virus vaccines (measles, mumps, rubella, varicella and yellow fever). Women should also avoid becoming pregnant within 1 month of having received one of

TABLE 9-3. HALF-LIVES OF SELECTED ANTIMALARIAL DRUGS

DRUG	HALF LIFE
Atovaquone	2–3 days
Chloroquine	Can extend from 6 to 60 days
Doxycycline	12–24 hours
Mefloquine	2–3 weeks
Primaquine	4–7 hours
Proguanil	14–21 hours
Pyrimethamine	80–95 hours
Sulfadoxine	150–200 hours

these vaccines because of theoretical risk of transmission to the fetus. However, no harm to the fetus has been reported from the unintentional administration of these vaccines during pregnancy. Table 9–4 summarizes use of each vaccine in pregnancy.

ROUTINE AND TRAVEL-RELATED IMMUNIZATIONS FOR PREGNANT WOMEN

Ideally, all reproductive-aged women should be up to date on their routine immunizations, whether or not they are planning a pregnancy. Therefore, in the event of an unplanned pregnancy, most women would be prepared if international travel were needed. The following information is intended for women who may require immunizations during pregnancy. Pregnant travelers may visit areas of the world where diseases eliminated by routine vaccination in the United States are still endemic and therefore, may require immunizations before travel.

Bacille Calmette-Guérin (BCG)
BCG vaccine, used outside the United States for the prevention of tuberculosis, can theoretically cause disseminated disease and thus affect the fetus. Although no harmful effects to the fetus have been

associated with BCG vaccine, its use is not routinely recommended for U.S. travelers. Skin testing for tuberculosis exposure before and after travel is preferable when the risk is high.

Diphtheria-Tetanus

The combination diphtheria-tetanus immunization should be given if the pregnant traveler has not been immunized within 10 years, although preference would be for its administration during the second or third trimester.

Hepatitis A

Pregnant women without immunity to hepatitis A virus (HAV) need protection before traveling to developing countries. HAV is usually no more severe during pregnancy than at other times and does not affect the outcome of pregnancy. There have been reports, however, of acute fulminant disease in pregnant women during the third trimester, when there is also an increased risk of premature labor and fetal death. These events have occurred in women from developing countries and might have been related to underlying malnutrition. HAV is rarely transmitted to the fetus, but this can occur during viremia or from fecal contamination at delivery. Immune globulin (IG) is a safe and effective means of preventing HAV, but immunization with one of the HAV vaccines gives a more complete and prolonged protection. The effect of these inactivated virus vaccines on fetal development is unknown and is expected to be low; the production methods for the vaccines are similar to that for IPV, which is considered safe during pregnancy.

Hepatitis B

The hepatitis B vaccine may be administered during pregnancy and is recommended for pregnant women at risk for hepatitis B virus infection. Exposed newborns need to be vaccinated and receive immune globulin as soon as possible.

Immune Globulin Preparations

No known fetal risk exists from passive immunization of pregnant women with immune globulin preparations. Administration of IG can be used pre-exposure as protection against hepatitis A or for postexposure management for other viral diseases if warranted.

TABLE 9-4. VACCINATION DURING PREGNANCY

VACCINE/IMMUNOBIOLOGIC		USE
Immune globulins, pooled or hyperimmune	Immune globulin or specific globulin preparations	If indicated for pre- or post-exposure use. No known risk to fetus.
Diphtheria-Tetanus	Toxoid	If indicated, such as lack of primary series, or no booster within past 10 years.
Hepatitis A	Inactivated virus	Data on safety in pregnancy are not available; the theoretical risk of vaccination should be weighed against the risk of disease. Consider immune globulin rather than vaccine.
Hepatitis B	Recombinant or plasma-derived	Recommended for women at risk of infection.
Influenza	Inactivated whole virus or subunit	All women who are pregnant in the second and third trimesters during the flu season; women at high risk for pulmonary complications, regardless of trimester.
Japanese encephalitis	Inactivated virus	Data on safety in pregnancy are not available; the theoretical risk of vaccination should be weighed against the risk of disease.
Measles	Live attenuated virus	Contraindicated; vaccination of susceptible women should be part of postpartum care.
Meningococcal meningitis	Polysaccharide	Indications for prophylaxis not altered by pregnancy; vaccine recommended in unusual outbreak situations.
Mumps	Live attenuated virus	Contraindicated; vaccination of susceptible women should be part of postpartum care.
Pneumococcal	Polysaccharide	Indications not altered by pregnancy.

TABLE 9-4. VACCINATION DURING PREGNANCY-CONT'D

VACCINE/IMMUNOBIOLOGIC		USE
Polio, inactivated	Inactivated virus	Indicated for susceptible pregnant women traveling in endemic areas or in other high-risk situations.
Rabies	Inactivated virus	Indications for prophylaxis not altered by pregnancy; each case considered individually.
Rubella	Live attenuated virus	Contraindicated; vaccination of susceptible women should be part of postpartum care.
Tuberculosis (BCG)	Attenuated mycobacterial	Contraindicated.
Typhoid (ViCPS)	Polysaccharide	If indicated for travel to endemic areas.
Typhoid (Ty21a)	Live bacterial	Data on safety in pregnancy are not available.
Varicella	Live attenuated virus	Contraindicated; vaccination of susceptible women should be considered postpartum.
Yellow fever	Live attenuated virus	Indicated if exposure cannot be avoided. Postponement of travel preferable to vaccination, if possible.

Influenza

Because of the increased risk for influenza-related complications, women who will be beyond the first trimester of pregnancy (>14 weeks gestation) during the influenza season of their travel destination should be vaccinated, when vaccine is available. Further, those with chronic diseases that increase their risk of influenza-related complications should be vaccinated, regardless of gestational dates. Data from influenza immunization of >2,000 pregnant women have not demonstrated an association with adverse fetal effects.

Japanese Encephalitis
No information is available on the safety of Japanese encephalitis vaccine during pregnancy. It should not be routinely administered during pregnancy, except when a woman must stay in a high-risk area. If not mandatory, travel to such areas should be postponed until after delivery and until the infant is old enough to be safely vaccinated (1 year).

Measles, Mumps, and Rubella
The measles vaccine, as well as the measles, mumps, and rubella (MMR) vaccines in combination, are live-virus vaccines and so they are contraindicated in pregnancy. However, in cases in which the rubella vaccine was unintentionally administered, no complications have been reported. Because of the increased incidence of measles in children in developing countries and because of the disease's communicability and its potential for causing serious consequences in adults, susceptible women should delay traveling until after delivery, when immunization can be given safely. If an unprotected (without a history of physician-diagnosed measles or without at least two doses of measles vaccine) pregnant woman has a documented exposure to measles, IG should be given within 6 days to prevent illness.

Meningococcal Meningitis
The polyvalent meningococcal meningitis vaccine can be administered during pregnancy if the woman is entering an area where the disease is epidemic. Studies of vaccination during pregnancy have not documented adverse effects among either pregnant women or neonates and have shown the vaccine to be efficacious. Based on data from studies involving the use of meningococcal vaccines administered during pregnancy, altering meningococcal vaccination recommendations during pregnancy is unnecessary.

Pneumococcal (PPV23)
The safety of pneumococcal polysaccharide vaccine during the first trimester of pregnancy has not been evaluated, although no adverse fetal consequences have been reported after inadvertent vaccination during pregnancy. Women with chronic diseases (such as asplenia, or metabolic, renal, cardiac, or pulmonary diseases), smokers, and immunosuppressed women should consider vaccination.

Poliomyelitis

The pregnant traveler must be protected against poliomyelitis. Paralytic disease can occur with greater frequency when infection develops during pregnancy. Anoxic fetal damage has also been reported, with up to 50% mortality in neonatal infection. If not previously immunized, a pregnant woman traveling to an area where polio still occurs should be advised to have at least two doses of vaccine one month apart before departure. There is no convincing evidence of adverse effects of inactivated poliovirus vaccine in pregnant women or developing fetuses. However, it is prudent to avoid polio vaccination of pregnant women unless immediate protection is needed.

Rabies

Because of the potential consequences of inadequately treated rabies exposure and because there is no indication that fetal abnormalities have been associated with cell culture rabies vaccines, pregnancy is not considered a contraindication to rabies postexposure prophylaxis. If the risk of exposure to rabies is substantial, preexposure prophylaxis may also be indicated during pregnancy.

Typhoid

No data are available on the use of either typhoid vaccine in pregnancy. The Vi capsular polysaccharide vaccine (ViCPS) injectable preparation is the vaccine of choice during pregnancy because it is inactivated and requires only one injection. The oral Ty21a typhoid vaccine is not absolutely contraindicated during pregnancy, but it is live-attenuated and thus has theoretical risk. With either of these, the vaccine efficacy (about 70%) needs to be weighed against the risk of disease.

Varicella

Women who are pregnant or planning to become pregnant should not receive the varicella vaccine. Nonimmune pregnant women should consider postponing travel until after delivery when the vaccine can be given safely. Varicella zoster immune globulin (VZIG) should be strongly considered within 96 hours of exposure for susceptible, pregnant women who have been exposed. However, VZIG may not be readily available overseas.

Yellow Fever

The safety of yellow fever vaccination during pregnancy has not been established, and the vaccine should be administered to a pregnant woman only if travel to an endemic area is unavoidable and if an increased risk for exposure exists. In these instances, the vaccine can be administered, and infants born to these women should be monitored closely for evidence of congenital infection and other possible adverse effects resulting from yellow fever vaccination. Although concerns exist, no congenital abnormalities have been reported after administration of this vaccine to pregnant women. Further, serologic testing to document an immune response to the vaccine can be considered, because the seroconversion rate for pregnant women may be lower than in other healthy adults.

If traveling to or transiting regions within a country where the disease is not a current threat but where policy requires a yellow fever vaccination certificate, pregnant travelers should be advised to carry a physician's waiver, along with documentation (of the waiver) on the immunization record.

In general, pregnant women should be advised to postpone travel to areas where yellow fever is a risk until after delivery, when vaccine can be administered to the mother without concern of fetal toxicity. Travelers with infants <9 months of age should be strongly advised against traveling to areas within the yellow fever-endemic zone (See Chapter 4, *Yellow Fever* section).

THE TRAVEL HEALTH KIT DURING PREGNANCY

Additions and substitutions to the usual travel health kit need to be made during pregnancy. Talcum powder, a thermometer, ORS packets, prenatal vitamins, an antifungal agent for vaginal yeast, acetaminophen, and a sunscreen with a high SPF should be carried. Women in the third trimester may be advised to carry a blood-pressure cuff and urine dipsticks so they can check for proteinuria and glucosuria, both of which would require prompt medical attention. Antimalarial and antidiarrheal self-treatment medications should be evaluated individually, depending on the traveler, her gestational age, itinerary, and her health history. Most medications should be avoided, if possible.

Bibliography

American College of Obstetricians and Gynecologists. ACOG Committee Opinion No. 282. Immunization during pregnancy. Obstet Gynecol. 2003;101:207–12.

American College of Obstetricians and Gynecologists. ACOG Committee Opinion No. 264. Air travel during pregnancy. Obstet Gynecol. 2001;98:1187–8.

Barish RJ. In-flight radiation exposure during pregnancy. Obstet Gynecol. 2004;103:1326–30.

Bia FJ. Medical considerations for the pregnant traveler. Infect Dis Clin North Am. 1992;6:371–88.

Bocie JD Jr., Miller RW. Childhood and adult cancer after intrauterine exposure to ionizing radiation. Teratology. 1999;59:227–33.

–MADELINE SUTTON

>>International Travelers with Disabilities

By law, U.S. air carriers must comply with highly detailed regulations affecting people with disabilities, which do not cover foreign carriers serving the United States. However, all US and non-US carriers are required to file annual reports of disability-related complaints with the US Department of Transportation (DOT). The DOT maintains a toll-free hotline (1-800-778-4838) 7 am to 11 pm Eastern time to provide real-time assistance in facilitating compliance with DOT rules and to suggest possible customer-service solutions at the point of service to the airline involved (including foreign carriers). Carriers may not refuse transportation to people on the basis of disability. Airlines may not require advance notice that a person with a disability is traveling; however, they may require up to 48 hours' advance notice for certain accommodations that require preparation time.

Internationally, the International Air Transport Association (IATA) member airlines voluntarily adhere to codes of practice that are very similar to US legislation that takes provisions of the International Civil Aviation Organization into consideration (see bibliography). Smaller airlines overseas may not be IATA members. Airlines are obliged to accept a declaration by a passenger that he/she is self-reliant. Medical certificates can be required only in specific situations, such as possible communicable disease, stretcher cases, oxygen requirement, or unusual behaviors possibly affecting the operation of the flight. When a disabled person requests assistance, the airline is obliged to provide access to the aircraft door (preferably by a level entry bridge), an aisle wheelchair, and a seat with removable armrests. Aircraft with <30 seats are generally exempt. Airline personnel are not required to transfer passengers from wheelchair to wheelchair, wheelchair to aircraft seat, or wheelchair to lavatory seat. Disabled passengers who cannot transfer themselves should travel with a companion or attendant, but carriers may not without reason require a person with a disability to travel with an attendant. Only wide-body aircraft with two aisles are required to have fully accessible lavatories, although any aircraft with >60 seats needs to have an on-board wheelchair, and personnel must assist with movement of the wheelchair from the seat to the area outside the lavatory. Wet-acid batteries in electric wheelchairs may require special separate stowage and require early arrival at the airport. Airline personnel are not obliged to assist with feeding, bodily functions, or providing medication to travelers. Internationally standardized codes for classifying disabled passengers and their needs are available in all computerized reservations systems. These passengers should use travel agents experienced in the use of the disability coding; it is critical that appropriate codes and inter-airline messages are sequentially entered for all flights. The delivering carrier is always responsible for a disabled passenger until a subsequent carrier physically accepts responsibility for that passenger.

Service animals are not exempted from compliance with quarantine regulations and so may not be allowed to travel to all international destinations. U.S. companies or entities conducting programs or tours on cruise ships have obligations regarding access for travelers with disabilities, even if the ship itself is of foreign registry.

The medical preparation of a traveler with a stable ongoing disability does not differ from that of any other traveler. The key to safe, accessible travel is that each anticipated international itinerary must be assessed on an individual basis, in consultation with specialized travel agencies or tour operators, as well as print and Internet resources with specific expertise in this area.

Useful links

MossRehab ResourceNet. http://www.mossresourcenet.org/travel.htm

New Horizons Information for the Air Traveler with a Disability. Full text at http://airconsumer.ost.dot.gov/publications/horizons.htm

Non-discrimination on the Basis of Disability in Air Travel. http://airconsumer.ost.dot.gov/rules/rules.htm>

Society for Accessible Travel and Hospitality. http://www.sath.org/index. html?section=Travel%20Tips%20and%20Access%20Information

Bibliography

A World of Options (A Guide to International Exchange, Community Service and Travel for Persons with Disabilities) Editor: Christa Bucks. 3rd edition. Published by Mobility International USA. Eugene, OR

Convention on International Civil Aviation. International Civil Aviation Organization. http://www.icao.org/cgi/goto_m.pl?/icao/en/ download.htm#Docs

—DAVID FREEDMAN

>>VFRs: Recent Immigrants Returning 'Home' to Visit Friends and Relatives

The term VFR usually refers to an immigrant, ethnically and racially distinct from the majority population of the country of residence, who returns to his/her homeland to **V**isit **F**riends and/or **R**elatives. Over the past 30 years, the patterns of migration to North America have shifted; most immigrants come from Asia, Africa, and Latin America; previously the predominant source of immigrants was Europe. Immigrants from developing countries have become an increasingly important group of travelers for two reasons. First, there are far more VFRs than ever before. In 2002, 10% of the U.S. population was foreign born, and in the same year 40% of all overseas journeys made by U.S. citizens were made by VFRs. Second, disease rates in this group have been shown to be considerably higher than in native-born Americans.

VFRs appear to be at greater risk for malaria, typhoid fever, cholera, and hepatitis A. In 2002, 45% of imported malaria cases in the United States were in VFRs. Data from GeoSentinel, the International Society for Travel Medicine/CDC sentinel surveillance network, show that VFRs are eight times more likely to acquire malaria than are U.S.-born tourists. Most imported malaria cases in VFRs, documented both in Europe and North America, have been in travelers returned from sub-Saharan Africa. Because of their partial immunity, these VFRs are much less likely to die from malaria; however, in the absence of repeated malaria infections, waning immunity puts them at risk for serious complications.

Recent studies have shown that most typhoid fever cases in United States are imported and that 77% of these occur in VFRs, mostly from South Asia, Southeast Asia, and Latin America. The risk of typhoid fever during travel to South Asia has been shown to be 25% higher among foreign-born U.S. citizens. Similarly, a review of imported cholera into the United States from 1992 to 1994 showed that 78% of cases occurred among VFRs, mostly from Latin America. A British study of travel-associated hepatitis A showed that VFR children <15 years of age were at highest risk of infection, and surprisingly, many were symptomatic; most cases were acquired in South Asia.

The cause for the increased rates of infectious disease among VFRs is multifactorial and may vary among the different ethnic groups. VFRs may not seek pre-travel health advice, or they may seek advice from friends and relatives or even from physicians in their communities who may not understand the risks. In addition, VFRs may fail to use appropriate prevention measures, which may stem from living conditions abroad that include lack of control over food hygiene and water purification and inadequate protection against insects. Many VFRs believe that they will not contract infections such as malaria because they consider themselves immune.

For many VFRs newly arrived to North America or Europe, cost is one of the most important contributors to failure to obtain pre-travel health advice. This factor is particularly relevant to heads of large families who wish to return to visit their countries of origin with their children. Other barriers to pre-travel health advice include language issues, access to the health-care system, and concern over immigration status. Finally, studies have shown that primary-care physicians have not emphasized sufficiently the need for VFRs to take the same precautions as U.S.-born travelers to developing countries, failing to recognize that VFRs are at increased risk for travel-related infectious diseases, even though they grew up in countries where these diseases are commonplace and attract little attention.

In counseling VFRs, health-care providers must first convince them that they may be at risk for serious infection, not only because of waning immunity, but also because of the ever-changing patterns of disease and drug resistance in their home country. Travel immunization requirements for VFRs are the same as those for U.S.-born travelers. However, the health-care provider should establish whether the immigrant traveler has had his or her childhood immunizations or has a history of vaccine-preventable diseases. In the absence of documentation of childhood immunizations, the adult traveler should be considered to be unimmunized, and a full series of childhood vaccinations should be provided. Several recent studies have shown that adolescent and adult immigrants from developing countries may still be susceptible to hepatitis A, particularly if they have been living in the middle or upper end of the socioeconomic scale before immigrating to the United States. If time and costs permit, serologic testing for both hepatitis A and B may be worthwhile. Otherwise, it may be more practical to administer both vaccines. Immigrants from some developing regions of the world, notably Southeast Asia and Latin America, may also be susceptible to varicella, because this infection occurs at an older age in these areas. In the United States, approximately 90% of children will have had varicella vaccine or infection with chickenpox by the age of 10; at the same age, only 40%–60% of children in these regions are immune to this infection. Varicella infection in adults carries a much higher morbidity and mortality than when it occurs in children. Using the pre-travel consultation to ensure that travelers are not susceptible to varicella by documenting immunity or providing vaccination is an important way of preventing future serious illness.

With respect to malaria chemoprophylaxis, VFRs should be advised that older drugs such as chloroquine, proguanil, and pyrimethamine are often no longer effective. This advice is particularly important for travelers to sub-Saharan Africa, where the risk of *Plasmodium falciparum* malaria is high. Travelers should be encouraged to purchase their medications in North America, where the quality of the drugs can be assured, and to avoid obtaining conflicting advice from overseas practitioners who may not be aware of the impact of drug-resistant malaria on a traveler with waning immunity. One recent study in Southeast Asia showed that 38% of antimalarial drugs purchased locally were counterfeit or substandard.

Bibliography

Bacaner N, Stauffer B, Boulware DR, et al. Travel medicine considerations for North American immigrants visiting friends and relatives. JAMA. 2004;291:2856–64.

Barnett ED, Christiansen D, Figueira M. Seroprevalence of measles, rubella, and varicella in refugees. Clin Infect Dis. 2002;35:403–8.

Behrens RH, Collins M, Botto B, et al. Risk for British travellers of acquiring hepatitis A. BMJ. 1995;311:193.

Schlagenhauf P, Steffen R, Loutan L. Migrants as a major risk group for imported malaria in European countries. J Travel Med. 2003;10:106–7.

Steinberg EB, Bishop R, Haber P, et al. Typhoid fever in travelers: who should be targeted for prevention? Clin Infect Dis. 2004;39:186–91

—JAY KEYSTONE

Index

Note: Page numbers followed by the letter f refer to figures; those followed by the letter t refer to tables.

A

Accidents
   falls, 401–405
   pediatric, 443–444
   traffic, 403–404
Acupuncture, for motion
   sickness, 378
Acetaminophen
   for dengue fever, 122
   for sunburn, 381
Acetazolamide, for acute
   mountain sickness, 387
Acquired immunodefi-
   ciency syndrome
   (AIDS), 96–99. *See also*
   Human immunodefi-
   ciency virus (HIV) infection.
   and risk to travelers, 96
   influenza vaccine and,
      178–179
   MMR vaccine and, 217
   occurrence of, 96
   yellow fever vaccine and,
      316–317
Acute illness, vaccination
   during, 13–14, 217
Acute mountain sickness,
   385–388
Acyclovir, for varicella, 301
A/C/Y/W-135 meningococ-
   cal vaccine, 222–223,
   224t. *See* Meningococcal
   vaccine.
Adoption, international,
   464–472
   general information,
      464–465
   measles outbreaks asso-
      ciated with, 213, 471
   medical examinations in
      after arrival in United
      States, 466–472
      overseas, 465–466
      screening for infec-
         tious diseases in,
         467–469
      vaccinations during,
         470–472

Advance Processing of
   Orphan Petition, application for, 465
Advisory Committee on
   Immunization Practices
   (ACIP), recommenda-
   tions of, 8
Aedes aegypti, 118. *See also*
   Dengue fever.
Aeromonas hydrophila,
   causing travelers' diarrhea, 279
Afghanistan, 326
   diphtheria in, 124
   hepatitis E in, 169
   leishmaniasis in, 183
   malaria risk in, 326
   poliomyelitis in, 243
   rabies in, 247
   tuberculosis in, 80
   yellow fever vaccine re-
      quirements in, 326
African sleeping sickness.
   See African trypanosomiasis.
African tick-bite fever,
   254, 255t, 259
African trypanosomiasis,
   100–101
AIDS. *See* Acquired im-
   munodeficiency syn-
   drome (AIDS).
Air pollution, 400
Air travel, 414–418
   after scuba diving, 393
   cabin air in, 415
   cabin pressure in, 414
   deep venous thrombosis
      associated with, 415
   disinsection in, 418
   during pregnancy,
      488–489
   environmental control
      systems in, 415–416
   for children, 442–443
   for disabled passenger,
      499–500
   in-flight disease trans-
      mission in, 416–418
Aircraft cabin air, 415

Aircraft cabin pressure, 414
Airport security radiation
   exposure, during preg-
   nancy, 488
Alaska, cruise ship travel
   to, 420
Albania, 326
   diphtheria in, 124
   tick-borne encephalitis
      in, 141
   yellow fever vaccine re-
      quirements in, 326
Albendazole, for giardiasis,
   147
Alcohol abuse, in traffic
   accidents, 404
Algeria, 326
   African trypanosomiasis
      in, 100
   diphtheria in, 124
   leishmaniasis in,
      183
   malaria risk in, 326
   plague in, 233
   yellow fever vaccine re-
      quirements in, 326
Allergic reactions. *See also*
   Hypersensitivity.
   to influenza vaccine,
      177–178
   to insect stings, epineph-
      rine for, 410
   to measles vaccine,
      215–216
   to poliomyelitis vaccine,
      245
   to varicella vaccine,
      298
Altitude
   exposure to, after scuba
      diving, 393
   high, travel to, during
      pregnancy, 489
Altitude illness, 385–388
   in pediatric travelers,
      387, 444
Amantadine, for influenza,
   179
Amebiasis, 102–103
   treatment of, 285–286

American Samoa, 364
American trypanoso-
miasis in, 104
ciguatera poisoning in,
395
yellow fever vaccine re-
quirements in, 364
American Society of Trop-
ical Medicine &
Hygiene (ASTM&H),
travel website of, 4
American trypanoso-
miasis, 104–105
Amphotericin B
for coccidioidomycosis,
113
for histoplasmosis,
173
Ampicillin, for meningo-
coccal disease, 225
*Anaplasma phagocy-
tophilum,* 259. *See also*
Ehrlichiosis.
Anaplasmosis, 258t
Andorra, 326
Anemia, air travel and, 414
Aneruptive fever, 256t
Angola, 326
African trypanosomiasis
in, 100
malaria risk in, 326
plague in, 233
yellow fever in, 309t
yellow fever vaccine re-
quirements in, 326
Anguilla, yellow fever
vaccine requirements
in, 326
Animal(s), service, quar-
antine regulations re-
garding, 500
Animal bites, 408–410.
*See also specific animal
bites.*
in pediatric travelers,
442
Animal importation,
426–430
of African rodents and
civets, 429
of bats, 429
of cats, 427
of dogs, 426–427
requirements for,
428t–429t
of monkeys, 427

Animal importation–
cont'd
of restricted animals,
animal products, and
vectors, 427, 429
of turtles, 427, 429
Animal products and
vectors, importation of,
427, 429
Animal-associated
hazards, 408–410
Anopheles mosquito, 189.
See also Malaria.
Antibiotic prophylaxis
for meningococcal
disease, 223–224
for plague, 234
for travelers' diarrhea,
283–284
in immunocompro-
mised travelers,
481
Antibiotics
for *Haemophilus influen-
zae* type b meningitis,
150
for legionellosis,
182
for meningococcal
disease, 224–225
for pertussis, 130
for plague, 234–235
for travelers' diarrhea,
284
during pregnancy,
489–490
in children, 438–
439
in vaccines, hypersensi-
tivity to, 15–16
MMR vaccine interac-
tion with, 217
Antibody-containing
vaccines. *See also*
Vaccine(s).
recommended intervals
between administra-
tion of, and
measles/varicella vac-
cines, 12t–13t
Antifungal agents, for
coccidioidomycosis,
113
Antigua, yellow fever
vaccine requirements
in, 327

Antimalarial drugs,
200t–201t
acquired overseas,
208–209
adverse reactions and
contraindications to,
206–208
change of, as result of
side effects, 209
for breastfeeding
mothers, appropriate
for travel itinerary,
460
for pediatric travelers,
203–204, 205t, 439
administration of,
440
overdose of, 440
half-lives of, 492t
MMR vaccine inter-
action with, 217
tolerability of, 195, 197
use of
during breastfeeding,
206
during pregnancy,
204–205
Antimotility agents, for
travelers' diarrhea, 285
in children, 438
Anti-relapse therapy, for
malaria, 199, 203
Antiretroviral agents, 483
Antiviral agents,
influenza-specific, 179
Arabian Peninsula,
onchocerciasis in, 231
Aralen. *See* Chloroquine.
Arenaviral diseases,
302–303
Argentina, 327
coccidioidomycosis in,
112
malaria risk in, 327
VFRs in, 501
yellow fever in, 309t
yellow fever vaccine re-
quirements in, 327
Argentine hemorrhagic
fever, 303
Argonne diet, for jet lag,
374
Armenia, 327
malaria risk in, 327
Arterial gas embolism, in
divers, 391–392

Arthropod bites, 410
  protection against, 25
    in children, 440
Aruba, yellow fever vaccine
  requirements in, 327
Aspirin
  and Reye syndrome, 300
  for sunburn, 381
Atovaquone, half-life of,
  492t
Atovaquone/proguanil, for
  malaria, 195, 198, 200t
  adverse reactions and
    contraindications to,
    207
    in breastfeeding
      mothers, 206
  in children, 439
    dosages for, 204, 205t
  self-treatment with, 211t
Australia, 92f, 327
  ciguatera poisoning in,
    395
  disease distribution in,
    50t–52t
  hepatitis B in, 160
  histoplasmosis in, 172
  Japanese encephalitis
    risk in, 133t
  poisonous snakes in, 409
  scrub typhus in, 259
  sexually transmitted dis-
    eases in, 92
  travelers' diarrhea in,
    280, 281f
  tuberculosis in, 91
  typhus in, 259
  yellow fever vaccine
    requirements in,
    327
Austria, 328
  histoplasmosis in, 172
  tick-borne encephalitis
    in, 141
Azerbaijan, 328
  malaria risk in, 328
Azithromycin
  for travelers' diarrhea,
    284
    during pregnancy,
      490
    in children, 438
    in immunocompro-
      mised travelers, 482
  immunosuppressive
    effects of, 474

Azores, yellow fever
  vaccine requirements in,
  328

B

Bacille Calmette-Guérin
  (BCG) vaccine
  administration of, in
    breastfeeding
    mothers, 462t
  for tuberculosis, 289
  in internationally
    adopted children,
    468–469
  in pregnancy, 492–493
Bacterial pathogens,
  causing travelers' diarrhea, 278–279
Bahamas, 328
  ship registry in, 420
  yellow fever vaccine re-
    quirements in, 328
Bahrain, 328
Balkans, Crimean-Congo
  hemorrhagic fever in,
  304
Bangladesh, 328–329
  diphtheria in, 124
  hepatitis E in, 169
  Japanese encephalitis
    risk in, 133t
  leishmaniasis in, 183
  malaria risk in, 328
  rabies in, 247
  yellow fever vaccine re-
    quirements in,
    328–329
Barbados, yellow fever
  vaccine requirements in,
  330
Barbuda, yellow fever
  vaccine requirements in,
  327
Barotrauma, ear, in divers,
  391
Bartonella bacilliformis,
  260. See also Oroya
  fever.
Bartonella henselae, 260.
  See also Cat-scratch
  disease.
Bartonella quintana, 254.
  See also Trench fever.
Bats, importation of, 429
  rabies associated with,
  248

BCG vaccine. See Bacille
  Calmette-Guérin.
Belarus, 330
  radioactive contamina-
    tion in, 401
  tick-borne encephalitis
    in, 141
Belgium, 330
Belize, 330
  malaria risk in, 330
  yellow fever vaccine
    requirements in,
    330
Benin, 330
  malaria risk in, 330
  poliomyelitis in, 243
  yellow fever in, 309t
  yellow fever vaccination
    required by, 330
    proof of, 321t
Benznidazole, for Ameri-
  can trypanosomiasis,
  105
Benzodiazepines, for jet
  lag, 375
Bermuda, 330
Bhutan, 330
  diphtheria in, 124
  Japanese encephalitis
    risk in, 133t
  malaria risk in, 330
  yellow fever vaccine re-
    quirements in, 330
Bismuth subsalicylate
  contraindications to, 489
  for travelers' diarrhea,
    282–283, 284–285
Bites, animal, 408–410. See
  also specific animal bite.
  in pediatric travelers,
    442
Blood products
  antibody-containing
    MMR vaccine interac-
      tion with, 217
    varicella interaction
      with, 299
  testing for HIV antibod-
    ies in, 98
Blood transfusions
  in developing countries,
    40–41
  recommended interval
    between administra-
    tion of measles/vari-
    cella vaccines and, 12t

Boiling, of drinking water, 31–32
  prevention of HAV infection by, 158
Bolivia, 330–331
  malaria risk in, 330–331
  plague in, 233
  rabies in, 247
  tuberculosis in, 71
  yellow fever in, 308, 309t, 311f
  yellow fever vaccine requirements in, 330–331
Bolivian hemorrhagic fever, 303
Bora-Bora, yellow fever vaccine requirements in, 344. *See* French Polynesia.
Bordetella pertussis, 124. *See also* Pertussis.
Borrelia burgdorferi, 187–188. *See also* Lyme disease.
Bosnia and Herzegovnia, 331
  tick-borne encephalitis in, 141
Botswana, 331
  malaria risk in, 331
  plague in, 233
  poliomyelitis in, 243
  yellow fever vaccine requirements in, 331
Bovine spongiform encephalopathy, 106–109
  and risk to travelers, 107–108
  occurrence of, 106–107
  prevention of, 108–109
BRAT diet, for travelers' diarrhea, in children, 437–438
Brazil, 332
  coccidioidomycosis in, 112
  diphtheria in, 124
  leishmaniasis in, 183
  lymphatic filariasis in, 144
  malaria risk in, 332
  onchocerciasis in, 231
  plague in, 233
  rabies in, 247
  schistosomiasis in, 267f

Brazil–CONT'D
  yellow fever in, 308, 309t, 311f
  yellow fever vaccine requirements in, 332
Brazilian hemorrhagic fever, 303
Breast milk
  antimalarial drugs excreted in, 206
  expression of, 460
  storage of, 460, 461t
Breastfed infant
  traveling with, 461, 463
  use of antimalarial drugs in, 206
Breastfeeding
  as protection against travelers' diarrhea, 436, 463
  measles-mumps-rubella (MMR) vaccination while, 216
  travel decisions and, 459
  travel preparations while, 459–460, 461t
Breastfeeding mothers
  antimalarial drugs for, appropriate for travel itinerary, 460
  vaccination of, 460, 462t–463t
Brill-Zinsser disease, 254
British Indian Ocean Territory, 332
British Virgin Islands, 372
Brugia malayi, 144. *See also* Filariasis, lymphatic.
Brunei, 333
  Japanese encephalitis risk in, 133t
  yellow fever vaccine requirements in, 333
Bubonic plague, 233–234. *See also* Plague.
Bulgaria, 333
  histoplasmosis in, 172
Bunyaviral diseases, 303–304

Bureau of Citizenship and Immigration Services (BCIS), adoption requirements set by, 464, 465
Burkina Faso, 333
  malaria risk in, 333
  meningococcal disease in, 58, 220
  poliomyelitis in, 243
  yellow fever in, 309t
  yellow fever vaccination required by, 333
  proof of, 321t
Burma (Myanmar), 333
  diphtheria in, 124
  hepatitis E in, 169
  histoplasmosis in, 172
  Japanese encephalitis risk in, 133t
  malaria risk in, 333
  plague in, 233
  rabies in, 247
  yellow fever vaccine requirements in, 333
Burns, 405
Burundi, 333
  malaria risk in, 333
  yellow fever in, 309t
  yellow fever vaccine requirements in, 333

C

Cambodia, 334
  diphtheria in, 124
  Japanese encephalitis risk in, 133t
  malaria risk in, 334
  tuberculosis in, 78
  yellow fever vaccine requirements in, 334
Cameroon, 334
  malaria risk in, 334
  poliomyelitis in, 243
  yellow fever in, 309t
  yellow fever vaccination required by, 334
  proof of, 321t
Campylobacter jejuni, causing travelers' diarrhea, 278–279
Canada, 334
  bovine spongiform encephalopathy in, 107

Canada–CONT'D
cruise ship travel to, 420
norovirus infection in, 229
plague in, 233
severe acute respiratory syndrome in, 270
travelers' diarrhea in, 280, 281f
Canary Islands, 334
Cape Verde, 334
malaria risk in, 334
yellow fever in, 309t
yellow fever vaccine requirements in, 334
Cardiopulmonary disease, air travel and, 414
Caribbean
countries in, 62–63, 67f
cruise ship travel to, 420
disease distribution in, 50t–52t
hepatitis B in, 160
histoplasmosis in, 172
lymphatic filariasis in, 144
malaria in, 190
sexually transmitted diseases in, 68
travelers' diarrhea in, 280, 281f
typhoid fever in, 291
Cat(s)
as vector of disease, 256t
importation of, 427
Cat-flea rickettsiosis, 256t, 259
Cat-scratch disease, 254, 257t, 260
Cayman Islands, 335
Ceftriaxone, for meningococcal disease, 225
prophylaxis, 223
Central Africa
countries in, 53, 57f
disease distribution in, 50t–52t
plague in, 233
poliomyelitis in, 243
sexually transmitted diseases in, 59
travelers' diarrhea in, 280, 281f

Central African Republic, 335
malaria risk in, 335
poliomyelitis in, 243
yellow fever in, 309t
yellow fever vaccination required by, 335
proof of, 321t
Central America
adoptions from, 464
American trypanosomiasis in, 104
countries in, 61, 67f
cruise ship travel to, 420
disease distribution in, 50t–52t
histoplasmosis in, 172
malaria in, 190
sexually transmitted diseases in, 66
travelers' diarrhea in, 280, 281f
typhoid fever in, 291
Central Asia, plague in, 233
Central Intelligence Agency (CIA), travel website of, 5
Cephalosporins, for meningococcal disease, 225
Cerebral edema, high-altitude, 385–388
Cerebrovascular disease, air travel and, 414
Chad, 335
malaria risk in, 335
meningococcal disease in, 58
poliomyelitis in, 243
yellow fever in, 309t
yellow fever vaccine requirements in, 335
Chagas' disease. See American trypanosomiasis.
Chemical disinfection, of drinking water, 31, 32
Chemoprophylaxis, for malaria, 194–199, 200t–201t
adverse reactions and contraindications to, 206–208
changing drugs during, 209

Chemoprophylaxis–CONT'D
drugs acquired overseas in, 208–209
drugs used in, 200t–201t
during breastfeeding, 206
during pregnancy, 204–205
in areas with chloroquine-resistant P. falciparum, 198–199, 200t–201t
in pediatric travelers, 204
in pregnant women, 205–206
in areas without chloroquine-resistant P. falciparum, 197–198, 200t–201t
in pediatric travelers, 204
in immunocompromised travelers, 482
in pediatric travelers, 203–204, 205t
recommendations for, 197
tolerability of, 195, 197
Chickenpox. See Varicella.
Chiggers (mites), as vectors of disease, 256t–257t
Childhood vaccination. See also Vaccination; Vaccine(s).
modified (catch-up) scheduling of, for inadequately immunized pediatric international travelers, 447, 449t, 450–458
routine, 450–455
schedule for, 8, 448t–449t
Children. See Pediatric travelers.
Child-safety seat, FAA-approved, for air travel, 442
Chile, 335
norovirus infection in, 229
China, 336
Crimean-Congo hemorrhagic fever in, 304
diphtheria in, 124

China–CONT'D
hepatitis B in, 160
hepatitis E in, 169
histoplasmosis in, 172
Japanese encephalitis
risk in, 134t
malaria risk in, 336
measles in, 76, 471
plague in, 233
rabies in, 247
schistosomiasis in, 267f
scrub typhus in, 259
severe acute respiratory
syndrome in, 76, 270
tick-borne encephalitis
in, 141
tuberculosis in, 76
yellow fever vaccine re-
quirements in, 336
Chloramphenicol
for meningococcal
disease, 225
for plague, 234–235
Chlorine, water treatment
with, 31, 32
Chloroquine
for malaria, 195,
197–198, 200t
adverse reactions and
contraindications
to, 207
during pregnancy, 490
half-life of, 492t
resistance to, 195, 198
Cholera, 109–111
and risk to travelers,
110
prevention of, 110–111
treatment of, 111
Cholera vaccine, 110
booster schedule for,
11t
Christmas Island, yellow
fever vaccine require-
ments in, 337
Chronic disease, with
limited immune
deficits, in immuno-
compromised travelers,
475
Chronic health condi-
tions, exacerbation of
in air travelers, 414
in cruise ship travelers,
422–423
Ciguatera, sources of, 395

Ciguatera poisoning,
395–396
Ciprofloxacin, for travelers' diarrhea, 284
in immunocompro-
mised travelers, 481
Ciprofloxacin prophylaxis,
for meningococcal
disease, 223
Civets, African, importa-
tion of, 429
Clam-digger's itch. See
Schistosomiasis.
Clostridium tetani, 123. See
also Tetanus.
Clothing, prevention of
sunburn with, 380
Coccidioides immitis, 111,
112. See also Coccid-
ioidomycosis.
Coccidioidomycosis,
111–113
and risk to travelers,
112
prevention of, 113
treatment of, 113
Cocos (Keeling) Islands.
See Australia.
Colombia, 337
coccidioidomycosis in,
112
diphtheria in, 124
malaria risk in, 337
onchocerciasis in, 231
rabies in, 247
yellow fever in, 308,
309t, 311f
yellow fever vaccine re-
quirements in, 337
Commercial health kits,
37
Comoros, 337
malaria risk in, 337
Condoms
in HIV infection pre-
vention, 97–98
in sexually transmitted
disease prevention,
274
Congenital rubella syn-
drome, 263. See also
Rubella.
Congo, 338
Ebola hemorrhagic
fever in, 302
malaria risk in, 338

Congo–CONT'D
yellow fever in,
309t
yellow fever vaccination
required by, 338
proof of, 321t
Cook Islands, 338
Corals, 390
Corynebacterium diphthe-
riae, 123. See also Diph-
theria.
Costa Rica, 338
malaria risk in, 338
Côte d'Ivoire, 338
Ebola hemorrhagic
fever in, 59, 302
malaria risk in, 338
poliomyelitis in, 243
yellow fever in, 309t
yellow fever vaccination
required by, 338
proof of, 321t
Coxiella burnetii, 260. See
also Q fever.
Creutzfeldt-Jakob disease,
variant. See Bovine
spongiform encephalo-
pathy.
Crimean-Congo hemor-
rhagic fever, 304
Croatia, 338
tick-borne encephalitis
in, 141
Cruise ships, 420–423
CDC Vessel Sanitation
Program for, 421
illness or injury consid-
erations for, 422–
423
medical facilities
aboard, 421–422
preventive health mea-
sures for, 423
transmission of disease
on, 422
Cryptosporidiosis,
114–115
treatment of, 285
Cryptosporidium, in drinking water, filters to
remove, 33
Cryptosporidium parvum,
114. See also Cryp-
tosporidiosis.
causing travelers' diar-
rhea, 279

Cryptosporidium parvum—CONT'D
screening for, in internationally adopted children, 469
Cuba, 338
dengue fever in, 118
Culex tritaeniorhyncus, 131. *See also* Japanese encephalitis.
Culex vishnui, 131. *See also* Japanese encephalitis.
Curaçao. *See* Netherlands Antilles.
Cyclophosphamide, immunosuppressive effects of, 474
Cyclospora cayetanensis, 116. *See also* Cyclosporiasis.
causing travelers' diarrhea, 279
Cyclosporiasis, 116–117
treatment of, 285
Cyclosporine, transplant-related immunosuppressive effects of, 475
Cyprus, 338
Cytomegalovirus prophylaxis, recommended interval between administration of measles/varicella vaccines and, 13t
Czech Republic, 338
tick-borne encephalitis in, 141

D

Death overseas, 424–425
Decompression illness, in divers, 391–392
Deep venous thrombosis, associated with air travel, 415
DEET, 26–27
adverse reactions to, 27
leishmaniasis prevention with, 184
malaria prevention with, 194
plague prevention with, 234
toxicity of, 26–27
use of
during pregnancy, 491
for pediatric travelers, 440–441

DEET–CONT'D
yellow fever protection with, 312
Dehydration
avoidance of, 383
in pediatric travelers, assessment and treatment of, 436, 437t
Democratic Republic of Congo, 339
Ebola hemorrhagic fever in, 59, 302
malaria risk in, 339
Marburg hemorrhagic fever in, 302
plague in, 233
yellow fever in, 309
yellow fever vaccination required by, 339
proof of, 321t
Dengue fever, 117–122
and risk to travelers, 118, 121
clinical presentation of, 121–122
distribution of
in Eastern Hemisphere, 120f
in Western Hemisphere, 119f
occurrence of, 117–118
prevention of, 122
treatment of, 122
Dengue hemorrhagic fever. *See* Dengue fever.
Denmark, 339
tick-borne encephalitis in, 141
Depression, risk of, 406–407
Dexamethasone
for acute mountain sickness, 387
for high-altitude cerebral edema, 387
Diamox. *See* Acetazolamide.
Diarrhea
in pediatric travelers, 435–439. *See also* Pediatric travelers, diarrhea in.
travelers', 278–286. *See also* Travelers' diarrhea.

Diego Garcia, *See* British Indian Ocean Territory.
Dientamoeba fragilis, causing travelers' diarrhea, 279
Dietary modification, for travelers' diarrhea, in children, 436–438
Diethylcarbamazine, for lymphatic filariasis, 145
Diethylmetatoluamide. *See* DEET.
Dimenhydrinate, for motion sickness, 377t, 378
in children, 443
Diphenhydramine, for motion sickness, 377t, 378
in children, 443
Diphtheria, 123
and risk to travelers, 125
clinical presentation of, 125
occurrence of, 124
treatment of, 129–130
vaccination for
adverse reactions to, 128
booster schedule in, 11t
in children older than 7 years, adolescents, and adults, 127–128
in infants and children younger than 7 years, 126–127
precautions and contraindications to, 128–129
Diphtheria-tetanus vaccine
catch-up scheduling of, in children 7 to 18 years, 449t
for breastfeeding mothers, 462t
in pregnancy, 493, 494t
Diphtheria-tetanus-pertussis (DTP) vaccine
adverse reactions to, 128
for children older than 7 years, adolescents, and adults, 127–128
for infants and children younger than 7 years, 126–127

Diphtheria-tetanus-
pertussis (DTP)
vaccine–CONT'D
for pediatric travelers,
448t–449t, 450–451
precautions and contra-
indications to,
128–129
Disabilities, travelers
with, 498–500
Disinsection, of in-bound
flights, 418
Divers Alert Network,
393–394
Diving, scuba, 390–394.
See also Scuba diving.
Djibouti, 339
malaria risk in, 339
yellow fever vaccine re-
quirements in, 339
Dog(s)
as vector of disease,
256t
importation of,
426–427
requirements for,
428t–429t
rabies in, 247
Dominica, yellow fever
vaccine requirements
in, 339
Dominican Republic, 339
diphtheria in, 124
malaria in, 190
malaria risk in, 339
vaccine-derived polio-
myelitis in, 243
Doxycycline
for malaria, 195, 198,
200t
adverse reactions and
contraindications
to, 207
for plague, 234
half-life of, 492t
Doxycycline prophylaxis,
for plague, 234
Drinking water, 31–35.
See also Water, drinking.
Drowning, 389
of pediatric travelers,
443
Drugs. *See* Medications;
*named drug or drug
group.*

E

Ear barotrauma, in divers,
391
Ear infections, air travel
and, 414
Ear pain, in children,
during air travel, 442
East Africa
countries in, 53–54,
57f
disease distribution in,
50t–52t
plague in, 233
sexually transmitted
diseases in, 59
travelers' diarrhea in,
280, 281f
East Asia
countries in, 74, 75f
disease distribution in,
50t–52t
sexually transmitted
diseases in, 76–77
East Timor, 339
malaria risk in, 339
yellow fever vaccine re-
quirements in, 339
Easter Island, 339
Eastern Europe
adoptions from, 464
countries in, 83, 87f
disease distribution in,
50t–52t
hepatitis B in, 160
malaria in, 190
sexually transmitted
diseases in, 89
travelers' diarrhea in,
280, 281f
Eastern Hemisphere,
malaria-endemic coun-
tries in, 193f
Ebola hemorrhagic fever,
302
health care–associated
transmission of, 305
in Central, East, and
West Africa, 59
Ectoparasites, screening
for, in internationally
adopted children,
469
Ecuador, 340
diphtheria in, 124
malaria risk in, 340

Ecuador, 340–CONT'D
onchocerciasis in,
231
plague in, 233
rabies in, 247
tuberculosis in, 71
yellow fever in, 308,
309t, 311f
yellow fever vaccine re-
quirements in, 340
Eflornithine, for West
African trypanosomia-
sis, 101
Egg protein, hypersensi-
tivity to
in vaccines, 15, 215
in yellow fever vaccine,
318
Egypt, 340
African trypansosomia-
sis in, 100
diphtheria in, 124
lymphatic filariasis in,
144
malaria risk in, 340
poliomyelitis in, 243
Rift Valley fever in, 304
schistosomiasis in, 267f
yellow fever vaccine re-
quirements in,
340–341
Ehrlichiosis, 258t, 259
El Salvador, 341
malaria risk in, 341
rabies in, 247
yellow fever vaccine re-
quirements in, 341
Embolism, arterial gas, in
divers, 391–392
Emphysema, in divers,
392
Encephalitis
Japanese, 131–139. *See
also* Japanese en-
cephalitis.
tick-borne, 140–143.
See also Tick-borne
encephalitis.
yellow fever vaccine–
associated, 313
Encephalopathy, bovine
spongiform. *See* Bovine
spongiform
encephalopathy.

Endemic typhus, 254,
255t, 259
Entamoeba dispar, 103
Entamoeba histolytica, 102.
See also Amebiasis.
causing travelers' diar-
rhea, 279
Enteric infections, in immunocompromised trav-
elers, 481–482
Environmental hazards,
400–402
Environmental Protection
Agency (EPA), repel-
lents registered by,
25–27
Ephedrine, for motion
sickness, 378
Epinephrine, for allergic
reactions to stings,
410
Equatorial Guinea, 342
malaria risk in, 342
yellow fever in, 309t
yellow fever vaccine re-
quirements in, 342
Equine rabies immune
globulin, 249. See also
Rabies vaccine.
Eritrea, 342
malaria risk in, 342
yellow fever vaccine re-
quirements in,
342
Erythema chronicum
migrans, 188
Escherichia coli
causing travelers' diar-
rhea, 278
Estonia, 342
tick-borne encephalitis
in, 141
tuberculosis in, 89
Ethiopia, 342
malaria risk in, 342
meningococcal disease
in, 58, 219
yellow fever in, 309t
yellow fever vaccine re-
quirements in, 342
Evacuation insurance, purchase of, 405

F

Falkland Islands, 342
Faroe Islands, 342

Federal quarantine regulations, 424
Fever, in post-travel
period, 43, 44
Fiji, yellow fever vaccine
requirements in, 343
Filariasis, lymphatic,
144–145
Filoviruses, 302
Finland, 343
tick-borne encephalitis
in, 141
Fish
biting and stinging,
390
poisoning by, 395–
397
Fleas, as vectors of disease,
255t–256t
Flinders Island spotted
fever, 256t, 259
Florida
ciguatera poisoning in,
395
cruise ship travel to, 420
Fluids. See also Rehydra-
tion therapy.
for heat-related illnesses,
383
for sunburn, 381
Fluoroquinolones, for travelers' diarrhea, 284, 438
in immunocompromised
travelers, 481–482
Food(s)
contamination of, 29
travelers' diarrhea
associated with, 282
radioactive contamina-
tion of, 401
recommended, for
pediatric travelers with
diarrhea, 437
Food poisoning, from
marine toxins, 394–398
Food-borne infections. See
also specific infection.
during pregnancy,
489–490
in Australia, 91
in Caribbean, 68
in Central America,
65–66
in Central, East, and
West Africa, 58
in East Asia, 76

Food-borne infections–
CONT'D
in Eastern Europe,
88–89
in Mexico, 65–66
in Middle East, 82
in North Africa, 55
in North America, 63
in Northern Asia, 88–89
in South Asia, 80
in South Pacific, 91
in Southeast Asia, 78
in Southern Africa, 60
in temperate South
America, 72–73
in tropical South
America, 71
in Western Europe, 86
Formula feeding, of pedi-
atric travelers with diarrhea, 436–437
France, 343
bovine spongiform en-
cephalopathy in, 106
histoplasmosis in, 172
French Guiana, 343
malaria risk in, 343
yellow fever in, 308,
309t, 311f
yellow fever vaccination
required by, 343
proof of, 321t
French Polynesia, 344
ciguatera poisoning in,
395
yellow fever vaccine re-
quirements in, 344
Frostbite, 384

G

Gabon, 344
Ebola hemorrhagic fever
in, 59, 302
malaria risk in, 344
yellow fever in, 309t
yellow fever vaccination
required by, 344
proof of, 321t
Galápagos Islands See
Ecuador
malaria risk in, 340
yellow fever vaccine re-
quirements in, 340
Gambia, The, 344
malaria risk in, 344–
345

Gambia–CONT'D
  yellow fever in, 309t
  yellow fever vaccine
    requirements in,
    344
Gamow bag, for altitude
  illness, 388
Gas(es), inert, absorption
  of, by divers, 392
Gas embolism, arterial, in
  divers, 391–392
Gelatin, hypersensitivity
  to, in yellow fever
  vaccine, 318
Gentamicin, for plague,
  234
Georgia, 344
  malaria risk in, 344
Germany, 345
  tick-borne encephalitis
    in, 141
Ghana, 345
  malaria risk in, 345
  poliomyelitis in, 243
  yellow fever in,
    309t
  yellow fever vaccination
    required by, 345
    proof of, 321t
Giardia, in drinking water,
  filters to remove, 33
Giardia intestinalis, 146.
  See also Giardiasis.
  causing travelers' diar-
    rhea, 279
  screening for, in inter-
    nationally adopted
    children, 469
Giardiasis, 146–147
  treatment of, 285
Gibraltar, 345
Ginger, for motion sick-
  ness, 378
Gingko biloba prophy-
  laxis, for acute moun-
  tain sickness, 388
Glucose-6-phosphate de-
  hydrogenase deficiency
  primaquine and, 199
  screening for, in inter-
    nationally adopted
    children, 470
Greece, 345
  tick-borne encephalitis
    in, 141

Greenland, 345
Grenada, yellow fever
  vaccine requirements
  in, 345
Grenadines (See Saint
  Vincent), yellow fever
  vaccine requirements
  in, 364
Guadelope, yellow fever
  vaccine requirements
  in, 345
Guam, 346
  Japanese encephalitis
    risk in, 136t
Guatemala, 346
  coccidioidomycosis in,
    112
  hepatitis B in, 160
  malaria risk in, 346
  onchocerciasis in,
    231
  rabies in, 247
  tuberculosis in, 66
  yellow fever vaccine
    requirements in,
    346
Guillain-Barré syndrome
  associated with in-
    fluenza vaccine,
    178
  associated with yellow
    fever vaccine, 313
Guinea, 346
  Lassa fever in, 303
  malaria risk in, 346
  poliomyelitis in, 243
  yellow fever in, 309t
  yellow fever vaccine re-
    quirements in,
    346
Guinea-Bissau, 346
  malaria risk in, 346
  yellow fever vaccine re-
    quirements in,
    346–347
Guyana, 347
  lymphatic filariasis in,
    144
  tuberculosis in, 71
  yellow fever in, 308,
    309t, 311f
  malaria risk in, 347
  yellow fever vaccine re-
    quirements in,
    347

H

Haemophilus influenzae
  type b, in meningitis,
  148. See also Meningo-
  coccal disease,
  Haemophilus influenzae
  type b.
Haemophilus influenzae
  type b (Hib) vaccine,
  149–150
  adverse reactions to,
    150
  dosage and schedule
    for, 149, 150t
  for immunocompro-
    mised travelers, 478t,
    480
  for pediatric travelers,
    448t–449t, 451–452
  precautions and contra-
    indications to, 150
Haiti, 348
  diphtheria in, 124
  malaria in, 190
    risk of, 348
  rabies in, 247
  tuberculosis in, 68
  vaccine-derived polio-
    myelitis in, 243
  yellow fever vaccine re-
    quirements in,
    348
Hajj, meningococcal
  disease in, 82, 220
Handwashing, travel
  health benefits of, 20
Hantavirus pulmonary
  syndrome, 304
Hawaii
  ciguatera poisoning in,
    395
  dengue fever in,
    118
Health advice, pre-travel,
  6–7
Health care, in foreign
  country, 37–42
  blood transfusions and,
    40–41
  health-seeking travel
    and, 41–42
  illness and, 39–40
  pretravel preparation
    and, 37–39

Health insurance coverage
in foreign countries,
37–38
special, purchase of, 405
supplemental, 38, 445
Health travel kit, 35–37
commercial, 37
pediatric, 445
Health-care providers, pre-
travel advice from, 6–7
Heat-related illness,
382–383
Helmets, use of, 405
in developing countries,
404
Hemorrhagic fever, viral,
302–306. See also Viral
hemorrhagic fevers.
Hemorrhagic fever with
renal syndrome, 304
Hepatitis A, 151–158
and risk to travelers, 152
clinical presentation of,
152
immune globulin for,
156–157, 157t
occurrence of, 151–152,
153f
prevention of, 152,
154–158
in children, 455
tips in, 158
Hepatitis A vaccine, 152,
154–158
administration of, in
breastfeeding mother,
462t
adverse reactions to, 157
booster schedule for, 11t
for pediatric traveler,
448t–449t, 455
HAVRIX, 156
licensed schedule for,
155t
immune response to,
154–155
IG interference with,
13
in pregnancy, 493, 494t
VAQTA, 156
licensed schedule for,
155t
Hepatitis B, 159–166
and risk to travelers,
160, 162

Hepatitis B–CONT'D
clinical presentation of,
162
occurrence of, 159–160,
161f
prevention of, 162–166
screening for, in internationally adopted chil-
dren, 467
transfusion-associated
risk of, 41
treatment of, 166
Hepatitis B vaccine,
162–166
accelerated scheduling
of, 14
adverse reactions to, 165
booster schedule for,
11t
catch-up scheduling of,
for children 7 to 18
years, 449t
for pediatric traveler,
448t–449t, 450
in pregnancy, 493, 494t
intravenous administra-
tion of, recommended
interval between ad-
ministration of
measles/varicella vac-
cines and, 13t
MMR vaccine interac-
tion with, 217
precautions and contra-
indications to, 158,
165–166
recommended doses for,
163, 164t
recommended interval
between administra-
tion of measles/vari-
cella vaccines and,
12t
TWINRIX, 154
licensed schedule for,
155t
varicella zoster, varicella
vaccine interaction
with, 299
postexposure prophy-
laxis with, 300
Hepatitis C, 167–168
screening for, in internationally adopted chil-
dren, 467–468

Hepatitis E, 169–171
clinical presentation of,
170
in pregnancy, 488
occurrence of, 169–170
prevention of, 170–171
Herpes B virus, monkeys
as source of, 409
Herpes zoster (shingles),
295. See also Varicella.
High-altitude cerebral
edema, 385–388
High-altitude pulmonary
edema, 385–388
Histoplasma capsulatum,
171. See Histoplasmosis.
Histoplasmosis, 171–173
and risk to travelers, 172
occurrence of, 172
prevention of, 172–173
Holy See, 331
Honduras, 348
coccidioidomycosis in,
112
hepatitis B in, 160
malaria risk in, 348
tuberculosis in, 66
yellow fever vaccine re-
quirements in, 348
Hong Kong, 348
severe acute respiratory
syndrome in, 76, 270
Human diploid cell rabies
vaccine, 248–249, 252t.
See also Rabies vaccine.
Human immunodeficiency
virus (HIV) infection.
See also Acquired im-
munodeficiency syn-
drome (AIDS).
in immunocompromised
travelers
asymptomatic, 475
countries restricting
entry of, 483
influenza vaccination
and, 178–179
measles-mumps-rubella
(MMR) vaccine and,
217
prevention of, 97–98
risk of
in travelers, 96, 97
transfusion-associated,
41, 98

Human immunodeficiency virus (HIV) infection–CONT'D
screening for, 99
in internationally adopted children, 468
transmission of, 97–98
tuberculin skin test and, 288
yellow fever vaccine and, 317
Human remains, importation or exportation of, 424–425
Hungary, 348
histoplasmosis in, 172
tick-borne encephalitis in, 141
Hydrocortisone cream, for sunburn, 381
Hydroxychloroquine sulfate, for malaria, 200t
adverse reactions and contraindications to, 207
Hyperbaric therapy, 392
Hypersensitivity. *See also* Allergic reactions.
as contraindication to yellow fever vaccine, 318
to vaccine components, 15–16, 215–216
Hyperthermia. *See* Heat *entries.*
Hypothermia, 383
prevention of, 384

I

Ibuprofen, for sunburn, 381
Ice, contamination of, 31
Iceland, 348
Idoquinol, for amebiasis, 103
IG. *See* Immune globulin (IG).
Immigrants, returning home to visit friends and/or relatives, 501–503
counseling of, 502

Immigrants, returning home to visit friends and/or relatives–CONT'D
increased rates of infectious diseases in, 502
travel immunization requirements for, 502–503
Immune deficits, chronic disease with, in immunocompromised traveler, 475
Immune globulin (IG)
administration of,
during pregnancy, 493, 494t
equine rabies, 249
for hepatitis A, 156–157, 157t
adverse reactions to, 157–158
intravenous, recommended interval between administration of measles/varicella vaccines and, 13t
MMR vaccine and, 10
rabies, 249, 252t
vaccine administration with, antibody response to, 10, 13
varicella zoster
for postexposure prophylaxis, 300
varicella vaccine interaction with, 299
Immune thrombocytopenic purpura, intravenous IG for, recommended interval between administration of measles/varicella vaccines and, 13t
Immunization. *See* Vaccination.
Immunocompromised travelers, 474–483
enteric infections in, 481–482
Hib vaccine for, 478t, 480
HIV-positive
asymptomatic, 475
countries restricting entry of, 483

Immunocompromised travelers–CONT'D
influenza vaccine for, 478t, 480
malaria prophylaxis in, 482
pneumococcal polysaccharide vaccine for, 479t, 480
poliomyelitis vaccine in, 245–246
practical considerations for, 482–483
reducing risk of disease in, 482
risk assessment in, 474
severe immunosuppression in
due to symptomatic AIDS/HIV, 475
non-HIV, 474–475
specific conditions in, 474–475
vaccination of, 477, 478t–479t, 479–483
host considerations in, 477
vaccine considerations in, 479–480
yellow fever vaccine for, 478t, 479–480
Immunosuppression
as contraindication to MMR vaccine, 216–217
as contraindication to varicella vaccine, 299
as contraindication to yellow fever vaccine, 316–317
medications causing, 474–475
Imodium. *See* Loperamide.
Importation, of human remains, 424–425
India, 348–349
diphtheria in, 124
hepatitis E in, 169
histoplasmosis in, 172
Japanese encephalitis risk in, 134t
leishmaniasis in, 183
malaria in, 190
risk of, 348

India–CONT'D
  plague in, 233
  poliomyelitis in, 243
  rabies in, 247
  scrub typhus in, 259
  traffic accidents in, 403
  typhoid fever in, 291
  yellow fever vaccine requirements in,
    348–349
Indonesia, 349
  cholera in, 110
  diphtheria in, 124
  hepatitis B in, 160
  hepatitis E in, 169
  histoplasmosis in, 172
  Japanese encephalitis
    risk in, 134t
  malaria risk in, 349
  plague in, 233
  rabies in, 247
  yellow fever vaccine requirements in, 349
Inert gases, absorption of,
  by divers, 392
Infants. See Pediatric travelers.
Influenza, 174–179
  and risk to travelers,
    174–175
  chemoprophylaxis for,
    179
  clinical presentation of,
    175
  occurrence of, 174
  prevention of,
    175–179
  treatment of, 179
Influenza vaccine, 175–179
  administration of, in
    breastfeeding
    mothers, 462t
  adverse reactions to, 177
  allergic reactions to,
    177–178
  antiviral agents as adjuncts to, 179
  composition of, 177
  dosing, timing and route
    of administration of,
    176–177
  for immunocompromised travelers, 478t,
    480
  for pediatric travelers,
    448t–449t, 454–455

Influenza vaccine–CONT'D
  Guillain-Barré syndrome
    associated with, 178
  in HIV-infected persons,
    178–179
  in pregnancy, 178, 494t,
    495
  inactivated, 454–455
    adverse reactions to,
      177
  live-attenuated, 454–455
    adverse reactions to,
      177
  precautions and contraindications to,
    178–179
  revaccination schedule
    for, 11t
Injury(ies), 402–407
  animal-associated,
    408–410
  intentional, 406–407
  motor vehicle, 403–404
  pedestrian, 403–404
  unintentional, 404–406
Insect bites, 410
  protection against,
    24–25
  in children, 440–441
Insect repellents, 25–27.
  See also specific repellent,
  e.g., DEET.
International adoption,
  464–472. See also Adoption, international.
International Air Transport
  Association (IATA), travelers with disabilities
  and, 499
International Association
  for Medical Assistance to
  Travelers (IAMAT), 39
International Certificate of
  Vaccination, for yellow
  fever, 319–321, 320f
  authorized signature on,
    321
  countries requiring, 321,
    321t
  exemptions from,
    321–322
  validation of, 320
International Civil Aviation
  Organization (ICAO),
  disinfection of in-bound
  flights as specified by, 418

International Health Regulations (IHR), WHO,
  5–6
International Society of
  Travel Medicine (ISTM), 4
International SOS, medical
  care provided by, 38
International transplantation guidelines, 42
International traveler. See
  Traveler(s).
Intestinal pathogens,
  screening for, in internationally adopted children, 469
Iodine, water treatment
  with, 32, 33t
Iodoquinol, for amebiasis,
  286
Iran, 350
  diphtheria in, 124
  histoplasmosis in, 172
  leishmaniasis in, 183
  malaria risk in, 350
  plague in, 233
  schistosomiasis in, 267f
Iraq, 350
  diphtheria in, 124
  leishmaniasis in, 183
  malaria risk in, 350
  tuberculosis in, 82
  yellow fever vaccine requirements in, 350
Ireland, 350
  bovine spongiform encephalopathy in, 107
  histoplasmosis in, 172
Isoniazid, for tuberculosis,
  290
Israel, 350
  hepatitis B in, 160
Italy, 350
  bovine spongiform encephalopathy in, 107
  histoplasmosis in, 172
  tick-borne encephalitis
    in, 141
Itraconazole, for histoplasmosis, 173
Ivermectin, for onchocerciasis, 232
Ivory Coast. See Côte
  d'Ivoire.
Ixodes persulcatus, 140. See
  also Tick-borne encephalitis.

Ixodes ricinus, 140. *See also* Tick-borne encephalitis.

J

Jamaica, yellow fever vaccine requirements in, 350
Japan, 350
  hepatitis B in, 160
  histoplasmosis in, 172
  Japanese encephalitis risk, 135t
  scrub typhus in, 259
  travelers' diarrhea in, 280, 281f
  tuberculosis in, 76
Japanese encephalitis, 131–139
  and risk to travelers, 132
  occurrence of, 132, 137f
  personal protection measures against, 139
  prevention of, 132, 138
  risk of, by country, 133t–136t
Japanese encephalitis vaccine, 132, 138
  administration of, in breastfeeding mothers, 462t
  adverse reactions to, 138–139
  booster schedule for, 11t
  for pediatric travelers, 457–458
  in pregnancy, 494t, 495
  precautions and contraindications to, 139
  recommended dose of, 138, 139t
  routes and schedule for, in infants and children 1 to 3 years, 138
Jellyfish, 390
Jet lag, 374–375
  in pediatric travelers, 442–443
Jordan, 350
  plague in, 233
  yellow fever vaccine requirements in, 350

K

Kawasaki disease, intravenous IG for, recommended interval between administration of measles/varicella vaccines and, 13t
Kazakhstan, 350
  hepatitis E in, 169
  plague in, 233
  tick-borne encephalitis in, 141
  tuberculosis in, 89
  yellow fever vaccine requirements in, 350
Kenya, 351
  malaria risk in, 351
  Marburg hemorrhagic fever in, 302
  plague in, 233
  Rift Valley fever in, 304
  yellow fever in, 309t
  yellow fever vaccine requirements in, 351
Kiribati, yellow fever vaccine requirements in, 351
Korea. *See* North Korea; South Korea.
Kuwait, 352
Kyrgyzstan, 352
  hepatitis E in, 169
  malaria risk in, 352

L

La Leche League International, 459
Lactation, as contraindication to yellow fever vaccine, 316
Laos, 352
  diphtheria in, 124
  Japanese encephalitis risk in, 135t
  malaria risk in, 352
  plague in, 233
  yellow fever vaccine requirements in, 352
Lariam. *See* Mefloquine.
Lassa fever, 302–303
  in international travelers, 305
  ribavirin for, 306

Latvia, 352
  tick-borne encephalitis in, 141
  tuberculosis in, 89
Lead poisoning, screening for, in internationally adopted children, 470
Lebanon, yellow fever vaccine requirements in, 352
Legionellosis, 180–182
  and risk to travelers, 181
  occurrence of, 180–181
  prevention of, 181–182
  treatment of, 182
Leishmania tropica, 183. *See also* Leishmaniasis.
Leishmaniasis, 183–185
  and risk to travelers, 183
  clinical presentation of, 184
  occurrence of, 183
  prevention of, 184–185
  treatment of, 185
Leptospira, 186. *See also* Leptospirosis.
Leptospirosis, 185–187
  and risk to travelers, 186
  prevention of, 186–187
  treatment of, 187
Lesotho, yellow fever vaccine requirements in, 352
Levofloxacin
  for sepsis, in immunocompromised travelers, 483
  for travelers' diarrhea, 284
Liberia, 352
  Lassa fever in, 303
  malaria risk in, 352
  ship registry in, 420
  yellow fever in, 309t
  yellow fever vaccination required by, 352
  proof of, 321t
Libya, 352
  African trypanosomiasis in, 100
  plague in, 233
  yellow fever vaccine requirements in, 352

Lice. *See* Louse.
Liechtenstein, 352
Lithuania, 353
  tick-borne encephalitis in, 141
  tuberculosis in, 89
Live-virus vaccines. *See also* Vaccine(s); *specific vaccine.*
  impaired immune response to, 9–10
  use of, in multiple sclerosis patients, 476
Lomotil, for travelers' diarrhea, in children, 438
Loperamide, for travelers' diarrhea, 285
  in children, 438
  in immunocompromised travelers, 481
Louse, as vector of disease, 255t, 257t
Lungs, overinflation of, in divers, 391–392
Luxembourg, 353
Lyme disease, 187–189
  prevention of, 188
  treatment of, 188–189
  vaccine for, 188
Lymphocytic choriomeningitis virus, 303
Lyssavirus. *See* Rabies.

M

Macao, 353
Macedonia, 353
Macrolides, for legionellosis, 182
Mad cow disease. *See* Bovine spongiform encephalopathy.
Madagascar, 353
  malaria risk in, 353
  plague in, 233
  Rift Valley fever in, 304
  vaccine-derived poliomyelitis in, 243
  yellow fever vaccine requirements in, 353
Madeira Islands, yellow fever vaccine requirements in, 353
Malaria, 189–211
  chemoprophylaxis for, 194–199, 200t–201t

Malaria–CONT'D
  adverse reactions and contraindications to, 206–208
  changing drugs during, 209
  checklist in, 196–197
  drugs acquired overseas in, 208–209
  drugs used in, 200t–201t
  during breastfeeding, 206
  during pregnancy, 204–205
  general recommendations in, 197
  in areas with chloroquine-resistant *P. falciparum,* 198–199, 200t–201t
    in pediatric travelers, 204
    in pregnant women, 205–206
  in areas without chloroquine-resistant *P. falciparum,* 197–198
    in pediatric travelers, 204
  in immunocompromised travelers, 482
  in pediatric travelers, 203–204, 205t
  recommendations for, 197
  tolerability of, 195, 197
  clinical presentation of, 191
  during pregnancy, 490–491, 492t
    emergency management of, 491
  in pediatric travelers, 439–440
  mefloquine-resistant, geographic distribution of, 202f
  occurrence of, 190–191, 192f, 193f
  personal protection measures against, 194
  prevention of, 194–201

Malaria–CONT'D
  relapse of, prevention of, 199, 203
  risk of
    by country, 326–372. *See also under specific country.*
    in immigrants returning home to visit friends and/or relatives, 501
    to travelers, 190, 191
  self-treatment of, 210, 211t
  transfusion-associated risk of, 41
  transmission of, 190
  treatment of, 209–210
Malaria hotline, 210–211
Malarone. *See* Atovaquone/proguanil.
Malawi, 353
  malaria risk in, 353
  plague in, 233
  yellow fever vaccine requirements in, 353
Malaysia, 354
  hepatitis E in, 169
  histoplasmosis in, 172
  Japanese encephalitis risk in, 135t
  malaria risk in, 354
  yellow fever vaccine requirements in, 354
Maldives, yellow fever vaccine requirements in, 354
Mali, 354
  malaria risk in, 354
  meningococcal disease in, 58, 219
  poliomyelitis in, 243
  yellow fever in, 309t
  yellow fever vaccination required by, 354
    proof of, 321t
Malta, yellow fever vaccine requirements in, 354
Mantoux tuberculin skin test. *See* Tuberculin skin test.
Marburg hemorrhagic fever, 302
Marine toxins, food poisoning from, 394–398

Maritime Providences,
scrub typhus in, 259
Marshall Islands, 354
Martinique, 354
Mauritania, 355
malaria risk in, 355
Rift Valley fever in, 304
yellow fever in, 309t
yellow fever vaccination
required by, proof of,
321t
yellow fever vaccination
requirements in, 355
Mauritius, 355
malaria risk in, 355
yellow fever vaccine re-
quirements in, 355
Mayotte, 355
malaria risk in, 355
Measles, 212–218
and risk to travelers,
213
in internationally
adopted children,
471
in-flight transmission
of, 417
occurrence of, 212–213
prevention of, 213–218
vaccination in, 214
adverse reactions
to, 215
precautions and
contraindications
to, 215–218
treatment of, 218
Measles vaccine
booster schedule for,
11t
live-attenuated, 214
recommended interval
between administra-
tion of varicella
vaccine and, 12t
Measles virus, spread of,
limiting, 213
Measles-mumps-rubella
(MMR) vaccine, 214,
227, 264–265
adverse reactions to,
215
booster schedule for,
11t
catch-up scheduling of,
in children 7 to 18
years, 449t

Measles-mumps-rubella
(MMR) vaccine–
CONT'D
during breastfeeding,
216
for pediatric travelers,
448t–449t, 452–
453
immune response to,
IG interference with,
10
in immunosuppressed
travelers, 216–217
in pregnancy, con-
traindications to,
216, 494t, 495
Meclizine, for motion
sickness, 377t
MEDEX travel assistance
services, 38–39
Mediastinal emphysema,
in divers, 392
Medical examinations, of
internationally adopted
children
after arrival in United
States, 466–472
by designated physician
overseas, 465–466
Medical facilities, aboard
cruise ships, 421–422
Mediterranean spotted
fever, 255t, 259
Mefloquine
for malaria, 195, 199,
201t
adverse reactions and
contraindications
to, 207–208
during pregnancy,
490
half-life of, 492t
Mefloquine-resistant
malaria, geographic dis-
tribution of, 202f
Melarsoprol, for African
trypanosomiasis, 101
Melatonin, for jet lag, 375
in pediatric travelers,
443
Meningitis
Haemophilus influenzae
type b, 148. See also
Meningococcal
disease, Haemophilus
influenzae type b.

Meningitis–CONT'D
meninigococcal,
219. See also
Meningococcal
disease, Neisseria
meningitidis.
pneumococcal, 236,
237. See also Pneu-
mococcal disease.
Meningitis belt, 219,
221f
Meningococcal disease,
219–225
Haemophilus influenzae
type b, 148–151
and risk to travelers,
148
clinical presentation
of, 148–149
occurrence of, 148
prevention of,
149–150, 150t
treatment of,
150–151
Neisseria meningitidis
and risk to travelers,
220
clinical presentation
of, 220, 222
in-flight transmission
of, 416
occurrence of,
219–220, 221f
prevention of,
222–224, 224t
Meningococcal vaccine
A/C/Y/W-135, 222–223,
224t
adverse reactions to,
224
precautions and
contraindications
to, 224
booster schedule for,
11t
for pediatric travelers,
457
Hib, 150t, 149150
in pregnancy,
494t, 496
6-Mercaptopurine,
immunosuppressive
effects of, 474
Methotrexate, immuno-
suppressive effects of,
474

Metronidazole
for amebiasis, 286
for giardiasis, 147, 285
Mexico, 67f, 356
American trypanoso-
miasis in, 104
coccidioidomycosis in,
112
cruise ship travel to,
420
dengue fever in, 118
disease distribution in,
50t–52t
hepatitis B in, 160
hepatitis E in, 169
malaria risk in, 356
norovirus infection in,
229
onchocerciasis in,
231
rabies in, 247
sexually transmitted dis-
eases in, 66
trench fever in, 254
typhus in, 254
Micronesia, 356
ciguatera poisoning in,
395
Middle East
countries in, 57f, 81
Crimean-Congo hemor-
rhagic fever in, 304
disease distribution in,
50t–52t
hepatitis B in, 160
hepatitis E in, 169
histoplasmosis in,
172
malaria in, 190
poisonous snakes in,
409
sexually transmitted dis-
eases in, 82
travelers' diarrhea in,
280, 281f
Military orders, travel on,
vaccination for, 323
Miquelon, 364
Mites (chiggers), as vectors
of disease, 256t–257t,
259
Mitoxantrone, transplant-
related immunosuppres-
sive effects of, 475
Moldova, 357
Monaco, 357

Mongolia, 357
diphtheria in, 124
hepatitis E in, 169
plague in, 233
tuberculosis in, 76
Monkeys
as source of herpes B
virus, 409
importation of, 427
Montenegro, See Serbia,
365
Montserrat, yellow fever
vaccine requirements in,
357
Moorea, yellow fever
vaccine requirements in,
344. See French Polyne-
sia.
Morocco, 357
malaria risk in, 357
schistosomiasis in, 267f
Mosquito bites. See also
specific infection, e.g.,
Malaria.
protection against,
24–27
during pregnancy,
491
in children, 440–441
preventive measures
in, 24–25
repellents in, 25–27
Motion sickness, 376, 378
medications for, 377t
Motor vehicle(s), renting,
in foreign country, 405
Motor vehicle injuries,
403–404
in pediatric travelers,
443
Mozambique, 359
malaria risk in, 357
plague in, 233
yellow fever vaccine re-
quirements in, 357
Multiple sclerosis, use of
live-virus vaccines with,
476
Mumps, 226–228
revaccination schedule
for, 11t
Mumps vaccine, live-attenuated, 227
Murine typhus, 255t,
259
Myanmar. See Burma

Mycobacterium tuberculosis,
218, 288. See also Tuber-
culosis.
Mycophenolate mofetil,
transplant-related
immunosuppressive
effects of, 475

N

Namibia, 357
malaria risk in, 357
plague in, 233
yellow fever vaccine re-
quirements in, 357
National Home Oxygen
Patients Association, 414
National Immunization
Program (NIP), 4
Natural disasters, 399–400
Nauru, yellow fever
vaccine requirements in,
358
N-diethylmetatoluamide.
See DEET.
Needles, sterile, use of,
98–99
Neisseria meningitidis, 219.
See also Meningococcal
disease, Neisseria menin-
gitidis.
Neomycin, in vaccines, hypersensitivity to, 15–16
Neorickettsia sennetsu. See
Ehrlichiosis.
Nepal, 358
diphtheria in, 124
hepatitis E in, 169
Japanese encephalitis
risk in, 135t
leishmaniasis in,
183
malaria risk in, 358
rabies in, 247
yellow fever vaccine re-
quirements in, 358
Netherlands, 358
ship registry in, 420
Netherlands Antilles,
yellow fever vaccine re-
quirements in, 358
Neurologic disease, yellow
fever vaccine–
associated, 313
Nevis, yellow fever vaccine
requirements in, 362,
363

New Caledonia, yellow fever vaccine requirements in, 358
New Zealand, 90, 91f, 358
  hepatitis B in, 160
  travelers' diarrhea in, 280, 281f
  tuberculosis in, 91
Nicaragua, 359
  coccidioidomycosis in, 112
  malaria risk in, 359
  tuberculosis in, 66
  yellow fever vaccine requirements in, 359
Nicotinamide adenine dinucleotide, for jet lag, 375
Nifedipine, for high-altitude pulmonary edema, 387
Nifurtimox, for American trypanosomiasis in, 105
Niger, 359
  malaria risk in, 359
  meningococcal disease in, 58
  poliomyelitis in, 243
  yellow fever in, 309t
  yellow fever vaccination required by, 359
    proof of, 321t
Nigeria, 359
  Lassa fever in, 303
  malaria risk in, 359
  meningococcal disease in, 58
  poliomyelitis in, 243
  yellow fever in, 309t
  yellow fever vaccine requirements in, 359
Nitazoxanide
  for cryptosporidiosis, 115, 285
  for giardiasis, 147, 285
Niue, yellow fever vaccine requirements in, 359
Nonhuman primates. See also Monkeys.
  importation of, 427
Nonpharmacologic therapies, for jet lag, 374
Norfolk Island, yellow fever vaccine requirements in, 359

Norovirus infection, 228–230
  and risk to travelers, 229
  prevention of, 229–230
  treatment of, 230
North Africa
  countries in, 53, 57f
  disease distribution in, 50t–52t
  hepatitis E in, 169
  plague in, 233
  sexually transmitted diseases in, 55
North America
  countries in, 61, 67f
  disease distribution in, 50t–52t
  hepatitis B in, 160
  sexually transmitted diseases in, 64
North Asian tick typhus, 255t
North Korea, 351
  hepatitis B in, 160
  Japanese encephalitis risk, 135t
  malaria risk in, 351
  scrub typhus in, 259
  tuberculosis in, 76
Northern Asia
  countries in, 83, 87f
  disease distribution in, 50t–52t
  sexually transmitted diseases in, 89
Northern Europe, travelers' diarrhea in, 280, 281f
Northern Mariana Islands, 359
Norwalk-like virus infection. See Norovirus infection.
Norway, 359
  histoplasmosis in, 172
  ship registry in, 420
  tick-borne encephalitis in, 141
  tuberculosis in, 86

O
Oman, 360
  Crimean-Congo hemorrhagic fever in, 304
  malaria risk in, 360

Oman—CONT'D
  yellow fever vaccine requirements in, 360
Onchocerca volvulus, 231. See also Onchocerciasis.
Onchocerciasis, 231–232
Oral rehydration solution (ORS) packets, availablity of, 436, 438
Oral rehydration therapy. See Fluids; Rehydration therapy.
Oriental spotted fever, 256t
Orientia tsutsugamushi, 259. See also Scrub typhus.
Oroya fever, 254, 257t, 260
Oseltamivir, for influenza, 179
Outbreak notice, of disease, 21, 22t
Oxamniquine, for schistosomiasis, 269
Oxygen, supplemental, inflight, 414

P
Pakistan, 360
  diphtheria in, 124
  hepatitis E in, 169
  histoplasmosis in, 172
  Japanese encephalitis risk in, 135t
  malaria risk in, 360
  poliomyelitis in, 243
  rabies in, 247
  yellow fever vaccine requirements in, 360
Palau, yellow fever vaccine requirements in, 360
Pan American Health Organization (PAHO), travel website of, 5
Panama, 360
  malaria risk in, 360
  yellow fever in, 309t
  yellow fever vaccine requirements in, 360
Papua New Guinea, 360
  diphtheria in, 124
  Japanese encephalitis risk in, 135t
  malaria risk in, 360

Papua New Guinea–
CONT'D
yellow fever vaccine re-
quirements in, 360
Paraguay, 361
coccidioidomycosis in,
112
diphtheria in, 124
malaria risk in, 361
yellow fever in, 309t
yellow fever vaccine re-
quirements in, 361
Parasitic pathogens
causing travelers' diar-
rhea, 279
screening for, in internationally adopted chil-
dren, 469
Paromomycin, for amebia-
sis, 103, 286
Pediatric health travel kit,
445
Pediatric travelers
accidents and, 443–444
air travel by, 442–443
altitude illness in, 387,
444
animal bites in, 442
breastfeeding, 461, 463.
See also Breastfeeding
entries.
diarrhea in, 435–439
antibiotics for,
438–439
antimotility agents for,
438
dehydration and, as-
sessment and treat-
ment of, 436, 437t
dietary modification
for, 436–438
management of, 286,
435–438
prevention of, 435
drowning death in, 443
FAA-approved child-
safety seats for, 442
identifying information
and contact numbers
for, 445
infection and infestation
from soil contact in,
441
Japanese encephalitis
vaccine for, routes and
scheduling of, 138

Pediatric travelers–CONT'D
jet lag in, 442–443
malaria chemoprophy-
laxis for, 203–204,
205t
malaria in, 439–440
measles vaccination for,
213
mosquito, tick, and fly
bites in, protection
against, 440–441
motion sickness in, 443
pneumococcal conjugate
vaccine for, recom-
mended regimens for,
in children under 5
years, 239t
rabies in, 442
schistosomiasis in,
443–444
sun exposure in,
444–445
travel safety for, 434–
445
vaccine recommenda-
tions for, 447,
448t–449t, 450–458.
See also specific vaccine.
vehicle-related accidents
in, 443
water-related illness and
injury in, 443–444
Pediculosis. *See* Louse.
Penicillin G, for meningococcal disease, 225
Penicillin prophylaxis, for
pneumococcal disease,
in infants with sickle-cell
hemoglobinopathy, 241
Penicillium marneffei, 482
Pentamidine, for West
African trypanosomiasis,
101
Pepto-Bismol. *See* Bismuth
subsalicylate.
Permethrin
as insect repellent, 25
Lyme disease prevention
with, 188
malaria prevention with,
194
Pertussis, 124
clinical presentation of,
126
in North America, 64
occurrence of, 124–125

Pertussis–CONT'D
treatment of, 130
vaccination for, *See also*
Diphtheria-tetanus-
pertussis (DTP)
vaccine.
adverse reactions to,
128
in children older than
7 years, adolescents,
and adults, 127–
128
in infants and children
younger than 7
years, 126–127
precautions and con-
traindications to,
128–129
Peru, 361
cholera in, 110
leishmaniasis in, 183
malaria risk in, 361
plague in, 233
rabies in, 247
tuberculosis in, 71
yellow fever in, 308,
309t, 311f
yellow fever vaccine re-
quirements in, 361
Philippines, 362
diphtheria in, 124
hepatitis B in, 160
histoplasmosis in, 172
Japanese encephalitis
risk in, 136t
malaria risk in, 362
rabies in, 247
schistosomiasis in, 267f
vaccine-derived polio-
myelitis in, 243
yellow fever vaccine re-
quirements in, 362
Physician waiver letters,
stating contraindications
to yellow fever vaccina-
tion, 322
Pitcairn Islands, yellow
fever vaccine require-
ments in, 362
Plague, 233–235
occurrence of, 233
prevention of, 234
treatment of, 234–235
Plague vaccine, 234
Plaquenil. *See* Hydroxy-
chloroquine sulfate.

Plasmodium, 189. *See also* Malaria.
Plasmodium falciparum, 189
drug-resistant, 195, 198, 204, 205–206
Plasmodium malariae, 189
Plasmodium ovale, 189, 195
malarial relapses involving, prevention of, 199, 203
Plasmodium vivax, 189, 195
malarial relapses involving, prevention of, 199, 203
Plesiomonas shigelloides, causing travelers' diarrhea, 279
Pneumococcal disease, 236–241
and risk to travelers, 236
clinical presentation of, 236–237
occurrence of, 236
prevention of
additional measures in, 241
vaccines in, 237–238, 240
precautions and contraindications to, 240
recommended regimens for, in children under 5 years, 239t
safety/side effects of, 240
treatment of, 241
Pneumococcal vaccine, 237–238, 238, 240
administration of, in breastfeeding mothers, 462t
booster schedule for, 11t
for immunocompromised travelers, 479t, 480
for pediatric travelers, 448t–449t, 453–454
in pregnancy, 494t, 496
recommended regimens for, in children under 5 years, 239t

Pneumonia, 236. *See also* Pneumococcal disease.
Pneumonic plague, 234
Pneumothorax, in divers, 392
Poisoning
ciguatera, 395–396
food, 394–398
in various settings, 405
lead, screening for, in internationally adopted children, 470
scombroid, 396–397
shellfish, 397–398
Poisonous snakes, 409–410
Poland, 362
tick-borne encephalitis in, 141
Poliomyelitis, 242–246
and risk to travelers, 243
occurrence of, 243
prevention of, 244–246
in adults, 244–245
in immunosuppressed travelers, 245–246
in infants and children, 244
in pregnancy, 245
precautions and contraindications to, 245
Poliovirus vaccine
allergy to, 245
booster schedule for, 11t
for adults, 244–245
for immunocompromised travelers, 245–246
for pediatric travelers, 448t–449t, 452
in pregnancy, 495t, 496
inactivated, 244
catch-up scheduling of, in children 7 to 18 years, 449t
live oral, 244
Pontiac fever, 181
Ports of entry, measures at, in animal importation, 430

Portugal, 362
histoplasmosis in, 172
yellow fever vaccine requirements in, 362
Post-travel period, 43–44
Praziquantel, for schistosomiasis, 269
Preconceptual vaccination, international travel and, 484
Prednisone
immunosuppressive effects of, 475
MMR vaccine contraindicated with, 216
pretravel treatment with, 476
Pregnancy
avoidance of insects during, 491
Bacille Calmette-Guérin vaccine in, 492–493
diphtheria-tetanus vaccine in, 493
hepatitis A vaccine in, 158, 493
hepatitis B vaccine in, 493
hepatitis E during, 488
IG administration during, 493
influenza vaccine in, 178, 494t, 495
Japanese encephalitis vaccine in, 494t, 495
malaria chemoprophylaxis in, 204–205, 490
malaria during, 490–491, 492t
emergency management of, 491
meningococcal vaccine in, 493
MMR vaccine in, contraindications to, 216, 495
pneumococcal vaccine in, 494t, 496
poliovirus vaccine in, 245, 495t, 496
rabies vaccine in, 465t, 496
radiation exposure during, 48, 488

Pregnancy–CONT'D
travel before, factors affecting decision to, 484–485
travel during
by air, 488–489
factors affecting decision to, 484–485
greatest risks in, 487–488
immunizations and, 491–492
routine and travel-related, 492–493, 494t–495t, 495–497
in areas with chloroquine-resistant *P. falciparum,* 205–206, 490
in areas with chloroquine-sensitive *P. falciparum,* 490
potential contraindications to, 486t
preparation for, 485, 487–488
recommendations for, 487
to high altitudes, 489
travel health kit during, 498
typhoid vaccine in, 495t, 496–497
vaccination during, 494t–495t
varicella vaccine in, contraindications to, 298, 495t, 497
yellow fever vaccine in, 316, 495t, 497
Pre-travel advice, for adoptive parents, 465
Primaquine
anti-relapse therapy with, 203
for malaria, 195, 199, 201t
adverse reactions and contraindications to, 208
half-life of, 492t
Primates, nonhuman. *See also* Monkeys.
importation of, 427

Probiotics, for travelers' diarrhea, 283
Proguanil. *See* Atovaquone/proguanil.
Promethazine, for motion sickness, 377t, 378
Puerto Rico, 362
Pulmonary edema, high-altitude, 385–388
Purified chick embryo cell rabies vaccine, 248–249, 252t. *See also* Rabies vaccine.
Purified protein derivative (PPD) testing, suppressed response in, vaccines and, 300
Pyrimethamine, half-life of, 492t

Q

Q fever, 254, 257t, 260
in North Africa, 55
Qatar, 363
Queensland tick typhus, 256t, 259
Quinacrine, for giardiasis, 147
Quinolones
for legionellosis, 182
for travelers' diarrhea, in immunocompromised travelers, 481

R

Rabies, 247–252
and risk to travelers, 247–248
countries indigenous, 248t
in pediatric travelers, 442
occurrence of, 247
prevention of, 248–249, 250t, 251, 252t
Rabies immune globulin, 249, 252t
Rabies vaccine
administration of, in breastfeeding mother, 462t
adverse reactions to, 251
for pediatric traveler, 458
in pregnancy, 495, 495t, 496

Rabies vaccine–CONT'D
postexposure, 252t
preexposure, 248–249, 252t
booster schedule for, 11t
criteria for, 250t
recommended interval between administration of measles/varicella vaccines and, 12t
Rabies vaccine adsorbed, 249, 252t
Radiation, exposure to, 400–402
during pregnancy, 488
"Red tides," shellfish poisoning associated with, 397
Rehydration therapy. *See also* Fluids.
for cholera, 111
for travelers' diarrhea, 285, 286t
during pregnancy, 489
in pediatric travelers, 435–436
Religious pilgrimages, health-seeking, 41–42
Repellents, 25–27. *See also* specific repellent, e.g., DEET.
Respiratory syncytial virus (RSV) prophylaxis, recommended interval between administration of measles/varicella vaccines and, 13t
Réunion, yellow fever vaccine requirements in, 363
Revaccination (booster) schedules, 11t
Reverse-osmosis water filters, 32–33
Reye syndrome, aspirin and, 300
Ribavirin, for Lassa fever, 306
Rickettsia africa, 259. *See also* African tick-bite fever.
Rickettsia akari, 260. *See also* Rickettsialpox.

Rickettsia australis, 259. *See also* Queensland tick typhus.
Rickettsia conorii, 259. *See also* Mediterranean spotted fever.
Rickettsia felis, 259. *See also* Cat-flea rickettsiosis.
Rickettsia honei, 259. *See also* Flinders Island spotted fever; Thai tick typhus.
Rickettsia prowazkeii, 254. *See also* Endemic typhus.
Rickettsia rickettsii, 259. *See also* Rocky Mountain spotted fever.
Rickettsia typhi, 259. *See also* Murine typhus.
Rickettsial infections, 253–254, 259–262. *See also specific infection.*
  and risk to travelers, 254, 259–260
  clinical presentation of, 260–261
  diagnosis of, 261
  epidemiologic features and symptoms of, 255t–258t
  prevention of, 261
  treatment of, 261–262
Rickettsialpox, 254, 256t, 260
Rickettsiosis
  cat-flea, 259
  tick-borne, 259–260
Rifampin, for tuberculosis, 290
Rifampin prophylaxis, for meningococcal disease, 223
Rifaximin, for travelers' diarrhea, 284
Rift Valley fever, 303–304
Rimantadine, for influenza, 179
River blindness. *See* Onchocerciasis.
Rocky Mountain spotted fever, 254, 255t, 259
Rodent plague, 233

Rodents, African, importation of, 429
Romania, 363
  histoplasmosis in, 172
  tick-borne encephalitis in, 141
Rota Island, yellow fever vaccine requirements in, 359
Rubella, 263–265
  occurrence of, 263
  prevention of, 264–265
Rubella vaccine, 264–265
  booster schedule for, 11t
Rubeola. *See* Measles.
Russia, 363
  Crimean-Congo hemorrhagic fever in, 304
  hepatitis B in, 160
  Japanese encephalitis risk in, 136t
  radioactive contamination in, 401
  tick-borne encephalitis in, 141
  tuberculosis in, 89
Rwanda, 363
  malaria risk in, 363
  yellow fever in, 309t
  yellow fever vaccination required by, 363
    proof of, 321t

S

Saba. *See* Netherlands; Netherlands Antilles.
Safety belts, for pregnant woman, 487
St Barthelemy, yellow fever vaccine requirements in, 345
St Christopher, yellow fever vaccine requirements in, 363
St Helena, yellow fever vaccine requirements in, 363
St Kitts and Nevis, yellow fever vaccine requirements in, 363
St Lucia, yellow fever vaccine requirements in, 363

St Martin, yellow fever vaccine requirements in, 345
St Pierre and Miquelon, 364
St Vincent and Grenadines, yellow fever vaccine requirements in, 364
Saipan, 359
  Japanese encephalitis risk in, 136t
Sakhalin Island, scrub typhus in, 259
Salmonella
  causing travelers' diarrhea, 279
  screening for, in internationally adopted children, 469
Samoa. *See* American Samoa.
Samoa (formerly Western Samoa), 364
San Marino, 364
Sand fly, as vector of disease, 257t
São Tomé and Principe malaria risk in, 364
  yellow fever in, 309t
  yellow fever vaccination required by, 364
    proof of, 321t
SARS. *See* Severe acute respiratory syndrome (SARS).
Saudi Arabia, 364
  Crimean-Congo hemorrhagic fever in, 304
  leishmaniasis in, 183
  malaria risk in, 364
  meningococcal disease in, 82, 220
  plague in, 233
  Rift Valley fever in, 304
  yellow fever vaccine requirements in, 364
Schistosoma, 266. *See also* Schistosomiasis.
Schistosomiasis, 266–269
  and risk to travelers, 266, 267f
  clinical presentation of, 266, 268

Schistosomiasis–CONT'D
occurrence of, 266
prevention of, 268–269
treatment of, 269
Scombroid poisoning,
396–397
Scopolamine, for motion
sickness, 376, 377t
Scrub typhus, 257t, 259
Scuba diving, 390–394
disorders associated
with, 391–392
prevention of, 393
treatment of, 393–394
flying after, 393
physical fitness and, 391
Seafood poisoning,
394–398
Seat belts, use of, 404
Sedatives, for air travel, in
children, 443
Senegal, 365
malaria risk in, 365
meningococcal disease
in, 58
yellow fever in, 309t
yellow fever vaccine re-
quirements in, 365
Sennetsu fever, 258t
Sepsis, levofloxacin for, in
immunocompromised
traveler, 483
Serbia, 365
Service animals. See
Animals, service.
Severe acute respiratory
syndrome (SARS),
270–272
as risk to travelers, 271
emergence of, 20–21
clinical presentation of,
271
in East Asia, 76
in-flight transmission of,
417–418
occurrence of, 270
prevention and treat-
ment of, 272
Sewage systems, disruption
of, 399
Sexually transmitted dis-
eases, 273–275
and risk to travelers, 274
in Australia, 91
in Caribbean, 68
in Central America, 66

Sexually transmitted dis-
eases–CONT'D
in Central, East, and
West Africa, 59
in East Asia, 76–77
in Eastern Europe, 89
in Mexico, 66
in Middle East, 82
in North Africa, 55
in North America, 64
in Northern Asia, 89
in South Asia, 80
in South Pacific, 91
in Southeast Asia, 78
in Southern Africa, 60
in temperate South
America, 73
in tropical South
America, 71
in Western Europe, 86
occurrence of, 273
prevention of, 274–275
treatment of, 275
Seychelles, yellow fever
vaccine requirements in,
365
Shellfish poisoning,
397–398
Shigella
causing travelers' diar-
rhea, 279
Shingles (herpes zoster),
295. See also Varicella.
Shipboard sanitation
inspections, 421
Sickle cell disease, air
travel and, 414
Sierra Leone, 365
Lassa fever in, 303
malaria risk in, 365
yellow fever in, 309t
yellow fever vaccine re-
quirements in, 365
Sildenafil, for high-altitude
pulmonary edema,
387–388
Simulium fly bites, 231
Singapore, 365
Japanese encephalitis
risk in, 136t
severe acute respiratory
syndrome in, 270
yellow fever vaccine re-
quirements in, 365
Sint Eustatius. See Netherlands Antilles.

Sinus infections, air travel
and, 414
Sirolimus, transplant-
related immunosuppres-
sive effects of, 475
Sleeping sickness, African.
See African
trypanosomiasis.
Slovakia, 365
tick-borne encephalitis
in, 141
Slovenia, 365
tick-borne encephalitis
in, 141
Smallpox, 276–277
Smallpox vaccine
administration of, in
breastfeeding mother,
463t
voluntary use of,
276–277
misuse of, 277
Snakebites, poisonous,
409–410
Sodium stibogluconate, for
leishmaniasis, 185
Soil- and water-associated
infections. See also
specific infection.
in Australia, 93
in Caribbean, 68, 70
in Central America, 66
in Central, East, and
West Africa, 59
in Eastern Europe, 89
in Mexico, 66
in Middle East, 82
in North Africa, 55
in North America, 64
in Northern Asia, 89
in South Asia, 81
in South Pacific, 93
in Southeast Asia, 79
in Southern Africa, 61
in temperate South
America, 73
in tropical South
America, 72
in Western Europe, 86
Soil contact, infection and
infestation from, in pediatric travelers, 441
Solomon Islands, 366
malaria risk in, 366
yellow fever vaccine re-
quirements in, 366

Somalia, 366
  malaria risk in, 366
  yellow fever in, 309t
  yellow fever vaccine requirements in, 366
South Africa, 366
  malaria risk in, 366
  travelers' diarrhea in, 280, 281f
  yellow fever vaccine requirements in, 366
South America
  adoptions from, 464
  American trypanosomiasis in, 104
  cruise ship travel to, 420
  histoplasmosis in, 172
  plague in, 233
  temperate
    countries in, 62, 69f
    disease distribution in, 50t–52t
    sexually transmitted diseases in, 73
  travelers' diarrhea in, 280, 281f
  trench fever in, 254
  tropical
    countries in, 61–62, 69f
    dengue fever in, 118, 119f
    disease distribution in, 50t–52t
    poisonous snakes in, 409
    sexually transmitted diseases in, 71
    yellow fever in, 308, 309t, 311f
    incidence of, 309
  typhoid fever in, 291
  typhus in, 254
  VFRs in, 501
South Asia
  countries in, 73–74, 75f
  disease distribution in, 50t–52t
  sexually transmitted diseases in, 80
  travelers' diarrhea in, 280, 281f
  VFRs in, 501

South Georgia, yellow fever vaccine requirements in, 342
South Korea, 351
  hepatitis B in, 160
  Japanese encephalitis risk, 135t
  malaria risk in, 351
  scrub typhus in, 259
  tuberculosis in, 76
South Pacific
  countries in, 89–90, 92f
  dengue fever in, 118, 120f
  disease distribution in, 50t–52t
  sexually transmitted diseases in, 92
  tuberculosis in, 91
South Sandwich Islands, yellow fever vaccine requirements in, 342
Southeast Asia
  countries in, 74, 75f
  dengue fever in, 118, 120f
  disease distribution in, 50t–52t
  malaria in, 190
  plague in, 233
  poisonous snakes in, 409
  sexually transmitted diseases in, 78
  VFRs in, 501
Southern Africa
  countries in, 53, 57f
  disease distribution in, 50t–52t
  norovirus infection in, 229
  plague in, 233
  sexually transmitted diseases in, 60
  travelers' diarrhea in, 280, 281f
Southwest Asia, hepatitis B in, 160
Spain, 366
  histoplasmosis in, 172
SPF (sun protection factor), in sunscreens, 380

Sri Lanka, 366
  Japanese encephalitis risk in, 136t
  malaria risk in, 366
  rabies in, 247
  travelers' diarrhea in, 280, 281f
  yellow fever vaccine requirements in, 366
Steroids
  immunosuppressive effects of, 475
  pretravel treatment with, 476
Stings, arthropod, 410
Storage, of breast milk, 460, 461t
Streptococcus pneumoniae, 236, 453. See also Pneumococcal disease.
Streptomycin, for plague, 234
Strongyloides stercoralis, screening for, in internationally adopted children, 469
Subcutaneous emphysema, in divers, 392
Sub-Saharan Africa
  hepatitis E in, 169
  lymphatic filariasis in, 144
  malaria in, 190, 191
  meningococcal disease in, 219, 220
  poisonous snakes in, 409
  poliomyelitis in, 243
  Rift Valley fever in, 304
  schistosomiasis in, 266, 267f
  yellow fever in, 308, 309t, 310f
  incidence of, 309
Sudan, 367
  Ebola hemorrhagic fever in, 59, 302
  leishmaniasis in, 183
  malaria risk in, 367
  meningococcal disease in, 58
  poliomyelitis in, 243
  yellow fever in, 309t
  yellow fever vaccine requirements in, 367

Sulfadoxine, half-life of, 492t
Sun protection factor (SPF), in sunscreens, 380
Sunburn, 378–381
    clinical presentation of, 379
    prevention of, 379–380
    treatment of, 381
Sunlight, exposure to
    damage caused by, 379
    jetlag and, 374, 442–443
    pediatric travelers and, 444–445
Sunscreens, 379–380
    for pediatric traveler, 444
Suramin, for African trypanosomiasis, 101
Suriname, 367
    malaria risk in, 367
    yellow fever in, 309t
    yellow fever vaccine requirements in, 367
Swaziland, 367
    malaria risk in, 367
    yellow fever vaccine requirements in, 367
Sweden, 367
    tick-borne encephalitis in, 141
    tuberculosis in, 86
Swimmer's itch. See Schistosomiasis.
Swimming
    in contaminated water, 30
    safety tips for, 389–390
Switzerland, 367
Syphilis, screening for, in internationally adopted children, 468
Syria, 367
    diphtheria in, 124
    leishmaniasis in, 183
    malaria risk in, 367
    yellow fever vaccine requirements in, 367

T

Tacrolimus, transplant-related immunosuppressive effects of, 475

Tahiti, yellow fever vaccine requirements in, 344. See French Polynesia.
Taiwan, 367
    severe acute respiratory syndrome in, 76, 270
    yellow fever vaccine requirements in, 367
Tajikistan, 368
    hepatitis E in, 169
    malaria risk in, 368
    scrub typhus in, 259
Tanzania, 368
    malaria risk in, 368
    plague in, 233
    Rift Valley fever in, 304
    yellow fever in, 309t
    yellow fever vaccine requirements in, 368
Temperate South America. See South America, temperate.
Temperature, extremes of, 382–384
Tetanus, 123–124
    clinical presentation of, 125–126
    occurrence of, 124
    treatment of, 130
    vaccination for
        adverse reactions to, 128
        in children older than 7 years, adolescents, and adults, 127–128
        in infants and children younger than 7 years, 126–127
        precautions and contraindications to, 128–129
Tetanus vaccine. See also Diphtheria-tetanus-pertussis (DTP) vaccine.
    booster schedule for, 11t
    recommended interval between administration of measles/varicella vaccines and, 12t
Tetracycline
    for plague, 234
    for travelers' diarrhea, in children, 438
Tetracycline prophylaxis, for plague, 234

Tetraglycine hydroperiodide tablets, water treatment with, 32
Texas, dengue fever in, 118
Thai tick typhus, 256t, 259
Thailand, 368
    diphtheria in, 124
    histoplasmosis in, 172
    Japanese encephalitis risk in, 136t
    malaria risk in, 368
    rabies in, 247
    yellow fever vaccine requirements in, 368
Thimerosal, in vaccines, hypersensitivity to, 15
Thrombosis, deep venous, associated with air travel, 415
Thymus disease, as contraindication to yellow fever vaccine, 315–316
Tick(s), as vectors of disease, 255t–256t, 258t
Tick bites, 141
    protection against, 142–143
    in children, 440–441
Tick-borne encephalitis, 140–143
    and risk to travelers, 141–142
    clinical presentation of, 142
    occurrence of, 141
    prevention of, 142–143
    treatment of, 143
Tick-borne encephalitis vaccine, 143
Tick-borne rickettsiosis, 256t, 259–260
    prevention of, 24–25
Tincture of iodine, water treatment with, 32, 33t
Tinian, yellow fever vaccine requirements in, 359
Tinidazole
    for amebiasis, 286
    for giardiasis, 147, 285
Tobago, 369
    yellow fever in, 309t
    yellow fever vaccine requirements in, 369

Togo, 368
  poliomyelitis in, 243
  yellow fever in, 309t
  yellow fever vaccination
    required by, 368
    proof of, 321t
Tokelau, 369
Tonga, yellow fever
  vaccine requirements
  in, 369
Toxins, marine, food poi-
  soning from, 394–398
Traffic accidents, 403–404
Transfusions, blood. *See*
  Blood transfusions.
Transplantation, interna-
  tional guidelines for, 42
Travel health information
  additional sources of,
  4–5
  other sources of, 3–4
Travel Health Online, 39
Travel health precaution,
  21, 22t
Travel health warning,
  23t, 24
Travel notice definitions,
  provided by CDC, 21,
  22t–23t, 24
Travelers' checklist, for
  malarious areas,
  196–197
Travelers' diarrhea,
  278–286
  antibiotics for, 284
    prophylactic,
    283–284
  antimotility agents for,
    285
  bismuth subsalicylate
    for, 282–283,
    284–285
  clinical presentation of,
    280, 282
  during pregnancy,
    489–490
  in children, 435–439.
    See also Pediatric
    travelers, diarrhea in.
  occurrence of, 280,
    281f
  oral rehydration
    therapy for, 285, 286t
  pathogens causing,
    278–280

Travelers' diarrhea–
  CONT'D
  prevention of, 282–284
  probiotics for, 283
  treatment of, 284–286
Travelers' Health Elec-
  tronic Mail, 3–4
Travelers' Health home
  page, 3
Travelers' Health Hotline,
  for faxed information, 3
Travelers' health kit,
  35–37
  commercial, 37
  during pregnancy, 498
Trench fever, 254, 257t,
  259
Trimethoprim-sulfa-
  methoxazole, for travelers' diarrhea, in chil-
  dren, 438
  prophylaxis for cy-
  closporiasis, 285
  for plague, 234
Trinidad, 369
  yellow fever in, 309t
  yellow fever vaccine requirements in, 369
Tropical South America.
  See South America,
  tropical.
Trypanosoma brucei, 100.
  See also African try-
  panosomiasis.
Trypanosoma cruzi, 104.
  See also American trypanosomiasis.
Tsetse fly bite, 100. *See
  also* African trypanosomiasis.
Tuberculin skin test
  and HIV infection, 288
  and MMR vaccination,
  218
  for internationally
  adopted children,
  468–469
Tuberculosis, 288–290
  and risk to travelers,
    288–289
  in Australia, 91
  in Caribbean, 68
  in Central America, 66
  in Central, East, and
    West Africa, 58

Tuberculosis–CONT'D
  in Eastern Europe, 89
  in Mexico, 66
  in Middle East, 82
  in North Africa, 55
  in North America, 64
  in South Asia, 80
  in South Pacific, 91
  in Southeast Asia, 78
  in Southern Africa, 60
  in temperate South
    America, 73
  in tropical South
    America, 71
  in Western Europe, 86
  in-flight transmission
    of, 416
  prevention of, 289–290
  screening for, in inter-
    nationally adopted
    children, 468–469
  treatment of, 290
  varicella vaccine contra-
    indicated in, 300
Tunisia, yellow fever
  vaccine requirements
  in, 369
Turkey, 369
  Crimean-Congo hem-
    orrhagic fever in, 304
  diphtheria in, 124
  histoplasmosis in, 172
  malaria risk in, 369
  tick-borne encephalitis
    in, 141
Turkmenistan, 369
  hepatitis E in, 169
  malaria risk in, 369
Turks and Caicos Islands,
  yellow fever vaccine requirements in, 370
Turtles, importation of,
  427, 429
Tuvalu, 370
Typhoid fever, 291–293
  risk of
    in immigrants return-
      ing home to visit
      friends and/or rela-
      tives, 501
  occurrence of, 291
  prevention of,
    292–293, 294t
  to travelers, 291
  treatment of, 293

Typhoid vaccine, 292
   administration of, in
      breastfeeding mother,
      462t–463t
   adverse reactions to,
      293, 294t
   booster schedule for, 11t
   dosage and schedule for,
      294t
   for pediatric traveler,
      456
   in pregnancy, 495t,
      496–497
   precautions and contra-
      indications to, 293
Typhus, 254, 255t, 259

U

U. S. Virgin Islands, yellow
   fever vaccine require-
   ments in, 372
Uganda, 370
   Ebola hemorrhagic fever
      in, 302
   malaria risk in, 370
   Marburg hemorrhagic
      fever in, 302
   plague in, 233
   yellow fever in, 309t
   yellow fever vaccine re-
      quirements in, 370
Ukraine, 370
   radioactive contamina-
      tion in, 401
   tick-borne encephalitis
      in, 141
Ultraviolet (UV) light, 378,
   444. See also Sunlight.
Unintentional injuries,
   404–406
   prevention of, 405–406
United Arab Emirates, 370
   Crimean-Congo hemor-
      rhagic fever in, 304
United Kingdom, 370
   bovine spongiform en-
      cephalopathy in, 106,
      107
   histoplasmosis in, 172
United States, 370
   animal importation into,
      426–427, 428t–429t,
      429–430
   bovine spongiform en-
      cephalopathy in, 107

United States–CONT'D
   coccidioidomycosis in,
      112
   histoplasmosis in, 172
   measles in, 212–213
   meningococcal disease
      in, 220
   plague in, 233
   severe acute respiratory
      syndrome in, 270
   travelers' diarrhea in,
      280, 281f
   typhus in, 259
United States Department
   of State, travel website
   of, 5
Uruguay, 370
U.S. Consulate, and transportation of human
   remains, 425
U.S. Immigration and Na-
   tionality Act, vaccination
   requirements of, 466
UV index, 380
Uzbekistan, 371
   hepatitis E in, 169
   malaria risk in, 371
   tuberculosis in, 89

V

Vaccination
   adverse events following,
      reporting of, 16
   booster schedules for,
      11t
   childhood
      modified (catch-up)
         scheduling of, for
         inadequately immu-
         nized pediatric in-
         ternational travelers,
         447, 449t, 450–458
      routine, 450–455
      schedule for, 8,
         448t–449t
   during pregnancy,
      491–492, 494t–
      495t
   routine and travel-
      related, 492–493,
      494t–495t, 495–497
   Medical Contraindica-
      tion to, 322
   of acutely ill person,
      13–14

Vaccination–CONT'D
   of immigrants, U.S. Im-
      migration and Nation-
      ality Act requirements
      regarding, 466
   of immunocompromised
      travelers, 477,
      478t–479t, 479–483
      host considerations in,
         477
      vaccine considerations
         in, 479–480
   of internationally
      adopted children,
      470–472
   preconceptual, interna-
      tional travel and, 484
   recommendations for,
      8–16
   scheduling of, for last-
      minute traveler, 14–15
   spacing of, 9–10, 13–16
Vaccine(s). See also specific
   vaccine.
   administration of
      IG preparations and,
         10, 13
      recommended inter-
         vals between, for an-
         tibody-containing
         products vs.
         measles-containing
         or varicella vaccines,
         12t–13t
      simultaneous, 9–10
         yellow fever vaccine
            and,
            318
   components of, hyper-
      sensitivity to, 15–16
   for international travel, 7
   in children, 447,
      448t–449t, 450–458
   missed doses of, 10
Vaccine Adverse Events
   Reporting System
   (VAERS), website for, 16
Vaccinia (smallpox)
   vaccine
   administration of, in
      breastfeeding mother,
      463t
   voluntary use of,
      276–277
   misuse of, 277

Valley fever. *See* Coccidioidomycosis.
Vanuatu, 371
malaria risk in, 371
Varicella, 295–301
occurrence of, 296
prevention of, 297–300
risk of
in immigrants return-
ing home to visit
friends and/or rela-
tives, 503
to travelers, 296–297
treatment of, 301
Varicella vaccine, 297–298
adverse reactions to,
298
booster schedule for,
11t
catch-up scheduling of,
in children 7 to 18
years, 449t
efficacy of, 297
for HIV-infected chil-
dren, 299
for pediatric traveler,
448t–449t, 453
in pregnancy, con-
traindications to,
298, 495t, 497
postexposure prophy-
laxis with, 300
precautions and contra-
indications to,
298–300
recommended interval
between administra-
tion of measles
vaccine and, 12t
recommended intervals
between administra-
tion of, and antibody-
containing vaccines,
12t–13t
use of salicylates and,
299–300
Varicella zoster immune
globulin
for postexposure pro-
phylaxis, 300
varicella vaccine inter-
action with, 299
Vector-borne infections.
See also specific infection.
avoidance of, during
pregnancy, 491

Vector-borne infections–
CONT'D
in Australia, 90–91
in Caribbean, 68
in Central America, 65
in Central, East, and
West Africa, 56, 58
in East Asia, 76
in Eastern Europe, 88
in Mexico, 65
in Middle East, 81–82
in North Africa, 55
in North America, 63
in Northern Asia, 88
in South Asia, 79–80
in South Pacific, 90–91
in Southeast Asia,
77–78, 78
in Southern Africa, 60
in temperate South
America, 72
in tropical South
America, 70–71
in Western Europe, 84,
86
prevention of, 24–25
Venezuela, 371
coccidioidomycosis in,
112
dengue fever in, 118,
119f
malaria risk in, 371
onchocerciasis in, 231
schistosomiasis in,
267f
yellow fever in, 308,
309t, 311f
yellow fever vaccine re-
quirements in, 371
Venezuelan hemorrhagic
fever, 303
Venom, snake, 410
Venous thrombosis, deep,
associated with air
travel, 415
Vessel Sanitation
Program, CDC, 421
VFR. *See* Visit friends
and/or relatives (VFR).
Vibrio cholerae, 109, 110.
See also Cholera.
causing travelers' diar-
rhea, 279
Vibrio parahaemolyticus,
causing travelers' diar-
rhea, 279

Vietnam, 371
diphtheria in, 124
histoplasmosis in, 172
Japanese encephalitis
risk in, 136t
malaria risk in, 371
plague in, 233
rabies in, 247
yellow fever vaccine re-
quirements in, 371
Violence-related injuries,
406
Viral hemorrhagic fevers,
302–306
and risk to travelers,
304–305
arenaviral, 302–303
bunyaviral, 303–304
filoviral, 302
occurrence of, 304
prevention of, 305–306
treatment of, 305–306
Viral pathogens, causing
travelers' diarrhea,
279–280
Virgin Islands, 372
Viscerotropic disease,
yellow fever vaccine–
associated, 314
Visit friends and/or relatives (VFR), immigrants
returning home to,
501–503
counseling, 502
increased rates of infec-
tious diseases in, 502
travel immunization re-
quirements for,
502–503
Vitamin A, supplemental,
for infants with
measles, 218

W

Waiver letters, from physician, stating contraindi-
cations to yellow fever
vaccination, 322
Wake Island, 372
Water
contaminated
chemical compounds
in, 400
swimming in, 30
travelers' diarrhea as-
sociated with, 282

Water–CONT'D
drinking
boiling of, 31–32
chemical disinfection of, 31, 32
filters for, 32–35
treatment of, 31–35
schistosome-infested, exposure to, 268–269
Water filters, 32–35
reverse-osmosis, 32–33
selection, operation, and maintenance of, 34
travelers' guide to, 34
Water safety, recreational, 389–390
Water systems, disruption of, 399
Water-borne infections. *See also specific infection.*
during pregnancy, 489–490
in Australia, 91
in Caribbean, 68
in Central America, 65–66
in Central, East, and West Africa, 58
in East Asia, 76
in Eastern Europe, 88
in Mexico, 65–66
in Middle East, 82
in North Africa, 55
in North America, 63
in Northern Asia, 88
in pediatric travelers, 443–444
in South Asia, 80
in South Pacific, 91
in Southeast Asia, 78
in Southern Africa, 60
in temperate South America, 72–73
in tropical South America, 71
in Western Europe, 86
West Africa
countries in, 54, 57f
disease distribution in, 50t–52t
Lassa fever in, 303
poliomyelitis in, 243
sexually transmitted diseases in, 59

West Africa–CONT'D
travelers' diarrhea in, 280, 281f
yellow fever in, 309
Western Europe
countries in, 83–84, 85f
disease distribution in, 50t–52t
hepatitis B in, 160
sexually transmitted diseases in, 86
travelers' diarrhea in, 280, 281f
Western Hemisphere
eradication of poliomyelitis in, 243
malaria-endemic countries in, 192f
Western Sahara, 372
malaria risk in, 372
Whooping cough. See Pertussis.
World Health Organization (WHO)
disinsection of in-bound flights as specified by, 418
travel information website of, 4–5
World Health Organization (WHO)/International Health Regulations (IHR), 5–6
Wuchereria bancrofti, 144. *See also* Filariasis, lymphatic.

Y

Yellow book, online version of, 3
Yellow fever, 308–323
and risk to travelers, 308–309, 312
in unvaccinated traveler, risks of illness and death due to, 312
occurrence of, 308, 309t, 310f–311f
prevention of, 312–323
personal protection measures in, 312
vaccination in, 312–318. *See also* Yellow fever vaccine.
exemptions from, 321–322

Yellow fever–CONT'D
for travel on military orders, 323
treatment of, 323
Yellow fever vaccine, 312–313
administration of, in breastfeeding mother, 463t
adverse reactions to, 313–314
booster schedule for, 11t
country requirements and CDC recommendations for, 326–372. *See also under specific country.*
for immunocompromised travelers, 478t, 479–480
for pediatric travelers, 455–456
in pregnancy, 495t, 497
international regulations requiring proof of, 319–321, 321t. *See also* International Certificate of Vaccination.
precaution(s) and contraindication(s) to, 315–318, 322
age as, 315
hypersensitivity as, 318
immunosuppression as, 316–317
lactation as, 316
pregnancy as, 316
simultaneous administration of of other vaccines and drugs as, 318
thymic disease as, 315–316
Yellow Fever Vaccine Registry, 4
Yemen, 372
diphtheria in, 124
malaria risk in, 372
onchocerciasis in, 231
plague in, 233
rabies in, 247
Rift Valley fever in, 304
tuberculosis in, 82
yellow fever vaccine requirements in, 372

Yersinia enterocolitica,
   causing travelers' diarrhea, 279
Yersinia pestis. See
   Plague.

Z

Zambia, 372
   malaria risk in, 372
   plague in, 233
Zanamivir, for influenza,
   179
Zimbabwe, 372
   malaria risk in,
      372

Zimbabwe–CONT'D
   Marburg hemorrhagic
      fever in, 302
   plague in, 233
   yellow fever vaccine re-
      quirements in, 372
Zolpidem, for jet lag, 375
Zoonotic infections. *See
   also specific infection.*
   in Australia, 91
   in Caribbean, 68
   in Central America, 66
   in Central, East, and
      West Africa, 59
   in East Asia, 77

   in Eastern Europe, 89
   in Mexico, 66
   in Middle East, 82
   in North Africa, 55
   in Northern Asia, 89
   in South Asia, 80–81
   in South Pacific, 91
   in Southeast Asia, 79
   in Southern Africa, 61
   in temperate South
      America, 73
   in tropical South
      America, 71
   in Western Europe, 86